TRANSPARENCY, POWER, AND INFLUENCE IN THE PHARMACEUTICAL INDUSTRY

Policy Gain or Confidence Game?

Edited by Katherine Fierlbeck, Janice Graham, and Matthew Herder

There is plenty of controversy surrounding pharmaceuticals, but it cannot be denied that the pharmaceutical industry is both socially beneficial and profitable. Regulators are expected to ensure that the economic success of the industry does not come at the expense of public safety, yet they have also assumed a cooperative role by providing advice on regulation and by targeting unmet medical needs. Concerns over regulatory standards, conflicts of interest, and the manipulation of information on drug safety and effectiveness have led to public mistrust and a greater need for transparency between the pharmaceutical industry and government regulators.

Transparency, Power, and Influence in the Pharmaceutical Industry evaluates the progress made in holding the pharmaceutical industry responsible for creating transparency in the industry, from development to market. The contributors to this volume examine the various mechanisms introduced to make the regulatory process more informative and situate these efforts within the larger project of enhancing the safety of drugs, vaccines, and other products.

KATHERINE FIERLBECK is the McCulloch Professor of Political Science at Dalhousie University, with a cross-appointment as a professor of community health and epidemiology.

JANICE GRAHAM is a professor of pediatrics (infectious diseases) and medical anthropology, university research professor, and director of the Technoscience and Regulation Research Unit at Dalhousie University.

MATTHEW HERDER is the director of the Health Law Institute and an associate professor of medicine and law at Dalhousie University.

Transparency, Power, and Influence in the Pharmaceutical Industry

Policy Gain or Confidence Game?

EDITED BY KATHERINE FIERLBECK,
JANICE GRAHAM, AND MATTHEW HERDER

UNIVERSITY OF TORONTO PRESS
Toronto Buffalo London

ISBN 978-1-4875-2903-1 (cloth)   ISBN 978-1-4875-2906-2 (EPUB)
ISBN 978-1-4875-2904-8 (paper)   ISBN 978-1-4875-2905-5 (PDF)

Library and Archives Canada Cataloguing in Publication

Title: Transparency, power, and influence in the pharmaceutical industry : policy
   gain or confidence game? / edited by Katherine Fierlbeck, Janice Graham, and
   Matthew Herder.
Names: Fierlbeck, Katherine, editor. | Graham, Janice Elizabeth, 1958–, editor. |
   Herder, Matthew, editor.
Description: Includes bibliographical references and index.
Identifiers: Canadiana (print) 20210159006 | Canadiana (ebook) 2021015912X | ISBN
   9781487529031 (cloth) | ISBN 9781487529048 (paper) | ISBN 9781487529055 (PDF) |
   ISBN 9781487529062 (EPUB)
Subjects: LCSH: Pharmaceutical policy – United States. | LCSH: Pharmaceutical policy –
   European Union countries. | LCSH: Pharmaceutical policy – Canada.
Classification: LCC RA401.A1 T73 2021 | DDC 362.17/82 – dc23

Funding for the Jean Monnet Network on Health Law and Policy was supported by the
European Union's Erasmus+ Programme. | The European Commission support for the
production of this publication does not constitute endorsement of the contents, which
reflects only the views of the authors, and the Commission cannot be held responsible
for any use that may be made of the information contained therein. | Funding for this
project was made possible in part by the Canadian Institutes of Health Research, Grant
PJT 156256, "Beyond Transparency in Pharmaceutical Research and Regulation." | The
research workshop for this book was hosted by the MacEachen Institute for Public Policy
and Governance at Dalhousie University.

University of Toronto Press acknowledges the financial assistance to its publishing
program of the Canada Council for the Arts and the Ontario Arts Council, an agency of
the Government of Ontario.

With the support of the
Erasmus+ Programme
of the European Union

CIHR | Canadian Institutes of
     | Health Research
IRSC | Instituts de recherche
     | en santé du Canada

MacEachen
INDEPENDENT. INFORMED.

Canada Council   Conseil des Arts
for the Arts   du Canada

ONTARIO ARTS COUNCIL
CONSEIL DES ARTS DE L'ONTARIO
an Ontario government agency
un organisme du gouvernement de l'Ontario

Funded by the   Financé par le
Government   gouvernement
of Canada   du Canada

Canadä

Contents

1 Introduction 3
KATHERINE FIERLBECK, JANICE GRAHAM, AND MATTHEW HERDER

2 Transparency, Pharmaceuticals, and the Problem of Policy
Change 13
KATHERINE FIERLBECK

3 Data Transparency and Pharmaceutical Regulation in Europe:
Road to Damascus, or Room without a View? 63
COURTNEY DAVIS, SHAI MULINARI, AND TOM JEFFERSON

4 The FDA and Health Canada: Similar Origins, yet Divergent Paths
and Approaches to Transparency 95
MARGARET E. MCCARTHY AND JOSEPH S. ROSS

5 Clinical Trial Data Transparency in Canada: Mapping the Progress
from Laggard to Leader 114
MARC-ANDRÉ GAGNON, MATTHEW HERDER, JANICE GRAHAM,
KATHERINE FIERLBECK, AND ANNA DANYLIUK

6 The Limits of Transparency and the Role of Essential
Medicines 129
NAV PERSAUD

7 Speak No Secrets: (Non)transparency in Health Canada's
Communications about Pharmaceutical Regulation 139
JOEL LEXCHIN

8 The Political Economy of Influence: Ghost-Management in the
Pharmaceutical Sector 159
MARC-ANDRÉ GAGNON

 9 Data Transparency and Rare Disease: Privacy versus Public
    Interest?   184
    KANKSHA MAHADEVIA GHIMIRE AND TRUDO LEMMENS

10 The European Registration of the Pandemic Influenza Vaccine
    Pandemrix: A Case Study of the Consequences of Poor Clinical Data
    Transparency   219
    TOM JEFFERSON

11 The Road Forward: How Researchers Can Sustain an Ethical and
    Transparent Health System   243
    RITA BANZI

12 Conclusion   261
    KATHERINE FIERLBECK, JANICE GRAHAM, AND MATTHEW HERDER

Contributors   277

Index   281

TRANSPARENCY, POWER, AND INFLUENCE IN THE PHARMACEUTICAL INDUSTRY

1 Introduction

KATHERINE FIERLBECK, JANICE GRAHAM,
AND MATTHEW HERDER

Behind any approved therapeutic drug and vaccine are regulatory processes, practices, and policies that authorize their safety, efficacy, and quality. Government regulators evaluate the scientific evidence produced by scientists over years of laboratory experimentation, animal testing, and human clinical trials. This scientific evidence must stand up to rigorous methodological standards that meet all regulatory requirements, and we rely on our government regulatory authorities to marshal that process behind the scenes.

Scientific evidence is, by its very nature, highly technical; it is not normally the subject of broad public discussion. As with car maintenance, it seems sensible for us simply to trust the experts to make sure, on our behalf, that things work safely and efficiently. The degree to which scientific data should be easily accessible for scrutiny thus seems irrelevant to most people. But is it? Most of us ride in cars, and we care that they run well and that our safety is not at risk. Similarly, most of us take prescription drugs: one recent survey found that three-quarters of Canadians took prescription medication in the past six months (Nanos, 2017). Those over sixty-five are the heaviest consumers of pharmaceutical products, with a quarter of seniors taking ten or more drug classes (Canadian Institute for Health Information, 2018). At the same time, as this volume explains, the evidentiary base for these drugs is problematic. Well-documented issues such as questionable clinical trial design, publication bias, and poor reporting of adverse events mean that we may be taking drugs that do not work or may, in fact, be more harmful to us than beneficial.

There are, of course, always a few dodgy mechanics. But when we suspect the quality of our car's servicing, we can take it to another garage for a second opinion. Imagine, then, if we were instead told by our mechanic that the mysterious inner workings of our car had been formally sealed off and that we should simply trust them: after all, they would have no interest in having us drive a poorly serviced car, as it would reflect badly on them. Imagine, too, that the government body in charge of regulating mechanics was in fact paid by the mechanics themselves to investigate service quality. We would be appalled. How would we know whether our mechanic was doing proper work? To whom were mechanics accountable? Would obvious conflicts of interest undermine the few safeguards we had against sketchy mechanics?

Yet that is precisely the way in which pharmaceutical regulation works. The scientific evidence compiled and submitted by large pharmaceutical corporations has historically been considered "confidential commercial information" (also known as "confidential business information") and thereby protected from public scrutiny. The government regulators who vet this information on behalf of the public are scientists and clinicians, but they are also bureaucrats, facing the same kinds of complications that all public servants confront: time pressures, political pressures, and limited resources. The process of regulation rarely delves deeply enough to reproduce or attempt to verify the laboratory or clinical trial results (for instance, the scientific claims in the sponsor's product submission). Yet, because the data used to support these scientific claims are considered to be confidential commercial information, neither are independent experts permitted to review and evaluate the data. In time, drugs that seriously harm enough individuals to raise alarm become the subject of lawsuits, and pharmaceutical firms may pay out billions of dollars in damages to individuals or class actions; but, for the most part, they are handled quietly out of court. In some rare cases, a harmful product may be withdrawn from the market, but knowledge by pharmaceutical watchdog groups of even serious adverse events largely goes unnoticed in the medical community and the wider public. As the contributors to this volume describe, the fact that citizens believe medicines are reasonably safe and that the medications work is based more on trust than on the scientific evidence.

During the twentieth century, several scandals rocked public confidence, thereby spurring political attention to therapeutic product safety. The visible birth defects embodied in the victims of thalidomide, prescribed in pregnancy during the late 1950s and early 1960s, forced legislative amendment of health regulations across many European jurisdictions and in Canada. The persistence of the US Food and Drug Administration (FDA) drug reviewer Dr. Frances Oldham Kelsey in withholding approval by requesting further scientific evidence for the safety of the tranquilizer being prescribed for morning sickness in other jurisdictions saved many lives in the United States and put a hero's face on the regulatory watchdog. Trust needed legal enforcement; but memories are short, and the FDA fell under increasing pressure by the 1970s to speed up its reviews as access to new and important drugs in the United

States was seen as "lagging" behind Europe (for more detail, see Richert, 2014). By the 1980s, the Reagan administration had put into place a series of regulatory measures that privileged speed over safety. Fast forward to the early 2000s, and the pendulum had swung back in the other direction. The *Journal of the American Medical Association* and the *New York Times*, among others, were again questioning this relationship of trust and investigating the nature of the relationship between the regulator and the regulated, the evidence presented by the latter to win marketing approval, and the relationship between producers and prescribers of licensed drugs. Appeasing no one, over time, regulatory agencies (especially in the United States, but elsewhere as well) have been attacked, on the one hand, for applying lax standards and letting dangerous and/or ineffective drugs on the market or, on the other hand, for slowing down progress and medical innovation to the detriment of patients and people in need. And through it all, several lines of argument have emerged.

One line of argument, most clearly evident in the United States, held that regulatory agencies were not effectively independent of corporate influence: the FDA depended upon corporate contributions to fund regulatory review and the very reports holding powerful firms to account; it was staffed by a "rotating door" of corporate executives unwilling to challenge corporate interests; and these staff were answerable to elected representatives who either were dependent upon corporate donations for re-election or had direct financial interests in the firms regulated by the agencies they controlled.

The second line of argument queried the way in which the evidence supporting the licensing of pharmaceuticals was gathered, presented, and even conceptualized. These criticisms noted that coding categories could be subjective or arbitrarily constructed; data could be collected selectively across research sites or combined in a way to produce a given result; negative primary outcomes could be buried; p-values could be manipulated; specious comparators or irrelevant populations could be employed; surrogate markers could be used in lieu of primary outcomes; large quantities of data could be mined for any apparent correlations; and so on. Individual testing sites lacked access to the entire database, making any significant trends noted locally spurious. In addition, the public dissemination of results was vulnerable to publication bias in which negative studies were buried; the pharmaceutical industry employed ghostwriters in place of independent academic authors; and editorial self-censorship stymied publication of provocative articles due to fear of litigation or loss of advertising revenue.

A third line of argument, focusing on the market promotion (rather than licensing) of pharmaceuticals, challenged the conflicts of interest that appeared to exist in the use of corporate funds for medical education and continuing medical education, the fashioning of a cadre of high-profile clinicians as key opinion leaders, the wide distribution of free samples by commercial detailing teams, the development of clinical guidelines by those receiving corporate funding, and the funding of patient advocacy groups or "social influencers" by pharmaceutical firms.

As several contributors to this volume describe, the most egregious instances of misrepresentation and conflicts of interest began to be addressed by public bodies and other organizations in the years following the extensive publication and discussion of these critiques. Clinical trial registries were established, and both funding agencies and publication venues stipulated some requirement to register new research. Public bodies such as EudraVigilance, the European Network of Centres for Pharmacoepidemiology and Pharmacovigilance (ENCePP), Sentinel, and the Canadian Network for Observational Drug Effect Studies (CNODES) were instituted in order to monitor drugs already on the market. Health technology assessment (HTA) agencies refined their capacity to evaluate the effectiveness of new drugs. Frameworks were put in place to monitor payments to physicians and other health-care professionals, as were clearer conflict-of-interest protocols for guideline development committees. The price of pharmaceuticals also became the subject for political discussion, leading to laws on pharmaceutical pricing transparency in several American states; antitrust investigations in the United Kingdom, the United States, and the European Union; the establishment of the European Integrated Price Information Database (EURIPID); and the formation of several joint purchasing groups in some Canadian federal jurisdictions.

But to what extent has this focus on requiring greater transparency actually made a difference? The claim that the pharmaceutical industry is unaccountable, and that too many people are being hurt because of this lack of accountability, did prompt several measures to make the pharmaceutical industry more transparent, especially regarding its presentation (and withholding) of evidence and its attempt to influence regulators, prescribers, and the wider public. This book is an attempt to evaluate the progress made in holding the pharmaceutical industry to account through greater transparency. The papers collected in this volume were presented at a workshop held in Halifax, Nova Scotia, in 2018, organized by the Jean Monnet Network for Health Law and Policy. The question put to the contributors was not whether there was legislative progress in achieving greater transparency in pharmaceutical regulation: that is an empirical question, and one can simply list the measures put into place to answer in the affirmative. Rather, the contributors were asked to provide more nuanced accounts of how actionable and meaningful these changes have been. Have these measures made the regulatory landscape safer? Has corporate behaviour become more accountable? Is the public safer because of these measures?

Or, to the contrary, are these regulatory measures largely symbolic and toothless, providing the appearance of accountability while making few substantive changes? Is the superficial embrace of transparency *itself* an impediment to more profound changes? Laws requiring registration and the reporting of clinical trials have been in place for over a decade in the United States, yet enforcement of these requirements is desultory and uneven. The European Medicines Agency (EMA) has attempted, in recent years, to provide much greater public access to clinical trial data than either the FDA or Health Canada, but its efforts have been repeatedly stymied by the European Commission and the European courts. Canada, meanwhile, enacted important changes in law in 2019 through the Protecting Canadians from Unsafe Drugs Act, known as Vanessa's Law, but not without innumerable obstacles that had to be overcome. The question, then, is whether the attempt to achieve greater transparency in pharmaceutical evidence, including regulatory decision-making, has been a success – or merely a shell game.

The starting point for this volume is a conceptual analysis of transparency as a means of achieving accountability. Modern methods of governance generally require accountability, but accountability itself is not necessarily dependent on transparency. Why, and how, has transparency become an integral component for contemporary pharmaceutical regulation? And what, exactly, do we mean by "transparency" per se? As Fierlbeck in chapter two argues, the idea of transparency must be understood as a set of relationships involving several kinds of conditions. These relationships are informed by the dynamics of power. "To understand the political nature of transparency relationships," she writes, "one must be able to identify with precision the material to be made transparent, the parties who are required to disclose it, those who have a right of access to this information, the conditions (formal or de facto) under which it is disclosed, and the mechanisms through which it is accessed." A partial and incomplete account of transparency (for example, one without an account of how information is to be accessed, or under what conditions, or to whom, and with what kind of enforcement sanctions) will give the appearance of transparency without much meaningful substance. The debate over transparency has thus become a discussion of the conditions within which transparency is situated, and this discussion is itself the locus for the exercise of power by those with an interest in greater or less disclosure. By providing a conceptual mapping of the various ways in which transparency can be achieved (and stymied), Fierlbeck presents tools for evaluating the effectiveness of transparency measures.

And by overlaying this mapping with a theory of power, she explains why and how political interests try to shape these measures in one particular way rather than another.

The next three chapters together provide a comparative analysis of the development of regulatory transparency across three federal jurisdictions. The insights of the social sciences here caution against the hope for the policy equivalent of a magic pill that can produce the desired results in all cases and at all times. The comparative discussion of how the attempt to require greater transparency in the pharmaceutical sector was undertaken in these jurisdictions (and the respective successes and barriers experienced by each) underscores the importance of understanding the unique institutional and political context of each jurisdiction. Why – and how – did each jurisdiction attempt to achieve policy change in pharmaceutical regulation? The EMA was, as Davis, Mulinari, and Jefferson write in chapter three, a pale shadow of the American regulatory agency until 2010. Using an advocacy coalition approach, the authors argue that a collection of civil society groups, academic journals, and key individuals managed to form an effective association that was able to push for greater clinical trial data transparency in the European Union. Why did this political change emerge at that particular time? The development of post-Maastricht institutions provide the backdrop: while the commercial orientation of the European Union as a business-friendly enterprise unsurprisingly legitimated the protection of clinical trial data as "confidential commercial information," the networked structure of EU technical bodies and social interest groups (which Greer and Brooks [2021] refer to as "termites" within the formal legislative structure of the European Union) provided a political counterbalance to the dominant business interests. It was the interweaving of these politically active interests with new EU institutions (such as the EU Ombudsman office and the Court of Justice of the European Union, with their newly configured powers and treaty bases) that provided an effective opposition to the established commercial interests pushing for the protection of commercial confidentiality.

In chapter four, McCarthy and Ross investigate why the United States was able to achieve relatively early success in pharmaceutical data transparency despite the influence of corporate interests in policy-making. Prior to 1938, they note, patent medicine manufacturers were largely able to successfully evade government control because successful prosecution required state officials to prove intent to defraud. As is often the case, real tragedy was required to provide sufficient momentum for policy reform: the 1938 Food, Drug, and Cosmetic Act followed the deaths of over a hundred individuals who had consumed sulfanilamide – a commonly used drug – in a toxic new liquid formulation; and the 1962

Kefauver amendments requiring proof of safety and effectiveness were a consequence of babies born with deformed limbs due to thalidomide. As the authors argue, however, it was the wider legislative context of the United States which led to the regulatory specification that this clinical evidence should on principle be made available to the public. The establishment of the 1966 Freedom of Information Act, and the subsequent "open government" revisions to this legislation, allowed advocates to successfully push the FDA, however grudgingly, to provide much greater access to the clinical trial data upon which marketing approval was based. Using Canada as a comparator to support their argument, the authors observe that Canada's much weaker access to information legislation (largely the responsibility of each province) meant that the clinical data used in the approval process by Health Canada's Therapeutic Products Directorate were not amenable to scrutiny until very recently. The lesson here is that, to understand the ability of a jurisdiction to implement transparency mechanisms, one must have a solid understanding of the wider legislative context within which these mechanisms are embedded.

And yet Canada has now become a jurisdiction with one of the most transparent data regimes for pharmaceutical products. The nature of this transition is documented in more detail by Gagnon and colleagues in chapter five, which focuses on the way in which transparency was woven into the larger regulatory reforms in the restructuring of Canada's Food and Drug Act. As the authors describe, the parameters of these reforms – generally referred to as "Vanessa's Law" – were initially aimed at modernizing the safety provisions of the legislation. Once regulatory reform was initiated, however, stakeholders involved in the process of amending the legislation were able to persuade policy-makers to introduce measures providing for greater transparency. As the chapter explains, it took a pivotal judicial decision to substantiate the content of the new transparency provisions; but the potency of these measures has now been validated in law. The narrative of Canada's regulatory success corroborates theories of policy formation that stress the importance of establishing networks of influence and developing clear reform proposals that are "shovel ready" when a window of opportunity presents itself (see, for example, Cairney, 2016).

Following the theme of this book that the nature of transparency in pharmaceutical regulation is highly contextual and relational despite aspirations for harmonization, the remaining chapters examine more nuanced aspects of data transparency regulation across three jurisdictions. In chapter six, Persaud presents a sober account of how access to clinical studies has not lived up to expectations. He describes notable cases (paroxetine for depression, oseltamivir for influenza, doxylamine-pyridoxine for pregnancy-related nausea, and opioid prescribing) in which greater scrutiny of clinical data after the fact has had minimal impact on prescribing behaviour. He notes the lack of a "dose response" correlation in transparency (the assumption that every little advance will have some small improvement) and underscores the observation made in chapter two that it is crucial to understand the specific nature and context of transparency measures, as the wrong kind of implementation may simply reinforce the status quo while providing a false assurance that the problem has been addressed. Substantive transparency, for example, may require greater scrutiny of the evidence base prior to extensive marketing, rather than post facto openness, or an accessible record of the way in which drugs are marketed and promoted.

Similarly, limited and nebulous measures promising greater transparency should be viewed with caution. "Transparency" is an amorphous concept, even in relation to the specific application of pharmaceutical regulation. In chapter seven, Lexchin makes the distinction between transparency in rule-making, transparency in access to data, and transparency in the way in which rules are applied. Much literature addresses the first two areas, but very little exists focusing on the third. To this end, Lexchin investigates the transparency expectations for the regulators themselves: Who watches the watchers? Merely because rules governing access to data exist, do we really have a good sense of whether, and in what cases, these rules are being executed?

The conceptual mapping in chapter two makes the claim that relationships of transparency are inherently political. The way in which access to information is structured will favour some interests and disadvantage others. Established interests are not passive entities but active agents, and will engage in strategies that maximize their ability to achieve their desired outcomes. What are these tactical approaches? Who are the powerful political players here, and how do they attempt to shift the regulatory landscape in their favour? Gagnon, in chapter eight, explains the political dynamics that permit pharmaceutical interests to maintain their political dominance in the face of the greater regulatory embrace of data transparency. This process, he argues, is a subtle discursive strategy in which key players quietly shape the context of ideas in their favour. It can include framing what is meant by evidence in the first place, including clinical trial design, the use of publications in addition to clinical trials as evidence despite the existence of publication bias, the acceptability of non-disclosure of evidence to protect corporate research development, and so on. The strategy may include the undermining of evidence or voices that conflict with corporations' image or message. It can "capture" trusted voices (generally physicians) by providing financial or professional recompense to them only when the proper message is articulated. Or it can reach into the regulatory sphere itself and influence process and outcome either directly (for example, by financially supporting regulators) or indirectly (for example, through the revolving door mentioned earlier that brings regulators in from the corporate world, then sends them back to the corporate domain after their regulatory assignment has ended).

Political influence on the way in which transparency is operationalized in the pharmaceutical sector is important to understand but often difficult to grasp, given the subtle and indirect way in which it is constructed. It is this subtlety that arguably makes it so effective: in this relationship there is no heavy hand of corporate interest imposing its influence upon public agencies. Rather, it can be a process of shaping narratives such that public support materializes on one side rather than another. A complex reality can be framed as an either/or choice, with one option presented as clearly inferior. This manner of presentation, in turn, puts public pressure on governments to respond by formally supporting the preferred option. In chapter nine, Ghimire and Lemmens analyse one example of epistemic reductionism – the claim that we must choose between *either* clinical data transparency for rare disease trials *or* data privacy for research participants – in detail. They show how this dichotomy was constructed, and how this binary choice is in fact reconcilable. To the extent that treatments for rare diseases do *not* require strict data privacy, the attempt to mobilize public support to keep pharmaceutical data confidential is undermined.

The political complication underlying the push for public scrutiny of pharmaceutical data is that it is difficult to build popular support for a measure for which only those with a high level of technical training will have any direct interest. There are many issues that compete for the attention of politically engaged citizenry, and the issue of access to endless banks of data tables, coding schema, or methodology protocol documents is unlikely to provoke the public imagination. Yet, it is important to recognize the *indirect* public benefit of a formal regime of data scrutiny. Transparency is important because it is a mechanism of accountability that ensures the safety and effectiveness of drugs that people consume on the basis of trust. Pharmaceutical products that underperform (or lead to unanticipated harms) not only damage the health of individual citizens but, more worrisomely, undermine the social trust in the utility of drugs such as vaccines. A regime of transparency in which experts are able to check the work of other experts is in this way still greatly advantageous to the public at large. In chapter ten, Jefferson's original case study of the flu vaccine used during the H1N1 pandemic unravels the complex political dynamics underlying pharmaceutical regulation: Why does it happen that key information on the adverse effects of drugs is not disclosed? And what are the consequences? Given the issues that Jefferson identifies with the H1N1 vaccine and antivirals, it is worthwhile to consider the political pressure to produce biologics for COVID-19 as quickly as possible. These are not opportune conditions for the release of any drug or vaccine, and may contribute to serious adverse events when rolled out on a wide scale. The lesson from H1N1, according to Jefferson, is that the ability for the scientific community to collaborate and to scrutinize the scientific data while a drug is in production – especially when there is a political imperative to produce a vaccine as quickly as possible – may produce a much safer and more effective drug than one produced under conditions of data secrecy.

On a more positive note, Banzi, in chapter eleven, discusses the possibility of moving beyond a paradigm of data confidentiality. While many accounts of greater data transparency have been largely theoretical and aspirational, Banzi grounds the discussion of data access in the concrete experiences of Italy's Mario Negri Institute, which has rethought its policies and practices in order to embrace a more open and accountable relationship with scientific data. Finally, in chapter twelve, Fierlbeck, Graham, and Herder review the conclusions of the contributors and ask how, given the complex, intractable, and sometimes invisible obstacles to greater transparency, we should think strategically about transparency in the pharmaceutical sector.

REFERENCES

Cairney, P. (2016). *The politics of evidence-based policy-making.* London, UK: Palgrave Macmillan.
Canadian Institute for Health Information (CIHI). (2018). *Drug use among seniors in Canada,* 2016. Ottawa, ON: CIHI. Retrieved from https://www.cihi .ca/sites/default/files/document/drug-use-among-seniors-2016-en-web.pdf
Greer, S., & Brooks, E. (2021). Termites of solidarity in the house of austerity: Undermining fiscal governance in the European Union. *Journal of Health Politics, Policy, and Law, 46*(1). Advance online publication. https://doi.org /10.1215/03616878-8706615
Nanos. (2017). Prescription use survey summary. Retrieved from http:// innovativemedicines.ca/wp-content/uploads/2018/01/2017-nanos-survey.pdf
Richert, L. (2014). *Conservatism, consumer choice, and the Food and Drug Administration during the Regan era: A prescription for scandal.* Lanham, MD: Lexington Books.

2 Transparency, Pharmaceuticals, and the Problem of Policy Change

KATHERINE FIERLBECK

Situating the Debate over Transparency: Evidence, Accountability, and Power

The powerful allure of the scientific revolution in the seventeenth century was rooted in the epistemological certainty that scientific evidence provided in an increasingly factionalized and divisive political environment. As the religious wars sweeping Europe undermined political stability, the emphasis on empirical evidence and rigorous logical thinking challenged faith-based political legitimacy and demanded that those claiming authority should be held to account according to these new scientific standards. This relationship between evidence and accountability remains for us a clear and prudent one. However, the nature of evidence itself has become much more contested. And where the categories and methodologies determining the legitimacy of evidence are uncertain, disputed, or manipulated, then transparency becomes critical.

The political role for transparency as a form of accountability also grew as religious authority waned. In Bentham's classic account, God's "all seeing eye" was replaced by the social gaze, but the message was the same: you are being watched, so behave. The enemies of open scrutiny, wrote Bentham (1843, p. 310), may be collected into three classes: "the malefactor, who seeks to escape the notice of the judge; the tyrant, who seeks to stifle public opinion, whilst he fears to hear its voice; [and] the timid or indolent man, who complains of the general incapacity in order to screen his views."

Yet the hierarchical or "Weberian" structure of political governance adopted throughout the twentieth century articulated a system of political accountability that had little need for transparency. This form of vertical accountability focused on the clear allocation of roles and responsibilities in a top-down management structure (Weber, 1958).

As modern states became more complex due to the bureaucratic tasks they were expected to perform, technical decisions were relegated to a competent cadre of technocrats with a clearly defined scope of expertise. These units were organized in a strict hierarchical system that, in Westminster democracies, culminated in an elected official (the minister) accepting final responsibility for all bureaucratic decisions under his purview. The minister, in turn, was responsible to his party, which was answerable to the electorate. Accountability and confidentiality, in this manner, could comfortably coexist: as long as public well-being was secured, there was no reason that the small technical details subject to public governance needed to be exposed to public scrutiny.

Pharmaceutical regulation, requiring extensive technical expertise, fit this model particularly well. With so few individuals capable of evaluating the epidemiological data submitted to the regulatory authority, there appeared little reason to require this information to be publicly accessible. When clear public health crises appeared – such as birth defects linked to thalidomide prescriptions – elected public officials duly responded by requiring administrative and legislative reforms. The system of governance was in this way responsive; accountability in public health and safety did not require thoroughgoing transparency.

Or did it? With thalidomide, the response of some governments – such as Canada's – was much slower and more begrudging than that of others (Johnson, Stokes, & Arndt, 2018; Lexchin, 2018). And the presumption that the regulation of pharmaceuticals was merely a technical matter of scientific evaluation was sharply challenged in the public domain when, just over three decades later, litigation against large pharmaceutical corporations such as Pfizer and Merck for illegal marketing practices also exposed internal documents suggesting that public regulatory agencies were not protecting the public interest to the extent that many had assumed.

In terms of formal governance, the problem is that the Weberian, or hierarchical, model of accountability is increasingly ill-suited for pharmaceutical regulation in the context of contemporary industrial production and regulation. Structural and institutional shifts, as well as evolution in the nature of drug development, require a rethinking of the way in which public accountability of pharmaceutical licensing, marketing, and provision is conceived. As Aucoin and Heintzman (2000) argue, traditional approaches that rely primarily on centralized command and control systems, and that focus exclusively on ensuring compliance, have become increasingly ineffective in securing accountability. This is especially the case in complex policy areas where decision-makers "derive the responsibility for policy management within these sub-sectors to civil servants who, in turn, rely on interest groups and other pressure participants for information and advice" (Cairney, 2011, p. 12). As policy-makers increasingly defer for technical advice to those in the field, and outside of government, the traditional bureaucratic relationships of accountability become blurred.

Because these traditional mechanisms of accountability are increasingly ineffectual, it is imperative to employ a different process of formal answerability. Most regulators are increasingly working with the drug industry to determine which kinds of compounds should be developed and to navigate the complexities of formal submission for licensing. The function of regulators is not simply to act as an impartial arbiter of the safety of new compounds, but also to assist and facilitate the development of new products. This binary responsibility can serve to expedite access to new or improved drugs in the market, so there is arguably a public function being served as well as a commercial one. However, as the regulators increasingly work side by side with the regulated in the development of new pharmaceutical products, the likelihood of co-optation – of regulators seeing their mandate as responsibility to those developing drugs rather than those using them – continues to increase. Someone, in other words, must watch the watchers. To ensure the accountability of regulators to the public, a much more stringent standard of transparency is required.

The remainder of this chapter will first develop a conceptual mapping of the term "transparency": How ought we to think about relations of transparency? From whom (and to whom) is transparency required? What, precisely, ought to be transparent? Under which circumstances, and through what mechanisms? The purpose of this mapping exercise is to illustrate the complexity of transparency relations. By breaking down the transparency relationship into its component parts, we can see more precisely how it is that transparency can at the same time seem to be both facilitated and stymied. While this volume focuses specifically on clinical data, the conceptual mapping in this chapter expands the discussion of transparency in the pharmaceutical sector to make the point that the term "transparency" can be applied quite widely and that we must be clear exactly what it means when we use it. The second task of this chapter is to articulate a theory of power that can help to explain both why some success in achieving greater transparency occurs and why so many attempts at thoroughgoing reform fail. The discussion in this section rests squarely on discussions suggesting that the way in which ideas are framed influences policy implementation (see, for example, Béland 2009, 2019). It argues that, far from being a simple concept, "transparency" is an ideational battleground where political influence is determined by the ability to successfully define what is meant by the term itself.

What Do We Mean by "Transparency"?

Traditional definitions of transparency have been simple and descriptive: Birkinshaw (2006, p. 89), for example, defines transparency as "the conduct of public affairs in the open or otherwise subject to public scrutiny." Meijer (2014), however, understands transparency as a set of relations. I argue that transparency must be even further refined to denote a relationship that is *informed by conditions*. Some parties have an obligation to disclose information; others have the right to access it. The specific conditions under which this transaction occurs in a meaningful way must be stipulated. And, because this relationship exists between those with conflicting interests (and varying capacities to achieve them), it is also a relationship informed by the dynamics of power. To understand the political nature of transparency relationships, one must be able to identify with precision the material to be made transparent, the parties who are required to disclose it, those who have a right of access to this information, the conditions (formal or de facto) under which it is disclosed, and the mechanisms through which it is accessed. These relationships are outlined in schematic form in Table 2.1. Such relationships are also frequently contested ones: whether the scope of transparency is extended, to whom, under what conditions, and through what mechanisms, and even what reasons are given for limiting or augmenting the scope of transparency, are as much about the exercise of power as they are about technical or legal issues. To understand the way in which power is deployed in order to maintain existing relationships or to change them to the advantage of one party or another, one must also be able to identify how each political actor is able to use resources at their disposal. This exercise of power is not always explicit and, as section three of this chapter explains, the most effective exercise of power is often that which is best obscured.

The subject of pharmaceutical transparency is primarily, though not exclusively, clinical data. Pharmaceutical firms argue that their commercial advantage rests on their ability to prevent competitors from discovering relevant clinical information. Yet clinical data are also essential to clearly understand the health benefits and risks of drugs and devices. There is thus a tension between private and public interests over the disclosure of clinical data. A second category of disclosure focuses on conflicts of interest. The justification of transparency on this point is representational integrity: parties have duties to perform tasks impartially and professionally, and the existence of clear material incentives with the potential to compromise people's behaviour can be offset through careful scrutiny by others. The nature of these potential conflicts of interest vary according to professional roles, but they have in common

Table 2.1. Relationships of Transparency

Transparency of what?	Disclosed by whom?	Disclosed to whom?	Under what conditions?	How is information made accessible?
CLINICAL DATA				
Approved	Sponsor	Regulatory agency	Generally defined by regulatory authority, although some companies voluntarily disclose this information	Determined by regulatory authority
	Regulatory agency	Researchers, health-care professionals	Access with strict confidentiality	Responsive disclosure
		The public		
		Other levels of government	Only access to studies that have been concluded (no access to Phase I trials)	Proactive disclosure
Unapproved	Regulatory agency	Researchers	Access with strict confidentiality	Responsive disclosure (e.g., FOI requests)
		The public		
		Other levels of government	No conditions	Proactive disclosure (e.g., EPARs and AusPARs)
Post-approval	Sponsor	Regulatory agency		
	Regulatory agency	Researchers, clinicians	Access with strict confidentiality	Responsive disclosure
		The public		
		Other levels of government	No conditions	Proactive disclosure
	Health-care professionals	Regulatory agency	For adverse drug reactions, only new cases v. all cases encountered	
		Sponsor		

(Continued)

Table 2.1. (*Continued*)

Transparency of what?	Disclosed by whom?	Disclosed to whom?	Under what conditions?	How is information made accessible?
PROCEDURAL AND ADMINISTRATIVE OVERSIGHT				
Clinical trial inspections	Regulators	The public (includes health-care professionals)	Standing disclosure Release of reports only after third-party consultation	Individual site-based information Summary information
Regulatory justifications	Regulators	The public	Disclosing rationale for approving drugs Disclosing rationale for *not* approving drugs	Responsive disclosure (e.g., FOI requests) Proactive disclosure
Effectiveness of communication strategies for safety information	Regulators	The public		Responsive disclosure (e.g., FOI requests) Proactive disclosure
Advertising oversight	Regulators	The public		Responsive disclosure (e.g., FOI requests) Proactive disclosure

CONFLICTS OF INTEREST

Campaign financing	Elected officials	Institutions of representation The public	Direct political donations over a set amount	Data collected by electoral authorities and proactively posted on a publicly accessible online database
			Indirect funding of campaign issues (e.g., PACs)	Data collected by electoral authorities and accessible only via FOI request
			Communication with public office holders for payment with regard to legislative acts or awarding of contracts	
Lobbying	Elected officials	Institutions of representation The public	Communication with public office holders or civil servants for payment with regard to legislative acts or awarding of contracts	Registry of Lobbyists
Patient advocacy organizations	Group representatives	Regulatory agencies Patients The public	When making submissions to regulatory agencies or undertaking public campaigns	PAO website noting what funding received and how it was utilized; regulatory website for cases where PAOs have made a submission to regulators
Journals	Authors	Editors Readership	Upon publication of articles	Information published with article
	Editors Boards	Readership The public	Upon appointment and at regular intervals	On journal website

(Continued)

Table 2.1. (Continued)

Transparency of what?	Disclosed by whom?	Disclosed to whom?	Under what conditions?	How is information made accessible?
Institutional membership	Professional associations	Self-regulating professions Relevant patient groups Journal editors, readership (if published) The public	When funds are received (e.g., for conferences)	Conference materials; professional associations' websites
	Regulatory agency membership	State authority The public	Upon appointment and at regular intervals	Agency website
	HTA committee members	Regulatory agencies (state, institutional) Funding agencies (state, institutional)	Upon appointment and at regular intervals	Agency website
Direct contributions (in cash and in kind) given to health-care professionals	Sponsor	The state; the public	When contributions over a set amount are received	Website
	Health-care professionals	The state; the public	When contributions over a set amount are received	Website
Medical education	CME organizers	CME participants	All educational events funded directly or indirectly by commercial interests	In educational materials provided and on website
	Medical schools	University administration Medical students	All educational events funded by commercial interests	In educational materials provided and on website
PRICE AND SUPPLY				
List price	Sponsor	Wholesalers Pharmacies Health service providers The public		

Wholesale price	Wholesalers	Pharmacies Health service providers	Generally confidential	Shortages website
Rebates	Manufacturers Wholesalers Pharmacies		Generally confidential	
Availability of drugs	Sponsor	State authority (e.g., regulatory agency or department of health)	Manufacturing or quality issues; commercial or capacity decisions	
	State authority	Health-care provider	Drugs deemed "medically necessary"	Direct communication; "Dear Health-care Provider" letters to individual providers and on website
	State authority	The public	Drugs deemed "medically necessary"	Shortages website
Production of drugs	Manufacturing plants	Regulators	Manufacturers must supply information regarding production of compounds as set out by regulatory authorities	Submission of documents
				On-site inspection
	Regulators	The public	Standing disclosure	Individual site-based information
	Regulators	The public	Release of reports only after third-party consultation	Summary information

Notes: AusPAR = Australian public assessment report; CME = continuing medical education; EPAR = European public assessment report; FOI = Freedom of Information; HTA = health technology assessment; PAC = political action committee; PAO = patient advocacy organization the expectation of impartiality in, for example, making laws, rules, or guidelines; treating patients; or presenting accurate information. Transparency can also perform other tasks: it can, for example, facilitate predictable access to drugs or prevent price gouging. Even where conflicts of interest are not an issue, requiring that individuals or interests are clearly identified in the roles they play (for example, in testing, writing, or rule-making) is an important aspect in securing accountability for outcomes.

It is useful to unpack this table in more detail. The rest of this section explains the nature of these relationships in a more detailed manner.

Clinical Data

Within the context of pharmaceuticals, most discussions of transparency are articulated with reference to the disclosure of the clinical data used as a basis for licensing. But this randomized controlled trial (RCT) data itself has several component parts (Table 2.2), and a key issue has been precisely *which parts* of this RCT data ought to be disclosed. Even before data are collected, a protocol document establishes the operating procedures for the clinical trial. The Consolidated Standards of Reporting Trials (CONSORT) group, for example, has specified twenty-two different items within its checklist, including eligibility criteria for participants, precise details of the interventions, clearly defined primary and secondary outcomes, the determination of sample size, methods for randomization, blinding processes, statistical methods, baseline demographic and clinical characteristics of participants, adverse events, and the existence of ancillary analyses (CONSORT, 2010). These methodological standards serve as the ground rules for the process of data gathering. Standards are critical, as the way in which one chooses to collect data can itself shape the information one obtains. Shaping can happen, for example, by selecting certain kinds of individuals, by coding events in specific ways, by adding participants in at opportune times, by reorganizing subgroups, or by modifying the length of the period under investigation. All of these factors could make a difference in the results that are reported.

Once the study commences, information on each participant is collected through the use of a clinical case report form (CRF). The protocol document may provide a template of the CRF to be used in the study, including a justification of why (and how) specific kinds of information are to be collected. Completed CRFs are the raw data from which final results are extrapolated. The collection of this empirical data may be basic, but it is not necessarily simple. A poorly designed CRF, for example, may contain ambiguous or redundant information

Table 2.2. The Component Parts of Clinical Trial Data

Component	What it is	Contents	Disclosed to
Protocol document	A procedural document that sets out what the study will investigate and how it will be executed	May contain all or some of the following: • background and rationale • list of locations and investigators • study design (e.g., # of subjects, length of study, outcome measures) • methods (e.g., recruitment, eligibility criteria, randomization and blinding techniques) • statistical methodology • policy on adverse event reporting • data management (storage of data, etc.) • safety review (e.g., when to stop trial)	The protocol document, and any amendments, is normally part of the CSR that is submitted to the regulator. It may be reproduced in the CSR in full or in part.
Case report form	Discrete forms that record data from individual study subjects	Contains information on each study participant. Can be a single snapshot in time or can present multiple points of information taken over the duration of the study. When the data is submitted for analysis, information identifying the participant will be replaced by a unique study number.	Data on CRFs are compiled by researchers into data sets. Blank CRFs may be included in study protocol and submitted in CSRs. Individual completed CRFs are rarely submitted to regulators, although they must be provided if requested. They are rarely made public.
Data sets	Aggregated data derived from CRFs	Each data set compiles CRF data addressing specific aspects of the study.	If data sets are submitted as part of the CSRs, they will be disclosed to regulators. If they are listed as appendices, they may or may not be part of the parcel submitted to regulators and/or to other researchers or the public.

(Continued)

Table 2.2. (*Continued*)

Component	What it is	Contents	Disclosed to
Clinical study report	A document presenting an interpretation of the data sets	CSRs generally contain some information on the study protocol, but the main content is the analysis of the data gathered throughout the study. CSRs may or may not contain data sets compiled from the trial.	CSRs are key documents submitted to regulators supporting the licensing of the product under review. Depending on the jurisdiction and the specific conditions, researchers and others may request access to the CSRs, or CSRs may be posted online and available to the public directly.
Journal article	A brief (ideally peer-reviewed) document, published in a professional periodical, that discusses study outcomes	Journal articles are highly compressed analyses of the data sets. They will only contain a small proportion of the data presented in the CSR.	Journal articles are generally considered to be publicly accessible, although individuals not affiliated to research institutions may encounter financial obstacles to easy access of these publications.

Notes: CRF = case report form; CSR = clinical study report

(Bellary, Krishnankutty, & Latha, 2014). In some cases, the information to be collected is easily quantifiable (blood pressure, heart rate, and so on); but in other cases, the information may depend upon reported feelings, sensations, or moods, and a clinician must exercise judgement in attempting to categorize this information. To this extent, a certain level of subjectivity already exists at the level of raw data entry.

Information compiled in individual CRFs is aggregated into data sets. These data sets are compiled according to the outcomes to be measured, as specified in the protocol document. Using the statistical methods also outlined in the protocol document, these data sets are analysed and the interpretation of the findings is presented in the clinical study report (CSR). The interpretation of data is a crucial aspect of the perceived success of a clinical trial. Here, again, the results involve a level of subjectivity that can result in selection bias. For example, exactly what results should be reported? Regulatory approval may be more likely if certain subgroup analyses were presented, while others were buried;

if secondary outcomes were positive, even if primary ones were not; or if adverse events were not reported or misleadingly coded.

The CSR, with its analysis of the results presented by the trial sponsor, is the primary document submitted to regulators for approval. In addition to interpretation of data sets, however, a good CSR will bring together other key pieces of information, such as the protocol, and any protocol amendments, and the statistical analysis plan. Precisely what is included in the CSR varies across jurisdictions. The information presented in CSRs is generally robust, but because the point of the CSR is to highlight "relevant" data, not all data may be contained in the report. Data can also be placed in appendices, which may or may not be as accessible as the main report (Doshi & Jefferson, 2013). Completed CRFs themselves are often not included in CSRs and are generally not required in the first instance by the regulators: one reason for this omission is the sheer volume of data involved in many studies, which is seen to place too heavy a burden on regulatory agencies. RCT sponsors making submissions to regulators must be able to produce both CRFs and full data sets if they are requested, although it is not always clear when, and for what reasons, this detailed information is sought by regulatory agencies.

Published articles in academic journals can also be part of the package of evidence submitted by pharmaceutical firms to regulators in support of their product. Yet, as Doshi and Jefferson (2013) observe, the "compression of information" presented in published articles means there is rarely enough detail from which to effectively evaluate either the methods or the interpretation of the data. Moreover, positive outcomes are much more frequently published than negative ones, and this publication bias underlying published submissions may distort the actual effectiveness of a drug (Bourgeois, Murthy, & Mandl, 2010; Ioannidis, Munafò, Fusar-Poli, Nosek, & David, 2014).

The argument for greater transparency in clinical data rests upon the utility of being able to verify the information submitted by those with a clear interest in a particular outcome. The efficacy of new pharmaceutical products in practice tends to be lower than predicted values, and the adverse events often tend to be higher. Access to the data under review permits greater scrutiny of the information, leading to a more accurate understanding of the compound under review, and acts as a check against the distortion of data collected in RCTs. In a turn to regulatory transparency in the early 2000s, many jurisdictions established clinical trial registries. Sponsors wishing to commence an RCT were expected to register their study in advance, including both primary and second outcomes, and to report results upon completion. In this way, negative results or adverse outcomes could not be easily obscured. Largely because of the Food and Drug Administration (FDA) requirement that Phase II and III trials in the United States had to be registered with ClinicalTrials. gov (the largest registry), the growth of clinical trial registries has been considerable. Trial registration was reinforced by the decision of the International Committee of Medical Journal Editors (ICMJE) in 2004 requiring RCTs to be registered if the results were to be published in key medical journals. In February 2020, a US federal court ruled that clinical trial data transparency was not simply limited to data collected after 2017, and it directed sponsors to submit missing data for trials conducted between 2007 and 2017.

The European Union has its own registry, as do some individual European member states (including Germany, the United Kingdom, and the Netherlands). Canada has a clinical trials database, but not a registry; it does, however, participate in the United Kingdom's ISRCTN registry. The World Health Organization (WHO) also hosts an International Clinical Trials Registry Platform (ICTRP). Clinical trial registration has climbed steadily since the mid-2000s (Viergever & Li, 2015), but adherence is still problematic. Depending on the jurisdiction, researchers may only be required to register trials if they receive public funding or if they desire publication of research results in specific high-level journals. Even when studies are registered, there is uneven compliance in reporting the results of these studies (Anderson et al., 2015; Fleminger & Goldacre, 2018).

Clinical trial registries are useful in providing clinical data, but there are limitations to the utility of registries. Even when studies are registered, results may simply not be reported. In the European Union, for example, only 51 per cent of registered trials reported within the mandated twelve months (Goldacre et al., 2018). Sanctions for non-compliance are rare. Despite the requirement for data transparency in the United States, the FDA has never levied a fine for failing to disclose information, nor have the National Institutes of Health in the United States withheld grant funding for those failing to comply (Piller, 2020). Moreover, even when results are posted, the summary reports may not provide sufficient information to verify interpretation of clinical data.

The development of clinical trial registries has not dampened the demand that clinical data submitted for approval to regulatory agencies ought to be disclosed more widely, a measure strongly resisted by pharmaceutical firms. The European Union's drug regulator, the European Medicines Agency (EMA), has made considerable progress towards this end, releasing over 1.3 million pages of clinical study reports between October 2016 and April 2018. As Davis, Mulinari, and Jefferson (chapter three in this volume) describe, however, it has not been without setbacks, such as the suspension of the proactive release of these reports (prompted by the relocation of the EMA) and the limitation of access to older clinical study reports to EU citizens only.

In the United States, the FDA developed a clinical data summary pilot program in which portions of CSRs from up to nine new drug applications are posted, although critics have suggested that this information is "extremely limited in scope" (Bruckner, 2018). More importantly, a federal court ruling released in February 2020 stipulated that clinical trial sponsors must release the results of clinical trial data conducted prior to 2017 (which had previously been exempted from the requirement that trial results were to be made public on the ClinicalTrials.gov registry.) In 2014, Canada amended its Food and Drugs Act (Vanessa's Law) to permit greater access to clinical data. This amendment was supported in March 2017 by Health Canada's announcement to view unpublished drug data as public information not subject to commercial confidentiality. A slightly different model for access to clinical data can be found in data sharing websites, where research data is "banked" and can be accessed through application by other sets of researchers (for example, the Yale Open Data Access [YODA] project; see Krumholz & Waldstreicher, 2016).

The focus on clinical data transparency is primarily for pharmaceuticals that have been approved for use. Another issue is the extent to which information on drugs that have *not* been approved should be accessible. Again, it varies widely by jurisdiction. The European Union does post public assessment reports for drugs that have been refused a market authorization, as does Australia. By contrast, the FDA does not disclose information on compounds that have not been approved nor, more pointedly, "does the agency even notify the public that such rejections or withdrawals have occurred" (Almashat & Carome, 2017, p. 46).

Clinical data may also be compiled after compounds have been licensed. The most common instance of this practice is the reporting of adverse events from approved medications. The pathways of reporting will vary across jurisdictions, as does the ability to access this information. The European Union's pharmacovigilance system, EudraVigilance, is a collaborative effort between the European Commission, the EMA, and individual member states; and it extends beyond the European Union to the European Economic Area (EEA). Information is received from both marketed use and clinical trials. The system was launched in 2001 and, by 2017, had collected over 12 million individual case safety reports (Postigo et al., 2018). Public access to the EudraVigilance system was expanded in 2017, with restricted access on reports available to the general public (by age, sex, and EEA/non-EEA origin). Extended data sets are available to academic researchers by request, dependent upon signing a confidentiality undertaking. Since 2016, the FDA's Adverse Event

Reporting System (FAERS) has been supported by Sentinel, a web of electronic health-care databases. Information on adverse events submitted to FAERS is accessible to the public via an electronic dashboard. Likewise, Canada has a Vigilance Adverse Reaction online database that is accessible to the public. The issue here is how these data are collected: Who reports perceived adverse events, and to whom? To what extent do adverse events experienced by individuals consuming prescription drugs get listed by these databases?

The issue of precisely *which* clinical data ought to be publicly accessible is in this way more complicated than might appear at first glance. But data transparency, as noted earlier, must be understood as a relationship, and the question of accessibility *to whom* is also far from straightforward. The issue of who should have access to clinical data is also mediated by the question *under which conditions* should any party be able to claim access? Moreover, access to data can be circumscribed by the particular *mechanisms* through which data is accessed. For example, the EMA granted public access to clinical trial data under Policy 0043 (in accordance with Regulation 1049/2001), but the mechanism was reactive: the data was only available upon request. Under Regulation 536/2014 and Policy 0070 (effective October 2016), however, all RCT materials used by the EMA for approval were released proactively (subject to redactions where necessary). The EU General Court upheld the default assumption of open and free access to clinical data in February 2018 (Mezher, 2018), but in September 2019, the advocate general of the Court of Justice of the European Union ruled that disclosure of this information would harm the commercial interests of pharmaceutical companies and should be kept confidential (Coombes, 2019). Only in 2020 did the Court of Justice of the European Union reaffirm public access to documents submitted by firms seeking market authorization in the European Union.

In Canada, revisions to the Food and Drug Act (commonly called Vanessa's Law) stipulated that access to clinical trial data is at the discretion of the minister of health and must be accessible to identifiable individuals (for example, "a person from whom the Minister seeks advice" or "a person who carries out functions relating to the protection or promotion of human health or the safety of the public" [Canada, 2014, p. 4]). An attempt to access clinical data for the drug Diclectin in 2015 was successful under this act only after a strict confidentiality agreement was negotiated between the researcher and Health Canada. As chapter five in this volume describes, a federal court ruling in 2018 (*Doshi v. Attorney General of Canada*) ultimately supported the disclosure of clinical trial data without restrictive conditions. Physical obstacles can also affect accessibility: for example, the scrutiny of large data sets can be difficult if the data are provided on a restricted or poorly designed web access interface (see, for example, Le Noury et al., 2015). Other physical obstacles can simply consist of limited resources by regulatory agencies for responding to requests for data. For example, the FDA's Center for Drug Evaluation and Research receives about 3,500 Freedom of Information (FOI) requests per year, with a backlog of about 600 requests (Sager, 2018).

Finally, transparency relationships can exist between governments without public involvement. In such cases, while clinical data is not publicly available, it is accessible on a government-to-government basis. This practice is becoming more common in federal systems, where regulation, purchasing, and service provision functions may exist across governments. Such a relationship of data sharing may arise horizontally (between governments at a similar level) or vertically (between central and regional governments). Because of the resource-intensive nature of health technology assessment (HTA), for example, federal jurisdictions may find it more efficient to combine resources or jointly finance evaluative units for new drugs (for example, EUnetHTA in the European Union or CADTH in Canada) or for the monitoring of adverse events (such as EudraVigilance for EEA states, CNODES across Canada, or Sentinel in the United States).

Procedural and Administrative Oversight

The issue of pharmaceutical transparency extends well beyond access to clinical data. In another set of transparency relationships, the object of the relationship is not clinical data but rather the activity of regulatory agencies themselves, including the information they use to make important decisions. As Lexchin writes in chapter seven of this volume, "the way that the government applies the regulations in reaching a final decision needs to be communicated effectively and publicly, and the effectiveness of those communications in achieving their objectives needs to be evaluated to be sure that people understand what is being said and that the messages, if necessary, are having the desired effect." For example, how is it possible to know whether a regulator performs an appropriate number of clinical trial inspections and whether these inspections are productive? If the number is based on risk, then the criteria for higher-risk trials must be clearly stated, and the agency must have current information for trial sites. Reports must be posted publicly in a timely manner, with concise details given regarding non-compliance, required corrective actions, and follow-through.

Similarly, it is not simply clinical data per se but rather the clear and detailed explanation of the rationale for approval of pharmaceutical compounds (or the refusal to approve them) that is useful to know. This is particularly the case for expedited reviews, which may require more resources and have higher safety risks. What is the rationale for taking an action on safety, both in general terms (the criteria for issuing a safety warning) and in specific cases? Moreover, when such warnings are issued, how effective are these communications strategies? Many regulatory agencies have functions that go beyond drug approval and safety monitoring. Health Canada, for example, has formal authority over the commercial promotion of pharmaceuticals, but it has in practice conferred this authority to the Pharmaceutical Advertising Advisory Board (PAAB). And, as Lexchin notes in chapter seven, there is little public information given regarding the criteria used to consider complaints regarding breaches of promotion guidelines, the rationale used for taking action in specific cases, or the monitoring of compliance in these actions.

Conflicts of Interest

Another set of transparency relationships attempts to shed light on the interests of those who make policy decisions, represent certain constituencies, or espouse particular choices in treatments or guidelines. A conflict of interest can be understood as "a set of conditions in which professional judgement concerning a primary interest (such as a patient's welfare or the validity of research) tends to be unduly influenced by a secondary interest (such as financial gain)" (Thompson, 1993, p. 573). The reason such conflicts are problematic is that they have the potential to compromise the judgement of those making important decisions to the detriment of others to whom they may hold a duty of care or fair representation.

CAMPAIGN FINANCING

To the extent that elected officials benefit from the financial contributions of donors, for example, there is justifiable concern that they hold the donors' interests above those they have been elected to represent. Legislators establish the ground rules within which pharmaceutical firms operate; knowing how profoundly elected officials depend on the financial contributions of those subject to these rules can focus attention more squarely on the impartiality of the legislators. On this principle, the US Federal Election Commission oversees an online database of political contributions; websites like OpenSecrets.org and FollowTheMoney. org have accommodated this data into user-friendly interfaces that permit more precise scrutiny of the data. Using OpenSecrets.org, for example, one learns that pharmaceutical and health product corporations contributed US$29.3 million to all Senate and House candidates in the 2017–18 election cycle. The Republican Party benefited very slightly less than the Democratic Party (US$14.3 million versus US$14.9 million); the average contribution was higher in the Senate than in the House of Representatives; and the individual with the highest campaign contribution from pharmaceutical/health product donors was Bob Casey (D-PA) at US$540,192 (Center for Responsive Politics, 2018). A scan of FollowTheMoney.org permits one to track contributions by company: for example, one can determine that the pharmaceutical firm Wyeth made US$5.8 million in contributions to 1,203 filers over eleven years. (National Institute on Money in Politics, 2020). In addition to campaign contributions, political non-profit organizations or super political action committees (PACs) can engage in political spending without disclosing the source of funds. This practice is commonly referred to as "dark money." The spending on dark money is difficult to trace, as super PACs and similar groups can utilize funds for such functions as "media services" that do not have to be declared in tax filings as long as they remain issue-oriented and do not advocate explicitly for particular candidates by name. In this way, for example, members of the Pharmaceutical Research and Manufacturers of America (PhRMA) were able to contribute at least US$6.1 million to the organization American Action Network, which spent US$10 million on an advertising campaign advocating for the end to the US Affordable Care Act (Hancock, 2018). During the 2020 American electoral campaign, pharmaceutical corporations spent around US$11 million in campaign donations to 356 political officials via PACs (Facher, 2020).

LOBBYING

The contribution of lobbyists is a related issue: rather than contributing funds directly to political candidates, corporate and interest groups hire lobbyists to represent and promote their interests to elected officials. Again, many states have some form of mandated disclosure; the US data on lobbying are collected from the clerk of the House of Representatives and the secretary of the Senate. ProPublica organizes this data so that one can investigate what kind of activity is undertaken: in 2018, 2019, and 2020, for example, PhRMA hired the S-3 Group to lobby a number of key legislators on access to pharmaceuticals (ProPublica, 2020). OpenSecrets.org compiles its information slightly differently: in 2017, for example, it noted that PhRMA (including its subsidiaries We Work for Health and Partnership to Fight Chronic Disease) spent US$25.8 million on lobbying American officials (Center for Responsive Politics, 2017).

The activity of lobbyists in Canada is tracked rather differently. At the federal level, one can determine who (representing which interest) is lobbying whom on which issue; but there is no dollar value placed on this activity as in the United States. The kind of information that one can glean is thus quite different. One can see, for example, that Innovative Medicines Canada (IMC) and its affiliated partners had 108 interactions with "designated office holders" in Ottawa over a twelve-month period (Office of the Commissioner of Lobbying of Canada, 2020). Of IMC's eleven registered lobbyists, ten were active over this period. Fourteen government institutions were the focus of the lobbying activity. One interesting observation of this lobbying record is that the proportion of lobbying that focused on economic policy-making or trade units (Innovation, Service, and Economic Development; Finance Canada; Treasury Board; Global Affairs) far surpassed the lobbying interfaces with Health Canada. This finding supports the argument that, at a federal level, health policy is more importantly the purview of *fiscal* units rather than health-oriented ones. In this account, the interests of these fiscal units (economic and industrial development, international trade and competitiveness) are thus more likely the drivers of health policy at a federal level in Canada.

PATIENT ADVOCACY ORGANIZATIONS

Representational conflicts of interest also commonly arise when patient advocacy organizations (PAOs) receive funding from pharmaceutical companies. From their genesis in the 1980s as a strategy to pressure governments to expedite drug development for AIDS treatments, most large PAOs now receive funding from drug manufacturers (Batt, 2017; McCoy et al., 2017; Kang, Bai, Karas, & Anderson, 2019). A 2017 study found that 67 per cent of PAOs sampled in the United States received funding from for-profit companies, almost half of which were pharmaceutical, medical device, or biotechnology companies (Rose, Highland, Karafa, & Joffre, 2017). In the United Kingdom, a 2019 study noted that the pharmaceutical industry contributed over £57 million to PAOs between 2012 and 2020 (Ozieranski, Rickard, & Mulinari, 2019).

Patients' groups can be instrumental in getting drugs approved by regulatory agencies: in the case of Addyi, for example, industry-funded women's health groups were able to overturn the FDA's own internal reviewers, who recommended against approving the drug (Block & Canner, 2016). PAOs can also pressure governments to add new drugs to formularies by publicly "shaming" politicians with accusations of callous indifference to the obvious suffering of their constituents or by pointing out the seeming inequity of funding specialized drugs for some cancers, but not others. PAOs have also been active in voicing opposition to the attempt by governments to replace brand-name drugs on their formularies with generic and bio-similar alternatives. In Canada, for example, Crohn's and Colitis Canada organized a "No Forced Switch" campaign involving over 4,500 patients lobbying government officials not to impose the use of bio-similars in place of brand-name drugs. The organization received about 14 per cent of its CAN$14.9 million budget from brand-name pharmaceutical companies (Grant, 2018a). In Australia, 34 pharmaceutical firms distributed over AU$35 million to 230 organizations; those firms that spent the most had companies with drugs under review for public reimbursement (Fabbri, Swandari, Lau, Vitry, & Mintzes, 2019). PAOs are also increasingly involved in the decision-making process of health technology agencies: a 2019 study, for example, found that 72 per cent of the PAOs (38 out of 53) received funding from the manufacturer of the treatment under appraisal by the HTA agency (Mandeville et al., 2019).

The issue is not simply the active representation of the interests of corporate sponsors but also the potential for cautious self-censorship to avoid antagonizing commercial funders. Currently, most jurisdictions engage in some form of voluntary self-regulation, in which companies may or may not list the groups to which they provide funding. However, there is little monitoring for compliance. In 2017, the province of Ontario did enact legislation that would require pharmaceutical firms to disclose payments to PAOs (in addition to physicians), but this measure was suspended when a new government was returned and, by 2021, was still in abeyance. In 2018, *Kaiser Health News* compiled a database of corporate funding to PAOs in the United States. The database, "Pre$cription for Power," examined data from federal regulatory filings and websites for 594 PAOs and 14 large pharmaceutical firms. Notably, these companies spent almost twice as much supporting PAOs (US$116 million) as they did in direct lobbying (US$63 million) in 2015 (the first year for which data was available). One company, Bristol Myers Squibb, spent over US$20.5 million on PAOs, compared to US$2.9 million on direct government lobbying efforts (Kopp, Lupkin, & Lucas, 2018).

JOURNALS

In contrast to *representational* conflicts of interest (where the duty of representation may be compromised by competing interests), *professional* conflicts of interest are instances where the technical or clinical judgement of an individual may be compromised by competing interests they may have. One of the earliest formal protocols for the disclosure of competing interests was undertaken by medical journals (through the International Committee of Medical Journal Editors); the protocol requires authors to declare all relevant financial relationships (including, among other things, employment, affiliation, funding, consultancies, honoraria, stock ownership or options, expert testimony, royalties, and patents). Such financial conflicts do not preclude authors from publishing; the purpose of declaring competing interests is designed to allow readers "to interpret the information in the article accordingly in light of those disclosures" (Fontanarosa & Bauchner, 2017, p. 1768).

The point of ascertaining conflicts of interest is that financial biases can influence research results. The evidence, as Smith (2002) notes, increasingly shows that conflicts of interest have a strong influence on the interpretation of data. A 2004 survey of medical journals, for example, found competing interests for authors in 20 to 30 per cent of published manuscripts (depending on how conflicts of interest were defined); these manuscripts showed not only a strong association with positive study results but also an "extremely small" likelihood of correlating with negative results (Friedman & Richter, 2004). A 2017 study confirmed this relationship, noting that "financial ties were independently associated with positive clinical trial results" (Ahn et al., 2017, p. 6). Authorship conflict of interest guidelines are now standard practice. Less common, however, are conflict of interest policies for peer reviewers, editors, editorial boards, and publishers. One study found that over half of 713 medical journal editors had received payments from drug or device companies, some as high as US$1 million (Liu, Bell, Matelski, Detsky, & Cram, 2017; see also Kaestner & Prasad, 2017). Others have pointed out that some journals benefit considerably from reprint sales and thus have a clear financial interest in publishing large positive pharmaceutical studies. Lundh, Barbateskovic, Hróbjartsson, and Gøtzsche (2010) observe that 41 per cent of the *New England Journal of Medicine*'s profits in 2005–06 depended on reprint sales. The more a journal relies on these reprints, the more susceptible it may be to threats to pull a paper facing critical peer reviews. Given these conflicts of interest, suggest the authors, journals should publicly disclose their sources and amounts of income (Lundh et al., 2010).

Notwithstanding the greater awareness of conflicts of interest in publication and the greater prevalence of formal disclosure policies, progress in addressing conflicts of interest in medical journals might, as Smith (2002, p. 1375) declares, "be cruelly summarized as lots of rhetoric and not much action." While authors are generally required to disclose competing interests, there is much less uniformity on policies regarding peer reviewers, editors, boards, and publishers. Moreover, while information on author conflicts of interest are generally collected by a journal, this information is often not published by the journal. Cooper, Gupta, Wilkes, and Hoffman (2006) found that more than 40 per cent of the journals in their survey did not publicly disclose author conflict of interest statements, while Haivas, Schroter, Waechter, and Smith (2004) discovered that 37 per cent of the journals in their study did not intend to declare editors' financial interests, and 53 per cent would not disclose the financial interests of editorial board members. Finally, even where interests are disclosed, there is rarely any systematic process of verification of these declarations (Cooper et al., 2006). The process of verification, when performed at all, is generally undertaken by third parties rather than journals themselves. In 2018, for example, ProPublica and the *New York Times* cross-referenced the disclosure statements of José Baselga, chief medical officer of Memorial Sloan Kettering Cancer Center, with information from the Open Payment federal database, and found that Baselga failed to report industry funding in over half of almost 180 papers published since 2013 (Thomas & Ornstein, 2018).

INSTITUTIONAL MEMBERSHIP

A different category of transparency relationships focuses on professional associations that have a primary responsibility to make technical or clinical decisions as a matter of policy (as opposed to the treatment of identifiable individuals). These associations include clinical guideline committees, groups representing medical professionals, regulatory agencies, health technology assessment (HTA) bodies, and research institutions.

Clinical guidelines are "statements that include recommendations to optimize patient care that are informed by a systematic review of evidence and an assessment of the benefits and harms of alternate care options" (Sox, 2017). Treatment guidelines began to be formalized in the early 1980s, and have rapidly become more prevalent. Often the pharmaceutical industry stands to gain considerably from the articulation of these guidelines: by slightly adjusting the parameters of treatment, the proportion of individuals advised to take medications can rise significantly. The best-known example of this practice was the introduction of new recommendations for treating high cholesterol with statins. Guidelines issued by the American College of Cardiology and the American Heart Association in 2013 expanded the use of statins for those between 40 and 75 years of age by 25 to 30 per cent (Unruh, Rice, Vaillancourt Rosenau, & Barnes, 2016). More problematically, the attempt to articulate a clear balance between the harms and benefits of taking a drug can be highly subjective, as harms and benefits "seldom have the same unit of measure" (Sox, 2017, p. 1739).

In a study of the criteria developed for the Diagnostic and Statistical Manual of Mental Disorders (DSM)-IV and DSM-IV-TR between 1989 and 2004, Cosgrove, Krimsky, Vijayaraghavan, and Schneider (2006) found that, in six of the eighteen panels, more than 80 per cent of the panelists had financial ties to a pharmaceutical industry. A separate study determined that 90 per cent of the authors of psychiatric guidelines had financial relationships with pharmaceutical companies (Cosgrove, Bursztajn, Krimsky, Anaya, & Walker, 2009). The results were similar in a Danish study, which examined forty-five different clinical practice guidelines: of these, forty-three had been written by one or more authors with conflicts. Notably, these conflicts were disclosed in only one of the forty-five guidelines (Bindslev, Schroll, Gøtzsche, & Lundh, 2013). In response to growing concern, the US Institute of Medicine developed a set of recommendations in 2011 regarding conflicts of interest for those serving on guideline committees. Chief among these was the provision that chairs and co-chairs should have no competing interests, while committee members with conflicting interests should comprise a minority of the panel. Yet the application of these "guidelines on guidelines" has been mixed at best. In some cases, where guidelines on competing interests exist, this information may not be disclosed to the public (Sox, 2017). In other cases, the guidelines are simply ignored or are not verified. Jefferson and Pearson (2017) examined the membership of two key American guideline committees: one responsible for cholesterol guidelines, the other for hepatitis C treatment. While the 2011 guidelines on guideline development stated that chairs and co-chairs should not have any conflicts of interest, one of the three co-chairs openly declared competing interests. In addition, the study authors found even more undeclared conflicts of interest. For the hepatitis C committee, four of the six co-chairs declared financial competing interests; again, further research found additional undeclared conflicts of interest. In addition, a majority of members on this committee (twenty-one out of twenty-nine) had conflicts of interest.

Conflicts of interest exist not simply with those formulating guidelines but also with those responding to guideline development. When the US Centers for Disease Control and Prevention (CDC) released proposed guidelines for opioid prescribing in 2015, 158 organizations responded publicly to these draft guidelines. Unsurprisingly, those organizations with financial ties to opioid manufacturers were more likely to oppose the draft guidelines (Lin, Lucas, Murimi, Kolodny, & Alexander, 2017). Clinical practice guidelines are heavily accessed. Ioannidis (2018) points out that over half of the most-cited articles across all the sciences published in 2016 were focused on medical guidelines, disease definition, or disease statistics. The kinds of issues involved with the existence and disclosure of conflicts of interest in guideline publication are replicated in the governance boards of professional medical associations (Rothman et al., 2009), regulatory agencies (Lexchin & O'Donovan, 2010), HTA agencies (Frybourg, Remuzat, Kornfeld, & Toumi, 2015), and research institutes (Evans, 2010).

To address the issue of undisclosed bias in guideline development, the Guidelines International Network (GIN) has established a set of standards for the establishment of clinical guidelines (Qaseem et al., 2012). The *Canadian Medical Association Journal* (*CMAJ*) declared an intent to require all guidelines published in the journal from 2020 to meet these standards (Kelsall, 2019).

PAYMENTS TO HEALTH-CARE PROVIDERS

In light of increasing evidence that payments and gifts from pharmaceutical companies have a discernable impact upon physicians' prescribing habits (Wazana, 2000; Dana & Loewenstein, 2003; Pham-Kanter, Alexander, & Nair, 2012; Prescrire, 2015; Ornstein, Jones, & Tigas, 2016; Larkin et al., 2017; Goupil et al., 2019), there has been growing interest in documenting and measuring this relationship. Throughout the 2000s, these conflicts of interest began to be subject to several transparency measures in the United States. At the same time, a number of pharmaceutical firms accused of illegal marketing practices and kickback schemes agreed to disclose payments to physicians as part of their settlements. Data on physician payments were posted online, but the interface was cumbersome and awkward to use (Ornstein, 2017).

As part of the 2010 US Affordable Care Act (ACA), a provision (based on a failed 2007 bill known as the Physician Payments Sunshine Act) was passed into law. This provision (formally section 6002 of the ACA) requires drug and device manufacturers to report payments over US$10 (or annual cumulative payments over US$100) made to teaching hospitals and health-care professionals (including physicians, dentists, optometrists, podiatrists, osteopaths, and chiropractors). The "SUPPORT" Act, passed by Congress in 2018, extends reporting requirements to physician assistances, nurse practitioners, clinical nurse specialists, nurse anaesthetists, and nurse midwives.

These data are posted online by the Centers for Medicare and Medicaid Services (CMS) on an annual basis. Companies are subject to audits and fines, including US$150,000 for failure to report and US$1 million for knowing failure to report. No penalties were levied by the CMS for the first two full reporting cycles (2014 and 2015) in order to allow all parties to become familiar with the reporting provisions (given significant confusion over reporting obligations) and to encourage them to take advantage of the dispute resolution mechanisms permitting them to work such disputes out among themselves (Moore, 2016). Even so, no penalties have been levied to date after the expiration of this informal "grace period" (Centers for Medicare and Medicaid Services [CMS], 2018). The federal law does not preclude state-level transparency provisions; it merely sets a "floor" for transparency requirements. Eight states have transparency laws that predate section 6002 of the ACA. These laws do not tend to result in significant penalties; the only major breaches (for example, those addressed by Vermont's Prescribed Product Gift Ban and Disclosure Law) were self-reported (Sullivan, 2018).

In an effort to make the data submitted to the CMS more user-friendly, the non-profit group ProPublica developed two interactive websites utilizing CMS disclosure data. "Dollars for Docs" permits users to track both payments made by identifiable companies to specific individuals, for particular drugs and devices, and those made to identifiable doctors. This program lists the highest-earning doctors (one orthopaedic surgeon received US$29 million in 2018 alone) and the most-paid doctors (the top-ranked individual received 1,140 payments in the same year; Tigas, Jones, Ornstein, & Groeger, 2019). These data have provided interesting results: they show, for example, that some highly paid "experts" do not even have board certification in their stated area of expertise; that some recipients of industry payments had been sanctioned by their professional associations for abusive prescribing; and that faculty have received industry payments in contravention of university policies (Ornstein, 2017). The "Prescriber Checkup" website facilitates the analysis of physician prescribing practices. This tool highlights the correlation between industry payments and prescribing practices, with clear evidence showing not only that physicians receiving payments tend to prescribe more brand-name drugs but also that there is a "dose-response" correlation (the more funding received, the higher the prescribing rate; Ornstein, 2017).

Overall, the data collected in the United States between 2013 (a partial year of data collection) and 2016 (the last year of data released by the CMS) shows that, while the total value of payments increased slightly over the three years (US$7.86 billion to US$8.18 billion), the total number of records declined slightly from 12.02 million to 11.96 million (CMS, 2018). It is possible that the decline in payments could be related to the 33 per cent decrease in funding over this period given to doctors by makers of opioids (Ornstein & Jones, 2018).

Transparency laws governing industry payments to health-care providers in other jurisdictions are not as robust as the measures enacted in the United States under the ACA. In the European Union, only a small number of states (including France, Denmark, and Portugal) have transparency legislation regarding payments to health professionals.

Most states embrace voluntary codes of conduct put into place by the pharmaceutical industry (such as the European Federation of Pharmaceutical Industries and Associations [EFPIA] and the Association of the British Pharmaceutical Industry [ABPI]). Most self-regulatory schemes include "opt-out" clauses for recipients. Reporting thresholds vary (from 10 euros in France to 500 in the Netherlands); data access systems are variable at best; monitoring is complaint driven; and national systems do not readily permit cross-jurisdictional comparison (Fabbri, Santos, Mezinska, Mulinari, & Mintzes, 2018).

In Canada, the first pharmaceutical transparency law was passed in Ontario in 2017. Modelled after the Open Payments system in the United States, the legislation provided for a searchable online database comprised of industry payments to a wide variety of recipients (including long-term care homes, family health teams, and patient advocacy groups). Under the Health Sector Payment Transparency Act, 2019 was to be the first year of data collection, with online access beginning in 2020. However, the regulations supporting this legislation were not finalized before the provincial election in June 2018, and the new Conservative administration announced a moratorium while it embarked on a new process of "review and consultation" (Grant, 2018b).

MEDICAL EDUCATION SPONSORSHIP AND PAYMENTS

In 2007, the American Medical Student Association (AMSA) introduced a "scorecard" rating system into universities to highlight the degree of financial dependence of medical schools and teaching hospitals upon the pharmaceutical sector. Three years later, the US Institute of Medicine issued a report that declared that the system of continuing medical education (CME), "as structured today, is so deeply flawed that it cannot properly support the development of health professionals" (quoted in Nissen, 2015). A contemporaneous report found that, of US$2.4 billion spent on CME, 60 per cent was funded by commercial sources (Nissen, 2015). Steinman, Landefeld, and Baron (2012) optimistically noted that, while commercial support for CME had increased dramatically between 1998 and 2007, it had fallen from 2008 to 2010. Unfortunately, the reduction of direct industry funding for CME was more than offset by a significant increase in indirect funding. Accredited providers of CME reach out to medical education and communication companies (MECCs), which are generally independent for-profits firms funded largely by big pharmaceutical and medical device companies. These indirect payments from commercial entities to CME providers via MECCs are not subject to the US transparency laws governing conflicts of interest (Golestaneh & Cowan, 2017).

Transparency of sponsorship and direct payments in the education of medical students has shown equally poor progress. Despite voluntary codes of conduct enacted by the pharmaceutical industry prohibiting non-educational gifts to medical students, and despite increasingly numbers of medical schools and teaching hospitals adopting policies that limit access by drug and device companies, 57 per cent of the 721 fourth-year medical students surveyed reported receiving industry-sponsored gifts, and 40 per cent attended industry-sponsored lectures (Austad et al., 2013). The 2014 AMSA scorecard on conflicts of interest in medical schools assigned poorer ratings to institutions compared to 2013, although conclusions about trends over time cannot be made due to revisions in the 2014 methodology (Carlat, Fagrelius, Ramachandran, Ross, & Bergh, 2016). Canadian medical schools fared little better. A 2013 study of these schools' conflict of interest policies showed that a high number of these institutions had "permissive or no policies" in place for free samples, faculty involvement in companies' speakers' bureaus, and interaction with sales representatives (Schnier, Lexchin, Mintzes, Jutel, & Holloway, 2013).

HEALTH MEDIA

Citing the important role played by the media in interpreting scientific studies for the general public, a *British Medical Journal* (*BMJ*) editorial asked: Who watches the watchers? (Schwartz, Woloshin, & Moynihan, 2008). News organizations that report extensively on health-related issues (such as STAT, Vox, and National Public Radio [NPR]), for example, themselves receive funding from PhRMA (Schwitzer, 2017). The National Press Foundation, sponsored by pharmaceutical companies, offers all-expense-paid workshops for health-care journalists. Individual workshops, fellowships, or residencies for health journalists have also been financially supported by companies such as Purdue Pharma or by high-profile academic medical centres (Schwitzer, 2017). To the extent that such sponsors have specific goods and services to sell, there is a concern that participants may be given information (such as uncritical exposure to new technologies) with little analysis of benefits, harms, and costs (Jaklevic, 2018). Yet journalists are not obliged to be transparent about training events they may have attended that were funded by organizations about which they write.

More insidious is the role of pharmaceutical companies in providing journalists access to patients with particular conditions (Schwartz et al., 2008). For example, if a jurisdiction decides that an expensive but high-profile drug will not be publicly insured, journalists may be offered the contact details of individuals whose lives may be directly impacted by this policy decision. Such immediate human-interest stories generally receive a great deal of public attention, but journalists are unlikely to reveal the role of corporate public relations (PR) departments in the development of their articles. Social media presents another complicated issue for transparency, given the ability of medical professionals with financial conflicts of interest to freely discuss commercial products or services on these platforms without disclosing such conflicts (Tao, Boothby, McLouth, & Prasad, 2017; see also Persaud in chapter six).

Price and Supply

DRUG PRICING

The issue of price transparency for pharmaceuticals is another important transparency relationship. Beginning around 2014, high-priced "specialty" or "niche" drugs (focusing largely on hepatitis, autoimmune diseases, and oncology) became a cost driver of some concern to both public and private payers. By 2017, specialty drugs in the United States accounted for US$9.8 billion of the US$12.0 billion net new brand spending growth (IQVIA, 2018, p. 10). Other cost drivers for pharmaceuticals include an aging population, guideline changes for hypertensives, and increased usage of psychotropic medications. In the United States, an antitrust lawsuit involving forty-seven states claimed that extensive price-fixing by generic drug manufacturers (including a 3,400 per cent cost increase for albuterol, a decades-old asthma drug, and a 500 per cent increase in the price of EpiPens) was another major cost driver (Rowland, 2018).

The issue of price transparency is especially complicated because of the pricing structure for pharmaceuticals in most jurisdictions. There are at least three different prices for most drugs. The list price (or wholesale acquisition cost) is the initial price set by drug manufacturers. Large wholesalers can generally command a discount from the list price, but will then add their own markup to obtain a profit. This wholesale price (or pharmacy acquisition cost) is then paid by a pharmacy or pharmacy chain. Adding a markup, the pharmacy sets the "usual and customary" price. Some customers – especially those paying out of pocket – may pay this price. Often, rebates for generic drugs are offered by drug companies to pharmacies to expand manufacturers' market share of a drug produced by several different companies. These rebates may or may not be passed on as discounts to consumers. Most customers, however, will not pay the usual and customary price. If they have insurance, they may only be responsible for the co-pay or co-insurance specified by their plan. Or, they may be part of a co-pay assistance program (often involving manufacturers' coupons) that absorbs some of their (though not their insurer's) drug cost. What this system means is that different people may pay quite dissimilar prices for the same drug.

The diffuse and opaque nature of drug pricing makes it difficult to control overall costs. Consumers and payers alike find it difficult to determine what "reasonable" or "unreasonable" prices are, and the presence of multiple actors makes blame-shifting for high prices more common. Price transparency is seen as one way to control pharmaceutical costs. The mechanisms for pharmaceutical price transparency differ across jurisdictions. In the United States, two pieces of federal legislation (the Patient Right to Know Drug Prices Act and the Know the Lowest Price Act) were signed into law in October 2018. Both laws eliminate, in different contexts, restrictions upon pharmacists that prevent them from informing consumers of less-expensive choices. The same month, US Health and Human Services announced a proposal to oblige pharmaceutical companies to disclose in direct-to-consumer television commercials the list prices paid by Medicare and Medicaid programs for the advertised drug. PhRMA, the umbrella group for brand-name pharmaceuticals, opposed this measure, arguing that such information would be "too confusing" for patients. The measure passed in May 2019, but was then halted in a district court a day before it was to take effect on the grounds that the Department of Health and Human Services did not have the authority to compel pharmaceutical companies to disclose this information. This ruling has been appealed by the Department of Health and Human Services.

However, more far-reaching transparency laws have been enacted at the state level. In 2018 alone, twenty-four states passed thirty-seven bills aimed at rising drug prices (Pear, 2018). Most are similar to the 2017 price transparency laws passed by California and Nevada, but each state has its own specific set of requirements. Oregon, with one of the most sweeping transparency laws, requires drug manufacturers to file price reports for any new drug (or new price increases for existing drugs) above a specified threshold. Manufactures are obliged to disclose the costs related to research, develop, manufacture, market, and distribute the drug, as well as any other factor that necessitated the price increase. Total sales revenue must be stated, including net profit for the drug, as well as information on the highest price paid for the drug the previous year outside of the United States (Gudiksen, 2018). Many states have established rate-setting boards or pricing review boards to determine whether new or increased prices are excessive (Facher, 2018). California's price transparency law obliges pharmaceutical firms to give notice of price increases above 16 per cent at least sixty days in advance. Other states have required licensing of pharmacy benefit managers (PBMs), which allows government bodies to review PBM compensation and fee schedules and to determine whether rebate schemes contribute to rising costs (Cohen, 2018). Some of these states release this information on a public website; others do not.

In Canada, Health Canada proposed amendments to its Patent Medicines Regulations document in 2017 with an eye to cost control. Vocal opposition by industry stakeholders have to date delayed the regulations coming into force. At the provincial level, a proposal by the Ontario Medical Association for price transparency would use electronic health systems to permit physicians to ascertain the price of drugs (determined by provincial reimbursements to pharmacies) in real time (as they are considering prescriptions for patients) in order to choose the most affordable option for their patients (Gorfinkel & Lexchin, 2017; Ontario Medical Association, 2018).

In the European Union, as in Canada, small jurisdictions negotiating drug prices directly with pharmaceutical companies are placed at a distinct disadvantage. Larger jurisdictions can negotiate more competitive rates due to their size or their skill in brokering deals; but the final negotiated price is confidential, and smaller governments often pay higher prices. In response, public payers in federal systems have been developing collaborative mechanisms to engage in joint negotiation and to share information on prices and markets. In 2010, the Canadian provinces established the pan-Canadian Pharmaceutical Alliance in order to improve their negotiating strength. EU member states have also formed alliances regarding pharmaceutical strategy. In 2014, Belgium, the Netherlands, and Luxembourg established a pharmaceutical alliance; Austria joined "Beneluxa" in 2016, as did Ireland in 2018, giving the alliance a population base of 43 million people (Schmidt & Saldutti, 2018). Canada, too, expressed interest in joining Beneluxa. A key goal of the group is to increase price transparency to address rising drug prices. Based on this model, other European states have formed the Valletta group, the Central Eastern European and South Eastern Countries Initiative, the Southern European Initiative, the Nordic Pharmaceutical Forum, and the Baltic Partnership Agreement (Schmidt & Saldutti, 2018).

DRUG SUPPLY

In 1999, the worry that the year 2000 (Y2K) would cause massive disruptions in the electronic health infrastructure led the FDA to establish a Drug Shortage Program (DSP). While electronic systems remained unscathed, the DSP nonetheless proved quite valuable in identifying drug shortages that occurred for other reasons (Kweder & Dill, 2013). These include raw material shortages, manufacturing issues, voluntary recalls, "strategic business factors" (such as the discontinuation of unprofitable items), increases in demand for medications, and inventory management practices (De Oliveira, Theilken, & McCarthy, 2011). Because manufacturers were not routinely sharing information on potential shortages with the FDA on a voluntary basis as requested, the FDA Safety and Innovation Act was established in 2012 (Fox, Sweet, & Jensen, 2014). Under the new act, manufacturers are obliged to notify the FDA of potential shortages of "medically necessary" drugs six months in advance "or as soon as is practicable." Beyond "naming and shaming" companies that fail to notify the FDA of potential shortages in the appropriate time period, however, compliance mechanisms are limited. The FDA also has no authority to require companies to produce drugs or to distribute scarce drugs in any particular way. However, the FDA shortages website does list current information on existing shortages, all known sources of medically necessary drugs, and the expected duration of the shortage. The American Society of Health-System Pharmacists also hosts a discrete website listing drug shortages and related resources, and both bodies routinely share information to achieve "improved transparency and broad communication about shortages" (Fox et al., 2014, p. 370).

Like the United States, Canada found that voluntary disclosure of potential shortages was ineffective and cumbersome: more than half of the shortages owing to discontinuation prior to 2017, for example, were announced the day of the discontinuation (Donelle, Duffin, Pipitone, & White-Guay, 2018). While the House of Commons voted unanimously in 2012 to impose mandatory notification, this decision was rejected by the Harper administration (Donelle et al., 2018, p. 3). In 2017, the multistakeholder Steering Committee on Drug Shortages led to a restructuring of drug shortage reporting. The shortages website, which had previously been the responsibility of the pharmaceutical industry, was placed under the auspices of Health Canada (though contracted out). Like the FDA, Health Canada has no authority to enforce non-compliance of reporting responsibilities beyond publicizing the names of manufacturers who fail to comply. Unlike the FDA, Health Canada does not systematically measure and report publicly and systematically on the nature of drug shortages. A single study by the C.D. Howe Institute found that, of close to 8,000 active drugs in Canada, 10 per cent had been in short supply at some point between 2013 and 2016. Interestingly, while generic injectable drugs were most commonly subject to shortages in the United States, the most common shortage in Canada was for oral drugs. Brand-name drug shortages were more likely in Canada than in the United States, although shortages of generics were still common (Donelle et al., 2018, pp. 11, 20). Canada's shortages website also provides much less information on alternatives and substitutes; nor do manufacturers reveal the sources of supply regarding each drug they produce.

Transparency regarding drug supply in the European Union is slightly more complicated. According to a 2013 survey of 161 hospital pharmacists, 42 per cent noted that information on drug shortages from manufacturers only came at the point of "no delivery"; 40 per cent said that information on drug shortages was "rarely or never" received from government (Pauwels, Simoens, Casteels, & Huys, 2015). The EMA subsequently established a public list of shortages, although the criteria for inclusion on the list are quite restrictive. The key reason for this restriction is that, while the EMA has authority for the approval of drugs, the issue of shortages is the responsibility of member states themselves. The EMA can only declare authority if shortages are linked to specific safety concerns or if shortages affect several member states. Many individual member states do have their own shortage lists, but they vary considerably across jurisdictions: the information required by each website differs from country to country, as does public accessibility. There is, in consequence, no comprehensive public list of drug shortages in the European Union (Torjesen, 2015). While individual member states have their own reporting requirements, drug manufacturers are not required to report potential shortages directly to the EMA. In December 2016, the EMA and the Heads of Medicines Agencies (HMA) organized a Task Force on the Availability of Medicine in order to develop a coordinated approach to drug shortages in Europe, including establishing a common definition of "shortage," developing industry guidelines for reporting shortages, and creating common metrics for measuring shortages (Mulero, 2018). However, a 2018 survey of hospitalists found that respondents believed drug shortages were becoming more, rather than less, troublesome (European Association of Hospital Pharmacists, 2018).

In sum, it is important to understand the particular context of each transparency relationship in order to identify not only the specific kind of transparency achieved but also why transparency is so often stymied. God and the devil are in the details; and the ability to determine precisely what ought to be subject to transparency, to whom, under what conditions, and through which mechanisms is a powerful manifestation of political influence. To understand the way in which these forms of influence are employed, it is useful to briefly consider the ways in which power and influence can be exercised within this context.

Power, Politics, and Policy-Making: The Mirage of Simple Policy Solutions

Some policy solutions work well because they reorganize processes or restructure institutions in a relatively neutral environment: in such cases, no one is particularly opposed to changing the status quo because no one is heavily invested in it (all participants may well benefit from moving away from a suboptimal system). In such cases, nothing greater than the weight of convention or the lack of imagination constitutes a barrier to change. In other instances, however, policy change may threaten both the immediate objectives of stakeholders and the overall level of influence that they enjoy. As Thomas Hobbes (1968), writing in 1651 during the turmoil of the English Civil War, observed, political actors endeavour to hold on to as much general power as possible to ensure their ability to achieve whatever their specific goals happen to be; the less stable the environment, the more rational it is to maximize influence by whatever means possible.

The larger and more robust social and commercial actors are, the more political influence they tend to have. When their interests are impacted by shifts in policy-making, these policy changes only very rarely (for example, in cases of nationalization) eliminate the underlying relationships of power. As in guerrilla warfare, overt battles simply become more clandestine and surreptitious; they are not eliminated. This state of affairs is why any hope for a quick, simple solution in pharmaceutical policy is misplaced. Powerful interests encountering policy "successes" (including ones embracing greater transparency) will not simply accept the new status quo if it undermines their interests. In Hobbesian fashion, they will actively seek to regain their lost influence however they can within the new structures or protocol. Policy advocates who seek a quick policy fix will be disappointed. Like weight loss, immediate gratification is unlikely, and long-term maintenance is essential.

The nature of power is such that it can often metamorphize quite effectively. To understand the fluidity of transparency relationships, it is useful to gain a better sense of power relationships. How is power configured? How is it possible to ascertain whether power exists? To the extent that the analysis of politics is a "science," one can examine the empirical evidence presented by observable decision-making processes: for example, identifying the winners in electoral campaigns, the way in which formal legislation or regulation is structured, or the pattern of public funding are all means of measuring who has influence and who does not. Most examinations of pharmaceutical policy are performed on this axis of analysis. But not all power is visible. As many political scientists have argued (for example, Lukes, 1974), there also exist "hidden" forms of power where vested interests attempt to maintain their influence by creating obstacles to participation or by keeping certain issues off the public agenda. Here influence is exercised by excluding, minimizing, or delegitimizing competing interests. While these competing interests may not themselves have sufficient power to effectively challenge dominant interests or alter the status quo, they are nonetheless aware of what their interests are and understand that their lack of influence means their own objectives cannot be met.

A more insidious form of power relations operates by "influencing, shaping or determining" individuals' perception of what their interests are (Lukes, 1974, p. 27), the impression of whether goals are achievable, and even the nature of reality (for example, by shaping the evidentiary basis for what is or is not "true"). This form of "invisible power" is exercised in part through control of the institutions that shape and create meaning: these include not only formal institutions like laws or government bodies, but also informal institutions such as the media or popular culture. Ideas and experiences are constructed such that perceptions and beliefs are (often unconsciously) internalized and held instinctively and uncritically. The classic articulation of invisible power was Franz Fanon's analysis of Martinique, where colonial attitudes about racial inferiority were internalized by the local population (Fanon, 1963), thereby facilitating and reinforcing the structures of colonial governance. Contemporary accounts of inconspicuous power, like that of Gagnon (chapter eight in this volume), focus upon the discursive construction of ideas and attitudes through the deliberate framing of particular narratives.

The ability of jurisdictions to achieve transparency in pharmaceutical policy can thus be understood more precisely by seeing policy-making as a process that occurs in a highly politicized environment in which vested interests attempt to maintain or regain their influence through formal or "visible" mechanisms (lobbying or campaign funding), "hidden" strategies (agenda setting), and "invisible" techniques (the construction of narratives).

These three dynamics of power operate simultaneously. As Table 2.3 summarizes, transparency initiatives (as just described in the previous discussion) have frequently had limited impact because of the way in which they have been implemented. But what explains *why* these measures are executed in these particular ways? It could be the result of lobbying (visible power); structuring the political debate so that some concepts ("confidential commercial information") are privileged over others (public safety); or constructing a narrative in which individuals (as patients, voters, and consumers) themselves internalize the agenda of the pharmaceutical industry ("transparency threatens innovation, which diminishes the possibility of a cure for my disease").

In contemporary states defined by commercial and democratic values, subtler forms of power relations can be the most potent. They can also be the most difficult to confront. Whether individuals are consumers purchasing advertised goods or citizens casting votes, their choices are accepted as legitimate and final. It thus becomes important to influence

Table 2.3. Achievements in, and Barriers to, Greater Transparency

Achievement	Barrier	Example
The requirement of transparency is accepted in principle	Measures are voluntary rather than mandated	Reporting COIs
	Guidelines are vague rather than defined	No precise explanation of what COIs are, or when they should be reported, or what kind of information should be disclosed
	Guidelines exist for direct relationships but not for indirect ones	No COI guidelines for PAOs, PACs, and other astroturfing groups
Transparency measures are mandated	No means exist to verify compliance	Reporting COIs
	No means exist to enforce compliance	Reporting drug shortages
	Information required to be disclosed is vague or limited	COIs are stated without disclosing amounts or from whom the funds are given
	Insufficient resources are provided to make information accessible	Public posting of redacted CSRs
	Poor oversight of how well the disclosure mechanisms are working	Reports on performance of regulatory authority not accessible
		Rationale for decisions of regulatory authority not accessible
	Statute is enacted, but the regulatory framework supporting the legislation is delayed or not put into place	Ontario's Health Sector Payment Transparency Act
	Policy achievements at one level are subsequently challenged or undermined at another level	Vertical: EMA decisions overturned by European Council
		Horizontal: initiatives of Departments of Health blocked by Departments of Finance
Information is disclosed	Only in the aggregate ("summary" information)	Industry payments to health-care providers
		RCT data

(Continued)

Table 2.3. (*Continued*)

Achievement	Barrier	Example
	Only to certain authorized individuals or bodies	Access limited solely to vetted researchers or citizens of a specific jurisdiction
		Information is only shared at a government-to-government level
	Only under certain conditions	Requirement to sign confidentiality agreement as condition of access
	Processes used to access information are unwieldy	Reactive (request-based) systems of disclosure
	Physical mechanisms used to access information are unwieldy	Poorly designed or restrictive electronic websites or portals
	Significant exceptions are put into place	Expansive definition of what constitutes "confidential commercial information"
	Disclosure is temporary	COI information regarding industry funding is deleted as soon as collaboration ends
	Information isn't easily comparable across jurisdictions	Definition of "drug shortage"
	Data "dumps" mix key data files with large amounts of unimportant information	Government websites with health performance statistics filled with "low-level" data (such as popular baby names)

Notes: COI = conflict of interest; CSR = clinical study report; PAC = political action committee; PAO = patient advocacy organization; RCT = randomized controlled trial

individuals in their capacity both as consumers and voters, and it is here where powerful interests increasingly focus their attention and resources. Table 2.4 sets out examples of strategies that can be used to undermine public support for greater transparency.

Power relations that are based on ideas are effective precisely because they are insidious and unobtrusive. They can easily be denied, as the very standards of proof demanded for scientific validity (clear, quantifiable evidence of linear causality; replicability; predictability) are very difficult to substantiate conclusively. Policy-making in contemporary representative political systems depends on a number of factors, but a key variable

Table 2.4. How Power Can Be Exercised through Discursive Techniques

Strategy	Example
Epistemic reductionism (structuring ways of understanding the world into binary choices, ensuring that one of these choices is manifestly unacceptable)	There is an intelligent mainstream population who understand that vaccinations are safe and useful, and a fringe group of "anti-vaxxers" who believe vaccines lead to autism and other ailments. Anyone who questions the safety and effectiveness of vaccines belongs to the group of nutty conspiracy theorists and should not be taken seriously
Framing issues on a specific (often binary) set of outcomes in a zero-sum manner	Greater transparency is posed as a threat to innovation, choice, or timely access Greater transparency in clinical trials for rare drugs will undermine patient data confidentiality
Framing issues on a specific (often binary) set of values	"Freedom of speech" is prioritized as more important than any negative consequences of advertising "off-label" drugs for conditions that have not been approved
Burying or downplaying the effects of policy choices	Focusing on individual patient choice while neglecting the collective sustainability of the health-care / health insurance system
Normalizing practices	Greater transparency of COI countered or diminished by presenting previously hidden practices as acceptable ("everyone does it")
Gaslighting	As data is disclosed, the certainty of conclusions based on this data is undermined (data is accessible, but people don't trust it)
Methodological challenges	The credibility or authority of methodological techniques resulting in critical analyses is challenged
Poisoning the well	The credibility or authority of individuals using released data to present critical analyses is undermined
Redefining concepts in order to neutralize their significance	"Conflict of interest" is defined widely (e.g., "intellectual conflicts of interest") in order to distract from the specific power relationship underlying financial conflicts of interest
Structuring of choice	Stakeholders voluntarily choose to give up transparency due to other incentives presented (e.g., competitive prices given only if confidentiality clauses in contract are accepted)

Note: COI = conflict of interest

is policy-makers' judgement regarding public sensibility (specifically, the likelihood that voters will hold a government responsible for its actions or lack of actions). Health crises (tainted blood, pandemics, HIV-AIDS, thalidomide prescribing) are so politically volatile because of citizens' perceptions of immediate threats to their physical well-being. Constructivist strategies simply manipulate this relationship between citizens and their public representatives by framing narratives that attempt to structure individual behaviour on a large scale with the expectation that individuals will, of their own accord, push their elected representatives to make particular policy decisions (or to dissuade them from making others). It is extremely difficult, if not impossible, to prove conclusively that it was *this* set of constructed narratives that caused *that* set of individual behaviours. Most individuals tend not to accept that their behaviour was due to manipulation; they will generally claim they have acted on their own volition. And individuals generally do make rational choices in response to the evidence they have in front of them; they simply do not always perceive that the environment within which they make conscious and defensible choices can be deliberately constructed (see, for example, Lakoff, 2009).

The construction of choices is a pervasive aspect of commercial society: on a small scale, it is simply the realm of advertising, which presents choices for our consumption. But when resources are carefully and deliberately used in order to shape "scientific" knowledge, within which consumer choices are then embedded, the scope for individual volition becomes quietly and surreptitiously circumscribed. The narrative surrounding weight loss and sugary beverages is one well-documented example of this discursive strategy. In response to policy advocates who successfully pushed for soda taxes, Coca-Cola financially supported Global Energy Balance Network, which constructed a pervasive message to the public that "lack of physical activity is responsible for obesity – not diet, and certainly not soft drinks" (Nestle, 2015, p. 92).

In this way, one must remain aware that "transparency" itself is not merely a simple policy end point, but rather a tool that can be employed in a larger contest over power and influence. Indeed, transparency, as a policy response, can itself serve as a means of deliberately framing the legitimacy of policy choices. As Grundy, Habibi, Schnier, Mayes, and Lipworth (2018) describe, for example, the establishment of clinical data transparency in Australia was accepted only in order to *prevent* a more rigorous regulatory regime. The acceptability of transparency, they argue, reinforced the underlying idea that "the burden of responsibility for assessing the adverse outcomes of conflict of interest" was on those consuming the products, rather than on those producing them. The move to transparency was not debated as a choice between greater regulation or more transparency; rather, it was viewed as a positive-sum solution that allowed "governments to appear responsive to public concerns and health-related industries to appear credible and compliant" (Grundy et al., 2018, p. 515). Other alternatives – such as thoroughgoing regulation or a clinical trial regime that was fully public – were silently pushed off the agenda given the "win-win" policy solution on the table.

Transparency in and of itself is part of a useful set of solutions to address the lack of accountability on the part of those producing and licensing pharmaceutical products that pose risks of which the public is unaware. But it has its limitations. One must, in addition, strive to be conscious of the ways in which power relations are exercised by influential commercial interests. As noted earlier, transparency can be used in "risk management" strategies to offload risk to consumers: if they are aware of the limited safety or efficacy of natural health products, for example, then they – rather than the state or society – assume the risks of using the products.

Conclusion

Transparency, argues Dror (1999), itself acts like a drug: in correct doses it heals; in excessive amounts, it kills. Transparency should not be viewed as a simple solution: it has its own drawbacks. Loewenstein, Cain, and Sah (2011) argue that disclosing conflicts of interest can make agents more comfortable in giving bad advice, while others hold that greater transparency can lead to greater cynicism and delegitimacy. Kanter, Carpenter, Lehmann, and Mello (2019) provide some empirical justification for this claim, showing that widespread public disclosure of industry payments *decreased* public trust in physicians and the medical profession. Moreover, greater transparency assumes that the data made more accessible will in fact be accessed: yet there is evidence in many instances to show that this is not in fact the case (Meijer, 2014). Wilson (2014) notes that the mere presentation of conflicts of interest does not itself provide us with the tools to evaluate the implications of these conflicts. Too much transparency, observe Greer, Wismar, Figueras, and McKee (2016, p. 32), "can simply drive politics and decision-making underground," or it can backfire by giving well-resourced lobby groups "more time to prepare campaigns and start to influence policy."

Nonetheless, as newer mechanisms of governance move away from strict vertical systems of accountability to softer forms of horizontal governance, older forms of accountability become increasingly impracticable. Particular manifestations of transparency will of necessity vary across time, jurisdiction, and sector. And transparency relationships can be undermined or left ineffectual through the specific technicalities of their implementation. For this reason, it is important to examine the particular regulatory, institutional, and discursive contexts within which transparency mechanisms are realized. In President Obama's simple articulation, "a democracy requires accountability, and accountability requires transparency" (Obama, 2009).

REFERENCES

Ahn, R., Woodbridge, A., Abraham, A., Saba, S., Korenstein, D., Madden, E., ... Keyhani, S. (2017). Financial ties of principal investigators and randomized controlled trial outcomes: Cross sectional study. *BMJ, 356*, i6770. https://doi.org/10.1136/bmj.i6770

Almashat, S., & Carome, M. (2017). Withholding information on unapproved drug marketing applications: The public has a right to know. *Journal of Law, Medicine, & Ethics, 45*(2) supp., 46–9. https://doi.org/10.1177/1073110517750621

Anderson, M.L., Chiswell, K., Peterson, E.D., Tasneem, A., Topping, J., & Califf, R. (2015). Compliance with results reporting at clinicaltrials.gov. *New England Journal of Medicine, 372*(11), 1031–9. https://doi.org/10.1056/NEJMsa1409364

Aucoin, P., & Heintzman, R. (2000). The dialectics of accountability for performance in public management reform. *International Review of Administrative Sciences, 66*(1), 45–55. https://doi.org/10.1177/0020852300661005

Austad, K., Avorn, J., Franklin, J.M., Kowal, M.K., Campbell, E.G., & Kesselheim, A.S. (2013). Changing interactions between physician trainees and the pharmaceutical industry: A national survey. *Journal of General Internal Medicine, 28*(8), 1064–71. https://doi.org/10.1007/s11606-013-2361-0

Batt, S. (2017). *Health Advocacy Inc.: How pharmaceutical funding changed the breast cancer movement.* Vancouver, BC: UBC Press.

Béland, D. (2009). Ideas, institutions, and policy change. *Journal of European Public Policy, 16*(5), 701–18. https://doi.org/10.1080/13501760902983382

Béland, D. (2019). *How ideas and institutions shape the politics of public policy.* Cambridge, UK: Cambridge University Press.

Bellary, S., Krishnankutty, B., & Latha, M.S. (2014). Basics of case report form designing in clinical research. *Perspectives in Clinical Research, 5*(4), 159–66. https://doi.org/10.4103/2229-3485.140555

Bentham, J. (1843). An essay on political tactics. In J. Bowring (Ed.), *The works of Jeremy Bentham* (vol. 2, pp. 301–73). Edinburgh: William Tate.

Bindslev, J.B.B., Schroll, J., Gøtzsche, P.C., & Lundh, A. (2013). Underreporting of conflicts of interest in clinical practice guidelines: Cross sectional study. *BMC Medical Ethics, 14*(19), 1–7. https://doi.org/10.1186/1472-6939-14-19

Birkinshaw, P.J. (2006). Freedom of information and openness: Fundamental human rights? *Administrative Law Review, 58*(1), 177–218.

Block, J., & Canner, L. (2016, 8 September). The "grassroots campaign" for "female Viagra" was actually funded by its manufacturer. *The Cut.* Retrieved from https://www.thecut.com/2016/09/how-addyi-the-female-viagra-won-fda-approval.html

Bourgeois, F.T., Murthy, S., & Mandl, K.D. (2010). Outcome reporting among drug trials registered in clinicaltrials.gov. *Annals of Internal Medicine, 153*(3), 158–66. https://doi.org/10.7326/0003-4819-153-3-201008030-00006

Bruckner, T. (2018, 19 August). European Medicines Agency backtracks on transparency pledges, restricts access to key documents. *TranspariMed*. Retrieved from https://www.transparimed.org/single-post/2018/08/19 /european-medicines-agency-backtracks-on-transparency-pledges-restricts -access-to-key-drug

Cairney, P. (2011). *Understanding public policy: Theories and issues*. London, UK: Palgrave Macmillan.

Canada. (2014). Protecting Canadians from Unsafe Drugs Act (Vanessa's Law). S.C. 2014, c. 24.

Carlat, D.J., Fagrelius, T., Ramachandran, R., Ross, J.S., & Bergh, S. (2016). The updated AMSA scorecard of conflict-of-interest policies: A survey of US medical schools. *BMC Medical Education, 16*, 202. https://doi.org/10.1186 /s12909-016-0725-y

Center for Responsive Politics. (2017). Client profile: Pharmaceutical Research and Manufacturers of America. *OpenSecrets.org*. Retrieved from https://www .opensecrets.org/lobby/clientsum.php?id=D000000504&year=2017

Center for Responsive Politics. (2018). Pharmaceuticals/health products: Money to Congress – Summary. *OpenSecrets.org*. Retrieved from https://www .opensecrets.org/industries/summary.php?ind=H04&cycle=2018

Centers for Medicare and Medicaid Services (CMS), US Department of Health and Human Services. (2018). *Annual report to Congress on the Open Payments Program, April 2018*. Retrieved from https://www.cms.gov/About-CMS /Components/CPI/Downloads/PY16_2018-Open-Payment-Report-to -Congress.pdf

Cohen, J. (2018, 17 October). Improving drug price transparency: From removing pharmacy gag clauses to reforming the rebate system. *Forbes*. Retrieved from https://www.forbes.com/sites/joshuacohen/2018/10/17 /improving-drug-price-transparency-from-removing-pharmacy-gag-clauses-to -reforming-the-rebate-system/#42a7ce41303b

CONSORT. (2010). Checklist of information to include when reporting a randomised trial. Retrieved from http://www.consort-statement.org/media /default/downloads/consort%202010%20checklist.pdf

Coombes, R. (2019). European drug regulator fears return to days of data secrecy. *BMJ, 367*, i1633. https://doi.org/10.1136/bmj.l6133

Cooper, R., Gupta, M., Wilkes, M.S., & Hoffman, J.R. (2006). Conflict of interest disclosure policies and practices in peer-reviewed biomedical journals. *Journal of General Internal Medicine, 21*, 1248–52. https://doi.org/10.1111/j.1525-1497 .2006.00598.x

Cosgrove, L., Bursztajn, H., Krimsky, S., Anaya, M., & Walker, J. (2009). Conflicts of interest and disclosure in the American Psychiatric Association's clinical practice guidelines. *Psychotherapy and Psychosomatics, 78*(4), 228–32. https://doi.org/10.1159/000214444

Cosgrove, L., Krimsky, S., Vijayaraghavan, M., & Schneider, L. (2006). Financial ties between DSM-IV panel members and the pharmaceutical industry. *Psychotherapy and Psychosomatics, 75*, 154–60. https://doi.org/10.1159/000091772

Dana, J., & Loewenstein, G. (2003). A social science perspective on gifts to physicians from industry. *JAMA, 290*(2), 252–5. https://doi.org/10.1001/jama.290.2.252

De Oliveira, G.S., Theilken, L., & McCarthy, R.J. (2011). Shortage of perioperative drugs: Implications for anesthesia practice and patient safety. *Anesthesia & Analgesia, 113*(6), 1429–35. https://doi.org/10.1213/ANE.0b013e31821f23ef

Donelle, J., Duffin, J., Pipitone, J., & White-Guay, B. (2018). *Assessing Canada's drug shortage problem.* Commentary No. 515. C.D. Howe Institute. Retrieved from https://www.cdhowe.org/public-policy-research/assessing-canada%E2%80%99s-drug-shortage-problem

Doshi, P., & Jefferson, T. (2013). Clinical study reports of randomised controlled trials: An exploratory review of previously confidential industry reports. *BMJ Open, 3*(2), 1–9. https://doi.org/10.1136/bmjopen-2012-002496

Dror, Y. (1999). Transparency and openness of quality democracy. In M. Kelly (Ed.), *Openness and transparency in governance: Challenges and opportunities* (pp. 62–71). Maastricht: NISPAcee Forum.

European Association of Hospital Pharmacists (EAHP). (2018). EAHP's 2018 survey on medicines shortages to improve patient outcomes. Retrieved from https://www.eahp.eu/practice-and-policy/medicines-shortages/2018-medicines-shortage-survey

Evans, R.G. (2010). Tough on crime? Pfizer and the CIHR. *Healthcare Policy, 5*(4), 16–25. https://doi.org/10.12927/hcpol.2010.21778

Fabbri, A., Santos, A., Mezinska, S., Mulinari, S., & Mintzes, B. (2018). Sunshine policies and murky shadows in Europe: Disclosure of pharmaceutical industry payments to health professionals in nine European countries. *International Journal of Health Policy and Management, 7*(6), 504–9. https://doi.org/10.15171/ijhpm.2018.20

Fabbri, A., Swandari, S., Lau, E., Vitry, A., & Mintzes, B. (2019). Pharmaceutical industry funding of health consumer groups in Australia: A cross-sectional analysis. *International Journal of Health Services, 49*(2), 273–93. https://doi.org/10.1177/0020731418823376

Facher, L. (2018, 1 November). Drug pricing goes local: State lawmakers around the country are pledging to take on pharma, too. *STAT+.* Retrieved from https://www.statnews.com/2018/11/01/drug-pricing-goes-local/

Facher, L. (2020, 10 August). Pharma is showering Congress with cash, even as drug makers race to fight the coronavirus. *STAT.* Retrieved from https://www.statnews.com/feature/prescription-politics/prescription-politics/

Fanon, F. (1963). *The wretched of the earth.* C. Farrington (Trans.). New York, NY: Grove Press.

Fleminger, J., & Goldacre, B. (2018). Prevalence of clinical trial status discrepancies: A cross-sectional study of 10,492 trials registered on both clinicaltrials.gov and the European Union Clinical Trials Register. *PLOS One, 13*(3), e0193088. https://doi.org/10.1371/journal.pone.0193088

Fontanarosa, P., & Bauchner, H. (2017). Conflict of interest and medical journals. *JAMA, 317*(17), 1768–71. https://doi.org/10.1001/jama.2017.4563

Fox, E.R., Sweet, B.V., & Jensen, V. (2014). Drug shortages: A complex health care crisis. *Mayo Clinic Proceedings, 89*(3), 361–73. https://doi.org/10.1016/j.mayocp.2013.11.014

Friedman, L.S., & Richter, E.D. (2004). Relationship between conflicts of interest and research results. *Journal of General Internal Medicine, 19,* 51–6. https://doi.org/10.1111/j.1525-1497.2004.30617.x

Frybourg, S., Remuzat, C., Kornfeld, A., & Toumi, M. (2015). Conflict of interest in health technology assessment decisions: Case law in France and impact on reimbursement decisions. *Journal of Market Access & Health Policy, 3*(1), 25862. https://doi.org/10.3402/jmahp.v3.25682

Goldacre, B., DeVito, N., Heneghan, C., Irving, F., Bacon, S., Fleminger, J., & Curtis, H. (2018). Compliance with requirement to report results on the EU Clinical Trials Register: Cohort study and web resource. *BMJ, 362,* k3218. https://doi.org/10.1136/bmj.k3218

Golestaneh, L., & Cowan, E. (2017). Hidden conflicts of interest in continuing medical education. *The Lancet, 390*(10108), 2128–30. https://doi.org/10.1016/S0140-6736(17)32813-1

Gorfinkel, I., & Lexchin, J. (2017). We need to mandate drug cost transparency on electronic medical records. *CMAJ, 189*(50), e1541–2. https://doi.org/10.1503/cmaj.171070

Goupil, B., Balusson, F., Naudet, F., Esvan, M., Bastian, B., Chapron, A., & Frouard, P. (2019). Association between gifts from pharmaceutical companies to French general practitioners and their drug prescribing patterns in 2016: Retrospective study using the French Transparency in Healthcare and National Health Data System databases. *BMJ, 367,* i6015. https://doi.org/10.1136/bmj.l6015

Grant, K. (2018a, 23 October). How a blockbuster drug tells the story of why Canada's spending on prescriptions is sky high. *Globe and Mail.* Retrieved from https://www.theglobeandmail.com/canada/article-how-a-blockbuster-drug-tells-the-story-of-why-canadas-spending-on/

Grant, K. (2018b, 5 November). Ford PCs leave drug-company transparency law in limbo. *Globe and Mail.* Retrieved from https://www.theglobeandmail.com/canada/article-ford-pcs-leave-drug-company-transparency-law-in-limbo/

Greer, S.L., Wismar, M., Figueras, J., & McKee, C. (2016). Governance: A framework. In S.L. Greer, M. Wismar, & J. Figueras (Eds.), *Strengthening health system governance: Better policies, stronger performance* (pp. 27–56). Maidenhead, UK: Open University Press.

Grundy, Q., Habibi, R., Schnier, A., Mayes, C., & Lipworth, W. (2018). Decoding disclosure: Comparing conflict of interest policy among the United States, France, and Australia. *Health Policy, 122*(5), 509–18. https://doi.org /10.1016/j.healthpol.2018.03.015

Gudiksen, K. (2018). Spotlight on 2018 state drug legislation: Part 5 – Pricing transparency laws. *The Source on Healthcare Price & Competition*. Retrieved from https://sourceonhealthcare.org/ spotlight-on-2018-state-drug-legislation-part-5-pricing-transparency-laws/

Haivas, I., Schroter, S., Waechter, F., & Smith, R. (2004). Editors' declaration of their own conflicts of interest. *CMAJ, 171*(5), 475–6. https://doi.org/10.1503 /cmaj.1031982

Hancock, J. (2018, 30 July). Drug trade group quietly spends "dark money" to sway policy and voters. *Kaiser Health News*. Retrieved from https://khn.org /news/drug-trade-group-quietly-spends-dark-money-to-sway-policy-and-voters/

Hobbes, T. (1968). *Leviathan*. C.B. Macpherson (Ed.). Harmondsworth, UK: Penguin. (Original work published 1651)

Ioannidis, J.P.A. (2018). Professional societies should abstain from authorship of guidelines and disease definition statements. *Circulation: Cardiovascular Quality and Outcomes, 11*(10), e004889. https://doi.org/10.1161 /CIRCOUTCOMES.118.004889

Ioannidis, J.P.A., Munafò, M., Fusar-Poli, P., Nosek, B.A., & David, S.P. (2014). Publication and other reporting biases in cognitive sciences: Detection, prevalence and prevention. *Trends in Cognitive Science, 18*(5), 235–41. https:// doi.org/10.1016/j.tics.2014.02.010

IQVIA. (2018). 2018 and beyond: Outlook and turning points. Retrieved from https://www.iqvia.com/insights/the-iqvia-institute/reports/2018-and-beyond -outlook-and-turning-points

Jaklevic, M.C. (2018). 6 reasons journalists should just say no to Mayo Clinic's latest journalism "residency" program. *HealthNewsReview*. Retrieved from https://www.healthnewsreview.org/2018/12/6-reasons-journalists-should -just-say-no-to-mayo-clinics-latest-journalism-residency-program/

Jefferson, A.A., & Pearson, S.D. (2017). Conflict of interest in seminar hepatitis C virus and cholesterol management guidelines. *JAMA Internal Medicine, 177*(3), 352–7. https://doi.org/10.1001/jamainternmed.2016.8439

Johnson, M., Stokes, R.C., & Arndt, T. (2018). *The thalidomide catastrophe: How it happened, who was responsible and why the search for justice continues after more than six decades*. Exeter, UK: Onwards and Upwards Press.

Kaestner, V., & Prasad, V. (2017). Financial conflicts of interest among editorialists in high-impact journals. *Blood Cancer Journal*, *7*, e611. https://doi.org/10.1038/bcj.2017.92

Kang, S.-Y., Bai, G., Karas, L., & Anderson, G.F. (2019). Pharmaceutical industry support of US Patient advocacy organizations: An international context. *American Journal of Public Health*, *109*(4), 559–61. https://doi.org/10.2105/AJPH.2018.304946

Kanter, G., Carpenter, D., Lehmann, L.S., & Mello, M.M. (2019). US nationwide disclosure of industry payments and public trust in physicians. *JAMA Network Open*, *2*(4), e191947. https://doi.org/10.1001/jamanetworkopen.2019.1947

Kelsall, D. (2019). New *CMAJ* policy on competing interests in guidelines. *CMAJ*, *191*(13), e350–1. https://doi.org/10.1503/cmaj.190316

Kopp, E., Lupkin, S., & Lucas, E. (2018, 6 April). Patient advocacy groups take in millions from drugmakers. Is there a payback? *Kaiser Health News*. Retrieved from https://khn.org/news/patient-advocacy-groups-take-in-millions-from-drugmakers-is-there-a-payback/

Krumholz, H.M., & Waldstreicher, J. (2016). The Yale Open Data Access (YODA) Project – A mechanism for data sharing. *New England Journal of Medicine*, *375*(5), 403–5. https://doi.org/10.1056/NEJMp1607342

Kweder, S.L., & Dill, S. (2013). Drug shortages: The cycle of quantity and quality. *Clinical Pharmacology and Therapeutics*, *93*(3), 245–51. https://doi.org/10.1038/clpt.2012.235

Lakoff, G. (2009). *The political brain: A cognitive scientist's guide to your brain and its politics*. New York, NY: Penguin.

Larkin, I., Ang, D., Steinhart, J., Chao, M., Patterson, M., Sah, S., Wu, T., ... Loewenstein, G. (2017). Association between academic medical center pharmaceutical detailing policies and physician prescribing. *JAMA*, *317*(17), 1785–95. https://doi.org/10.1001/jama.2017.4039

Le Noury, J., Nardo, J.M., Healy, D., Jureidini, J., Raven, M., Tufanaru, C., & Abi-Jaoude, E. (2015). Restoring Study 329: Efficacy and harms of paroxetine and imipramine in treatment of major depression in adolescence. *BMJ*, *351*, h4320. https://doi.org/10.1136/bmj.h4320

Lexchin, J. (2018, 25 October). We need answers to the thalidomide tragedy – to ensure drug safety today. *National Post*. Retrieved from https://nationalpost.com/pmn/news-pmn/we-need-answers-to-the-thalidomide-tragedy-to-ensure-drug-safety-today

Lexchin J., & O'Donovan, O. (2010). Prohibiting or "managing" conflict of interest? A review of policies and procedure in three European drug regulation agencies. *Social Science & Medicine*, *70*(5), 643–7. https://doi.org/10.1016/j.socscimed.2009.09.002

Lin, D., Lucas, E., Murimi, I.B., Kolodny, A., & Alexander, C. (2017). Financial conflicts of interest and the Centers for Disease Control and Prevention's

2016 guideline for prescribing opioids for chronic pain. *JAMA Internal Medicine, 177*(3), 427–8. https://doi.org/10.1001/jamainternmed.2016.8471

Liu, J.J., Bell, C.M., Matelski, J.J., Detsky, A.S., & Cram, P. (2017). Payments by US pharmaceutical and medical device manufacturers to US medical journal editors: Retrospective observational study. *BMJ, 359*, i4619. https://doi.org/10.1136/bmj.j4619

Loewenstein, G., Cain, D.M., & Sah, S. (2011). The limits of transparency: Pitfalls and potential of disclosing conflicts of interest. *American Economic Review, 101*(3), 423–8. https://doi.org/10.1257/aer.101.3.423

Lukes, S. (1974). *Power: A radical view.* London, UK: Macmillan.

Lundh, A., Barbateskovic, M., Hróbjartsson, A., & Gøtzsche, P.C. (2010). Conflicts of interest at medical journals: The influence of industry-supported randomized trials on journal impact factors and revenue – cohort study. *PLoS Medicine, 7*(10), e1000354. https://doi.org/10.1371/journal.pmed.1000354

Mandeville, K.L., Barker, R., Packham, A., Sowerby, C., Yarrow, K., & Patrick, H. (2019). Financial interest of patient organisations contributing to technology assessments at England's National Institute for Health and Care Excellence: Policy review. *BMJ, 364*, k5300. https://doi.org/10.1136/bmj.k5300

McCoy, M.S., Carniol, M., Chockley, K., Urwin, J.W., Emanuel, E.J., & Schmidt, H. (2017). Conflicts of interest for patient-advocacy organizations. *New England Journal of Medicine, 376*, 880–5. https://doi.org/10.1056/NEJMsr1610625

Meijer, A. (2014). Transparency. In M. Bovens, R. Goodin, & T. Schillemans (Eds.), *The Oxford handbook of public accountability* (pp. 507–24). Oxford, UK: Oxford University Press.

Mezher, M. (2018, 6 February). EU court backs EMA in trio of transparency cases. *Regulatory Focus.* Retrieved from https://www.raps.org/news-and-articles/news-articles/2018/2/eu-court-backs-ema-in-trio-of-transparency-cases

Moore, T. (2016). Parting the clouds: Some thoughts on why CMS has not imposed civil monetary penalties for Sunshine Act violations. *Policy and Medicine Life Science Compliance Update, 2*(2). Retrieved from https://www.shb.com/-/media/files/professionals/m/mooretimothy/partingtheclouds.pdf

Mulero, A. (2018, 31 May). Mitigating drug shortages: FDA moves to address challenges. *Regulatory Focus.* Retrieved from https://www.raps.org/news-and-articles/news-articles/2018/5/mitigating-drug-shortages-fda-moves-to-address-ch

National Institute on Money in Politics (NIMSP). (2020). Wyeth Pharmaceutical has given $5,852,431 to 1,203 different filers spanning 11 years. *FollowTheMoney.org.* Retrieved from https://www.followthemoney.org/entity-details?eid=2904

Nestle, M. (2015). *Soda politics: Taking on big soda (and winning).* Oxford, UK: Oxford University Press.

Nissen, S.E. (2015). Reforming the continuing medical education system. *JAMA, 313*(18), 1813–15. https://doi.org/10.1001/jama.2015.4138

Obama, B. (2009). Memorandum for the heads of executive departments and agencies: Freedom of Information Act. Retrieved from https://obamawhitehouse.archives.gov/realitycheck/the-press-office/freedom-information-act

Office of the Commissioner of Lobbying of Canada. (2020). 12-Month lobbying summary – In-house organization. Retrieved from https://lobbycanada.gc.ca/app/secure/ocl/lrs/do/clntSmmry?clientOrgCorpNumber=371&sMdKy=1570377210339

Ontario Medical Association (OMA). (2018). Drug cost transparency: Real-time access to drug costs for physicians. Retrieved from https://www.oma.org/wp-content/uploads/DrugCostTransparencyPaperFinal2018-03-07.pdf

Ornstein, C. (2017). Public disclosure of payments to physicians from industry. *JAMA, 317*(17), 1749–50. https://doi.org/10.1001/jama.2017.2613

Ornstein, C., & Jones, R.G. (2018, 28 June). Opioid makers, blamed for overdose epidemic, cut back on marketing payments to doctors. *ProPublica.* Retrieved from https://www.propublica.org/article/opioid-makers-blamed-for-overdose-epidemic-cut-back-on-marketing-payments-to-doctors

Ornstein, C., Tigas, M., & Jones, R.G. (2016, 17 March). Now there's proof: Docs who get company cash tend to prescribe more brand-name meds. *ProPublica.* Retrieved from https://www.propublica.org/article/doctors-who-take-company-cash-tend-to-prescribe-more-brand-name-drugs

Ozieranski, P., Rickard, E., & Mulinari, S. (2019). Exposing drug industry funding of UK patient organisations. *BMJ,* 365, l1806. https://doi.org/10.1136/bmj.l1806

Pauwels, K., Simoens, S., Casteels, M., & Huys, I. (2015). Insights into European drug shortages: A survey of hospital pharmacists. *PLoS One, 10*(3), e0119322. https://doi.org/10.1371/journal.pone.0119322

Pear, R. (2018, 18 August). States rush in to rein in prescription costs, and drug companies fight back. *New York Times.* Retrieved from https://www.nytimes.com/2018/08/18/us/politics/states-drug-costs.html

Pham-Kanter, G., Alexander, G.C., & Nair, K. (2012). Effect of physician payment disclosure laws on prescribing. *Archives of Internal Medicine, 172*(10), 819–21. https://doi.org/10.1001/archinternmed.2012.1210

Piller, C. (2020). Transparency on trial. *Science, 367*(6475), 240–3. https://doi.org/10.1126/science.367.6475.240

Postigo, R., Brosch, S., Slattery, J., Van Haren, A., Dogné, J.-M., Kurz, X., … Arlett, P. (2018). EudraVigilance Medicines Safety Database: Publicly accessible data for research and public health protection. *Drug Safety, 41*(7), 665–75. https://doi.org/10.1007/s40264-018-0647-1

Prescrire. (2015). No-gift policy in medical schools: Demonstrated impact on prescribing behaviour. *Prescrire International, 24*(159), 111.

ProPublica. (2020). Lobbying by Pharmaceutical Research and Manufacturers of America (PhRMA). *ProPublica.* Retrieved from https://projects.propublica .org/represent/lobbying/r/301017376

Qaseem, A., Forland, F., Macbeth, F., Ollenschlager, G., Phillips, S., & Van der Wees, R. (2012). Guidelines International Network: Toward international standards for clinical practice guidelines. *Annals of Internal Medicine, 156*(7), 525–31. https://doi.org/10.7326/0003-4819-156-7-201204030-00009

Rose, S.L., Highland, J., Karafa, M.T., & Joffre, S. (2017). Patient advocacy organisations, industry funding, and conflicts of interests. *JAMA Internal Medicine, 177*(3), 344–50. https://doi.org/10.1001/jamainternmed.2016.8443.

Rothman, D.J., McDonald, W.J., Berkowitz, C.D., Chimonas, S.C., DeAngelis, C.D., Hale, R.W., ... Wofsy, D. (2009). Professional medical associations and their relationship with industry: A proposal for controlling conflict of interest. *JAMA, 301*(13), 1367–73. https://doi.org/10.1001/jama.2009.407

Rowland, C. (2018, 9 December). Investigation of generic "cartel" expands to 300 drugs. *The Washington Post.* Retrieved from https://www.washingtonpost .com/business/economy/investigation-of-generic-cartel-expands-to-300-drugs /2018/12/09/fb900e80-f708-11e8-863c-9e2f864d47e7_story.html

Sager, N. (2018, 13 November). CDER overview of transparency policy. Presented at Beyond Transparency in Pharmaceutical Research and Regulation, Silver Spring, MD.

Schmidt, M., & Saldutti, G. (2018, 22 August). Emerging collaboration in EU drug pricing and reimbursement: A Beneluxa case study. *PharmExec.com.* Retrieved from https://www.pharmexec.com/view/potential-disruption -pricing-and-reimbursement-pharmaceuticals-eu-beneluxa-case-study

Schnier, A., Lexchin, J., Mintzes, B., Jutel, A., & Holloway, K. (2013). Too few, too weak: Conflict of interest policies at Canadian medical schools. *PLOS One, 8*(7), e68633. https://doi.org/10.1371/journal.pone.0068633

Schwartz, L., Woloshin, S., & Moynihan, R. (2008). Who's watching the watchdogs? *BMJ, 337*, a2535. https://doi.org/10.1136/bmj.a2535

Schwitzer, G. (2017, 12 June). Conflicts of interest in health care journalism. Who's watching the watchdogs? We are. *HealthNewsReview.org.* Retrieved from https://www.healthnewsreview.org/2017/06/conflicts-of -interest-in-health-care-journalism-1-of-3/

Smith, R. (2002). Making progress with competing interests. *BMJ, 325*, 1375–6. https://doi.org/10.1136/bmj.325.7377.1375

Sox, H.C. (2017). Conflict of interest in practice guidelines panel. *JAMA, 317*(17), 1739–40. https://doi.org/10.1001/jama.2017.2701

Steinman, M., Landefeld, C.S., & Baron, R.B. (2012). Industry support of CME – Are we at the tipping point? *New England Journal of Medicine, 366*(12), 1069–71. https://doi.org/10.1056/NEJMp1114776

Sullivan, T. (2018, 6 May). Vermont fines 25 manufacturers for violations of the Vermont prescribed product gift ban and disclosure law. *Policy & Medicine.* Retrieved from https://www.policymed.com/2013/10/vermont-fines-25 -manufactures-for-violations-of-the-vermont-prescribed-product-gift-ban-and -disclosure-law.html

Tao, D.L., Boothby, A., McLouth, J., & Prasad, V. (2017). Financial conflict of interest among hematologist-oncologists on Twitter. *JAMA Internal Medicine, 177*(3), 425–7. https://doi.org/10.1001/jamainternmed.2016.8467

Thomas, K., & Ornstein, C. (2018, 13 September). Top Sloan Kettering cancer doctor resigns after failing to disclose industry ties. *New York Times.* Retrieved from https://www.nytimes.com/2018/09/13/health/jose-baselga-cancer -memorial-sloan-kettering.html

Thompson, D.F. (1993). Understanding financial conflicts of interest. *New England Journal of Medicine, 329*(8), 573–6. https://doi.org/10.1056 /NEJM199308193290812

Tigas, M., Jones, R.G., Ornstein, C., & Groeger, L. (2019). Dollars for docs: How industry dollars reached your doctors. *ProPublica.* Retrieved from https:// projects.propublica.org/docdollars/

Torjesen, I. (2015, 29 January). Drug shortages: It's time for Europe to act. *The Pharmaceutical Journal.* Retrieved from https://www.pharmaceutical-journal. com/news-and-analysis/features/drug-shortages-its-time-for-europe-to-act /20067701.article

Unruh, L., Rice, T., Vaillancourt Rosenau, P., & Barnes, A.J. (2016). The 2013 cholesterol guideline controversy: Would better evidence prevent pharmaceuticalization? *Health Policy, 120*(7), 797–808. https://doi.org/10.1016 /j.healthpol.2016.05.009

Viergever, R.F., & Li, K. (2015). Trends in global clinical trial registration: An analysis of numbers of registered clinical trials in different parts of the world from 2004 to 2013. *BMJ Open, 5*(9), 1–15. https://doi.org/10.1136/bmjopen -2015-008932

Wazana, A. (2000). Physicians and the pharmaceutical industry: Is a gift ever just a gift? *JAMA, 283*(3), 373–80. https://doi.org/10.1001/jama.283.3.373

Weber, M. (1958). Bureaucracy. In H.H. Gerth & C. Wright Mills (Eds.), *From Max Weber: Essays in sociology* (pp. 196–244). New York: Oxford University Press.

Wilson, M. (2014). Is transparency really a panacea? *Journal of the Royal Society of Medicine, 107*(6), 216–17. https://doi.org/10.1177/0141076814532744

3 Data Transparency and Pharmaceutical Regulation in Europe: Road to Damascus, or Room without a View?

COURTNEY DAVIS, SHAI MULINARI,
AND TOM JEFFERSON

Introduction

Incomplete or non-disclosure of the results of animal and clinical studies investigating the harms and benefits of new medical technologies threatens patient and public health since physicians and patients are unable to make informed decisions about the safest and most effective treatment strategies in the absence of full information. Conversely, data transparency and the unbiased reporting of research outcomes are critical for scientific and therapeutic progress as medical science and medical practice advance by building on, refining, and correcting previous knowledge. Yet, the research community has long been aware of deficiencies, distortions, and gaps in the dissemination and reporting of clinical trial results – including non-reporting of whole trials, time lag biases in publication, and biased or selective reporting of study outcomes (Chalmers, 1990, 2006; Dickersin, Chan, Chalmers, Sacks, & Smith, 1987; Dickersin & Rennie, 2003; Easterbrook, Gopalan, Berlin, & Matthews, 1991; Hemminki, 1980; Horton & Smith, 1999; Ioannidis, 1998; Jørgensen, Gøtzsche, & Jefferson, 2018; Lee, Bacchetti, & Sim, 2008; MacLean, Morton, Ofman, Roth, & Shekelle, 2003; McGauran et al., 2010; Melander, 2003; Rennie, 2004; Rising, Bacchetti, & Bero, 2009; Simes, 1986; Song et al., 2010; Turner, Matthews, Linardatos, Tell, & Rosenthal, 2008; Wieseler, Kerekes, Vervoelgyi, McGauran, & Kaiser, 2012; Jones et al., 2013; Wieseler et al., 2013). The risks of data secrecy are not just hypothetical. A number of studies have identified or confirmed serious health risks associated with widely prescribed drugs, which were not previously known to the medical community because data had been withheld from the public. Some examples include studies investigating the disputed benefits and harms of cox-2 inhibitors (Hrachovec & Mora, 2001; Mukherjee, Nissen, & Topol, 2001; Psaty &

Kronmal, 2007); antidepressants (Eyding et al., 2010; Le Noury et al., 2015; Whittington et al., 2004); muraglitazar (Nissen, Wolski & Topol, 2005); rosiglitazone (Nissen & Wolski, 2007; US Senate, Committee on Finance, 2010); gabapentin (Vedula, Bero, Scherer, & Dickersin, 2009); and oseltamivir (Jefferson, Jones, et al., 2014).

Reporting biases are possible because clinical trial data are in the possession of, and controlled by, study sponsors. In the case of medicines, the sponsor will almost always be a for-profit pharmaceutical company. However, in most jurisdictions, companies are legally required to submit data from animal and human studies to national and supranational drug regulatory bodies for independent review. The regulatory requirement includes submission of standardized clinical study reports (CSRs), which – in contrast to the highly condensed papers published in academic journals – are detailed reports containing full study protocols and amendments, statistical analysis plans, detailed information concerning the conduct of the trial, summarized efficacy and safety data on all outcomes, and individual anonymized patient data in the form of tabulations or listings. In principle, therefore, medicines regulators are in a unique position to facilitate access to scientific information about medicines for the benefit of patients, the medical community, and future research, and many of the studies just cited draw on data submitted to and/or accessed via government regulatory agencies. Some research has drawn on clinical trial data unearthed in the course of criminal and civil lawsuits in the United States (Egilman & Presler, 2006; Krumholz, Hines, Ross, Presler, & Egilman, 2007; Vedula et al., 2009) or data made public through voluntary initiatives on the part of individual companies (Simmonds et al., 2013). However, these forms of access are contingent on (rare) instances of litigation or wholly at companies' discretion. Comprehensive, reliable, and enforceable data transparency will only come through legislated initiatives that give citizens right of access to information held by public bodies (Mintzes, Lexchin, & Quintano, 2015).

In practice, where citizens' right of access exists, it has stopped short of direct access to original documents submitted by companies and has instead taken the form of access to regulators' evaluations of those documents. Most access to trial data has thus been selective and indirect as it has been "filtered" through a regulatory lens. The value of citizens' right of access to information is dependent, therefore, on three key characteristics of any drug regulatory regime. First, it will depend on the relative openness of a drug regulatory agency with respect to its scientific review and decision-making processes. Second, it depends on the extent to which regulators themselves receive full and comprehensive data from companies and on the thoroughness and independence of the regulators' scientific evaluations – that is, the extent to which regulators take a "deep dive" into company submissions, including whether they collect and examine raw data contained in case report forms (CRFs) or only look at company summaries, and whether and how frequently they conduct their own re-analyses of the data (Mulinari & Davis, 2017). And third, it depends on the extent to which regulatory standards and practices incentivize or mandate the generation of reliable information about the clinical outcomes that matter to patients, physicians, and health-care systems. For example, there is significant debate about the frequent failure of medicines regulators in North America and the European Union to require evidence on whether new cancer drugs extend survival or improve quality of life (Davis et al., 2017). These are important issues for regulators, but even more crucial for patients.

For most of the history of modern drug regulation, the US Food and Drug Administration (FDA) was seen as the model to which other medicines agencies should aspire in relation to two, at least, of the three dimensions outlined previously. With respect to the thoroughness of its scientific review processes, numerous studies have established that the FDA was exceptional in the degree to which it undertook rigorous, in-depth analyses of company data compared to other national or supranational regulatory bodies (Abraham, 1995; Davis & Abraham, 2013; Lexchin, chapter seven, this volume; Mulinari & Davis, 2017). The FDA is also unique in requesting submission of patient-level data sets in addition to the standard CSRs (McCarthy and Ross, chapter four, this volume). Access to patient-level data, in combination with relatively high levels of agency staffing, has enabled FDA reviewers to independently re-analyse the raw data submitted (albeit, re-analysis is not necessarily done on a routine basis). By contrast, European regulatory bodies, including the supranational European Medicines Agency (EMA), tend to rely heavily on company summaries of the data (Mulinari & Davis, 2017), may not be in possession of the full clinical trial data set (Jefferson & Doshi, 2014), and do not routinely request or examine patient-level data in the form of individual patient CRFs (Doshi, Dickersin, Healy, Vedula, & Jefferson, 2013).

Historically, the FDA has also surpassed most other medicines agencies (with the exception of some of the Nordic countries) with respect to the transparency of its scientific decision-making processes (Abraham, 1995; Abraham & Lewis, 2000; Davis & Abraham, 2013; Garattini, 2005; Lexchin & Mintzes, 2004; Prescrire, 2002, pp. 16–20; Vitry et al., 2008; Mulinari & Davis, 2017). The public can access copies of original agency reviews of company data, which also document scientific disagreements over the interpretation of data and how these were resolved. By contrast, researchers, independent drug bulletins, and European consumer health advocacy groups have criticized the EMA for its overly secretive approach since the agency was established in 1995 (Abraham & Lewis, 1998; Garattini & Bertele', 2001; Health Action International Europe et al., 2009; Prescrire, 2002, pp. 17–20). Official documents reporting the scientific basis of and processes underpinning EMA recommendations are relatively opaque. The EMA does not publish the original agency evaluations of company data (the "rapporteurs' reports"), and the meetings of its scientific committee – the Committee for Medicinal Products for Human Use (CHMP) – are not held in public, nor are full meeting transcripts made available. Instead, the EMA publishes "European public assessment reports" (EPARs), which provide highly summarized accounts of the data produced by the manufacturer, the rapporteurs' review of these data, and the basis for the CHMP's recommendation with respect to approval. Moreover, commentators have expressed concern over the superficiality and poor quality of reporting in the EMA's EPARs for over a decade (Barbui, Baschirotto, & Cipriani, 2011; Garattini, 2005; Garattini & Bertele', 2007; International Society for Drug Bulletins, 2001; Prescrire, 2002, pp. 17–20).[1]

Then, in 2010, the EMA announced a new policy on public access to EMA documents (European Medicines Agency [EMA], 2010b), which included a proposal to proactively release CSRs submitted by companies seeking a market authorization. This plan meant that researchers would have direct access to primary clinical trial data, rather than information selectively included in the summaries produced by regulators and companies. Political and legal support for the EMA's initiative followed. First came the adoption by the European Parliament in 2014 of important clinical trial transparency provisions as part of a new EU Regulation on Clinical Trials;[2] it was followed by rulings of the European Court of Justice on the scope of the so-called Transparency Regulation ([EC] No 1049/2001) in relation to documents held by the EMA (EMA, 2018). Both the regulation and the legal rulings appear to confirm principles articulated by the European Ombudsman (2010; discussed later): that clinical data to support marketing authorization cannot be presumed to be commercially confidential; that there should be a presumption in favour of public access; and that regulators or companies wishing to challenge such a presumption must provide concrete evidence as to how the release of specific documents would harm a company's commercial interests.

These policy and legal developments constitute a notable shift, such that the European Union now leads the United States with respect to the depth and breadth of citizens' right of access to clinical trial data, having previously lagged behind. The EMA's new policy is highly significant for public health since a number of studies have shown that "deep" data transparency, involving researcher access to full clinical study reports, is critical for proper evaluation of study results and for checking the accuracy of peer-reviewed journal articles, conference reports, and trial registry entries (Eyding et al., 2010; Hill, Ross, Egilman, & Krumholz, 2008; Jefferson, Jones, et al., 2014; Vedula et al., 2009; Wieseler et al., 2012). But it is also a significant departure from the EMA's previous treatment of clinical trial data (and other information submitted by companies) as strictly "confidential commercial information," and therefore raises important questions about the sociopolitical dynamics underlying recent developments.

In the following sections, we discuss pivotal events regarding, and map the relationships between, the activities of and the roles played by the key protagonists shaping these events. We argue that recent policy initiatives would not have occurred in the absence of a concerted effort on the part of a handful of civil society groups, academic journals, and individuals who formed a loose coalition to push for greater data transparency in the European Union. In attempting to understand the growth of this loose coalition of actors and its role in triggering and subsequently shaping the activities and policies of EU regulators and institutions, we identify four discrete but interconnected "streams" or series of events – each involving a distinct set of participants acting at member state, supranational, and international levels. Taken together, these four streams help to explain policy developments towards greater data transparency in the European Union. In addition, the continued and close engagement of those actors with unfolding events in the political sphere and at the institutional level has been critical in countering or diluting attempts by the pharmaceutical industry and the European Commission to undermine and reverse the new EU commitments.

From Laggard to Leader? Data Transparency in the European Union

The first stream involved a group of actors that joined together in March 2002 in the context of a major review of the legislative framework for governing pharmaceutical regulation and marketing in the European Union (described further on). The impetus was a determination by these civil society groups to resist what were seen as European Commission attempts to weaken pharmaceutical regulation in the interests of industry to the detriment of patients and public health (Bardelay & Kopp, 2002; Davis & Abraham, 2013; Medicines in Europe Forum [MiEF], n.d.; Prescrire, 2002, pp. 11–15). Around sixty organizations across twelve member states joined together in an informal network called the Medicines in Europe Forum (MiEF) to campaign for increased regulatory transparency, higher regulatory standards, and sustainable medicines pricing.[3] Core members of the group that led the early and subsequent campaigns include the consumer health advocacy organizations Health Action International (HAI), the European Public Health Alliance (EPHA), and the European Consumer Organisation (BEUC), as well as the International Society of Drug Bulletins (ISDB), *La Revue Prescrire*, and researchers like Silvio Garattini of the Mario Negri Institute in Milan, Italy (also a former member of the EMA committee responsible for human medicines). Individuals from these organizations have also played a key role in advocating for, monitoring, and engaging with the new EMA data transparency policy.

In 2001, the European Commission initiated a sweeping review of the existing regulatory framework for the authorization and post-market governance of medicines in Europe. This review culminated in 2004 with the adoption of a new regulation (Regulation 726/2004) and directive (Directive 2004/27/EC) by the European Parliament. At this time, responsibility for pharmaceuticals within the Commission lay with DG Enterprise, which was tasked with promoting the competitiveness of the European industry (Davis & Abraham, 2013, p. 81). Through its early advocacy activities between 2002 and 2004, while the complex European co-decision procedure unfolded, the MiEF gained an important understanding of and insights into the orientation of the Commission and complex legislative processes, as well as valuable experience in engaging with the formal institutions of the supranational European Union. Although Article 15 of the Treaty on the Functioning of the European Union, in conjunction with Regulation 1049/2001 (the so-called "Transparency Regulation"), granted the public a right to access European Parliament, Council, and Commission documents, important information held by the EMA (including conditions placed by the EMA on marketing authorizations, information on withdrawn applications, minority opinions within the CHMP, and information on the scientific basis for marketing authorizations granted via the mutual recognition procedure) was not being made public (Abraham & Lewis, 2000; Garattini & Bertele', 2001). Consequently, transparency was a central focus of MiEF's demands, and their petition to the president of the European Parliament in July 2002 included a demand for free access to scientific data from the results of clinical research on pharmaceuticals (including the data contained in post-marketing safety reports) (MiEF, n.d.).

When the new regulation and directive were introduced in 2004, the MiEF had managed to secure some key concessions, including important gains in terms of the obligations on national medicines agencies and the EMA with respect to increased transparency. Article 73 of Regulation

726/2004 required the EMA's Management Board to adopt arrangements for implementing the Transparency Regulation (Regulation 1049/2001). Transparency provisions were also extended to the national drug agencies of member states, and conditions attached to new marketing authorizations were to be made public along with the authorization, as well as the deadlines for fulfilling such obligations. However, while gains had been made at the legislative level, in practice the EMA interpreted its obligations with respect to transparency under Regulations 726/2004 and 1049/2001 extremely narrowly and continued to deny direct access to data submitted by companies and also to any regulatory evaluations beyond the highly summarized EPARs. Between 2005 and 2010, *Prescrire* submitted 142 requests to access documents held by the EMA. Whole or large parts of these requests were frequently denied, with the EMA citing its duty to protect the commercial interests and intellectual property rights of companies (Prescrire, 2010). Documents that were released were often heavily redacted. An example is the EMA's response to Prescrire's request for documents relating to the anti-obesity drug rimonabant. Public health researchers, independent drug bulletins, and consumer health advocates have had an understandable interest in scrutinizing the evidence base for anti-obesity drugs since most of these drugs have subsequently been shown to have low, and possibly clinically meaningless, efficacy and to pose unacceptable risks to patients' health (Gøtzsche & Jørgensen, 2011). Several anti-obesity drugs approved for marketing in the European Union were subsequently withdrawn for safety reasons. When Prescrire requested access to the Swedish rapporteur's report for the withdrawn drug rimonabant (Acomplia) in September 2008, the EMA initially refused the request on grounds that release of the document would undermine the protection of commercial interests. Following an appeal to the EMA's executive director at that time, Thomas Lönngren, the agency did finally provide Prescrire with the rapporteur's report. However, sixty-five pages of the sixty-eight page document had been systematically blacked out, including the date of the report, making the redacted document completely uninformative (Prescrire, 2009; Prescrire, 2010). The agency had also refused several requests for the periodic safety update reports (PSURs) for individual drug products, again citing protection of commercial interests (Prescrire, 2010). As late as June 2009, as evidenced by the release of its draft transparency policy, the EMA continued to give priority to the commercial interests of industry in a way that consumer health organizations like HAI argued was contrary to the spirit of the EU Transparency Regulation (Health Action International et al., 2009).

The starting point of the second sequence of events culminating in a change in EU policy also involved a request to the EMA for documentation pertaining to anti-obesity drugs. In June 2007, Peter Gøtzsche and other researchers from the Nordic Cochrane Centre applied to the EMA for access to the clinical study reports and protocols for fifteen trials undertaken with rimonabant and orlistat (Gøtzsche & Jørgensen, 2011). The EMA responded by invoking Article 3(2)(a) of Regulation (EC) No 1049/2001 on public access to documents held by the European Union, referring to the agency's obligation to protect commercial interests, and refused to release the documents (European Ombudsman, 2010). The Nordic Cochrane Centre appealed to Thomas Lönngren, who reiterated the EMA's position and informed the Cochrane researchers that they could lodge a complaint with the European Ombudsman, which they did (Gøtzsche & Jørgensen, 2011). Long drawn-out communications between the Ombudsman, the Cochrane researchers, and the EMA ensued, with the EMA continuing to insist that release of the data requested could "seriously harm the commercial interests" of the sponsors (European Ombudsman, 2010, point 75). To overcome this impasse, the Ombudsman visited the EMA to inspect the documents in question (Gøtzsche & Jørgensen, 2011).

The outcome of this process was critical to the way events unfolded in Europe. On 19 May 2010, the Ombudsman issued a draft recommendation that the EMA should grant the Nordic Cochrane Centre all the documents they had requested. In reaching this conclusion, the Ombudsman determined that the material he inspected did not contain intellectual property, trade secrets, or commercial confidences, but that, if the requested documents did contain information that fell within the scope of the commercial interests exception to Regulation (EC) No 1049/2001, the EMA had not established that they contained commercially confidential information, which if disclosed, might seriously harm the interests of the companies. Helpfully, in his final decision, the Ombudsman pointed out that case law of the European Community courts had established that the exceptions to the general right of access should be interpreted strictly and narrowly, that if an institution wished to rely on one of the exemptions it would need to provide a convincing explanation as to how granting access would "specifically and actually" undermine commercial interests, and that this threat should be reasonably foreseeable and not purely hypothetical (European Ombudsman, 2010, point 32).

On 7 June 2010, the European Ombudsman issued a press release in which he charged the EMA with maladministration for failing to grant access to the reports and protocols requested. The initial complaint, received by the Ombudsman on 8 October 2007, took three years to resolve – largely due to the obduracy of the EMA throughout the protracted negotiations (Gøtzsche & Jørgensen, 2011). Throughout that period, the Nordic Cochrane group's persistence and careful unpacking of the EMA's arguments and responses to the Ombudsman appeared crucial in influencing the Ombudsman's determination of "maladministration" on the part of the EMA (European Ombudsman, 2010). This finding, in turn, appeared to be a key trigger for the EMA. On 31 August 2010, the EMA performed an extraordinary about-turn, suddenly proclaiming that it agreed with the principle of providing to EU citizens the widest possible access to documents, that it shared the Ombudsman's reasoning, and that the Nordic Cochrane researchers would (finally) be granted access to the requested documents (European Ombudsman, 2010, points 89–91; Gøtzsche & Jørgensen, 2011). This positional shift was quite extraordinary given that, during each exchange up until the Ombudsman's June press release, the EMA had stubbornly reiterated its position that the clinical trial reports, analysis plans, and protocols in question were commercially sensitive and that release would undermine the commercial interests of the companies involved.

On 30 November 2010, the EMA announced a new, two-part policy on data transparency (EMA, 2010b). First, the EMA stated that, in reactively responding to written requests for documents, it was willing to release clinical study reports submitted by companies in support of marketing authorization applications. This part of the policy became known as Access Policy 0043 (EMA, 2010a). Second, the EMA indicated it would be adopting a policy of proactive disclosure of clinical trial data submitted to EMA by companies. The EMA's new commitment to proactive disclosure – known as Publication Policy 0070 – promised a new level of public access to industry documents and the possibility of independent scientific scrutiny of the evidence base for drugs approved after implementation of the policy (EMA, 2010c, 2019). By contrast, in 2013, the FDA made it clear it would not be considering the routine proactive release of such data (Moscicki, 2013). As suggested earlier, this approach marked a reversal of European regulators' long-standing position that data from clinical trials were commercially confidential and therefore exempt from the general right of citizens to access documents held by the institutions of the European Union.

The third stream involves a sequence of events and initiatives that forced EU policy-makers to consider the issue of publication bias and "missing data" more broadly. Individuals and organizations involved in this stream include the editors of the BMJ and PLoS Medicine, Cochrane researchers conducting systematic reviews of the anti-influenza drugs oseltamivir (Tamiflu) and zanamivir (Relenza), researchers from the Oxford Centre for Evidence-Based Medicine, and Iain Chalmers from the James Lind Alliance. The actors in this stream have, individually and together, campaigned to raise awareness of the various types of reporting bias and the threat these pose to evidence-based medicine.

In the mid-2000s, European political and regulatory institutions seemed relatively unaffected by widespread media coverage and public debate surrounding a number of high-profile cases where companies were found to have systematically and deliberately suppressed negative findings from drug trials (Kondro, 2004; New York State Court, 2004; Rennie, 2004; Teather & Boseley, 2004; US Senate, Committee on Finance, 2004; Wilde, Mathews, & Martinez, 2004; US Congress, House Committee on Government Reform, 2005a, 2005b; Armstrong, 2006). The controversy surrounding these cases, which had mainly come to light through US civil and criminal lawsuits and a series of US government investigations, prompted vigorous debate in the major medical journals and among ethicists, funding bodies, and also US policy-makers around (along with other issues) the problems of, and potential solutions to, publication bias (Abbasi, 2004; Turner, 2004; De Angelis et al., 2005; Groves, 2008; Krleža-Jerić et al., 2005; Krleža-Jerić, Lemmens, Reveiz, Cuervo, & Berol, 2011; Naci, Cooper, & Mossialos, 2015; World Health Organization [WHO], n.d.). However, controversies that ultimately led to legislative change in the United States in 2007, mandating prospective clinical trial registration under the Food and Drug Administration Amendments Act (Groves, 2008; Krleža-Jerić et al., 2011), appear to have had little impact in prompting policy change at the level of the supranational European Union and within the individual member states. Even the Mediator drug disaster in France, which hit French headlines in October 2010, appeared to have little impact on supranational EU medicines regulation, although it was an important trigger in prompting national level regulatory reform, including introduction of initiatives that significantly increased the transparency of the decision-making process (Prescrire, 2012).

By contrast, it was events surrounding a systematic review by the Cochrane Acute Respiratory Infections group that focused media and policy-makers' attention on the problems of publication bias and secrecy in medicines regulation in Europe – attention that included questions about the respective roles of the EMA, governments, and national and international health organizations in the approval and stockpiling of influenza drugs with unclear efficacy (Boseley, 2009; Cohen, 2009, 2012; Doshi, 2009; Godlee, 2009; Godlee & Clarke, 2009; Jefferson, Jones, Doshi, & Del Mar, 2009; Jefferson, Doshi, Thompson, & Heneghan, 2011; UK House of Commons, Committee of Public Accounts, 2014). In 2009, the UK National Institute for Health Research commissioned an update of the Cochrane systematic review of the neuraminidase inhibitors (NIs) in (otherwise) healthy adults. Coincidently, a paediatrician from Japan,

Keiji Hayashi, had challenged the Cochrane group with respect to a 2006 Cochrane review finding oseltamivir effective in reducing the complications of influenza. Hayashi pointed out that this conclusion was based on a single, manufacturer-funded meta-analysis of ten trials, of which only two were published in peer-reviewed journals (Doshi, 2009; Jefferson et al., 2011). Following failed attempts to access all the data on oseltamivir, the Cochrane's updated 2009 review of the NIs concluded that evidence for the drugs' efficacy in preventing complications was lacking. Yet, this attribute had been one of the main reasons for governments around the world stockpiling these drugs. The Cochrane researchers' experiences in trying to access full clinical trial data for the NIs led them to conclude that it was not sufficient for systematic reviews to be based on published papers (even assuming all studies undertaken were reported). Instead, they argued, reviews should be based on analysis of primary data from trials, particularly the original CSRs (Doshi, Jefferson, & Del Mar, 2012).

Although we have no direct evidence of this connection, it is possible that the high-profile Cochrane review in 2009 and its related inquiries increased pressure on the EMA in the context of the Ombudsman's investigation in 2010. Certainly, a 2009 joint investigation of the story by the *BMJ* and the UK television news program *Channel 4 News* (Cohen, 2009) ensured that the subject received attention beyond the medical press. And from 2012 onwards, the continued activities of these actors ensured that the problem of publication bias and missing trial data remained on the policy agenda. The *BMJ* continued to play a key role by following the Cochrane group's ongoing efforts to track down and verify the results from unpublished studies of the NIs, launching a linked "Open Data" campaign, and publishing and investigating similar cases involving reporting bias and missing data (Godlee, 2012; Godlee & Loder, 2010; Jackson, 2012; Lehman & Loder, 2012; Loder, Tovey, & Godlee, 2014; Payne, 2012; Wieseler, McGauran, & Kaiser, 2010). In January 2013, the AllTrials campaign was launched, calling for past and present clinical trials to be registered and their results shared. The campaign was founded by Ben Goldacre in collaboration with the Cochrane Collaboration, the James Lind Initiative, the Oxford Centre for Evidence-Based Medicine, Sense About Science, and the *BMJ* and *PLoS*. Within three years, AllTrials had garnered the support of over 80,000 people and around 600 organizations, thereby demonstrating widespread support for full data transparency and data sharing. Also important was a letter signed by fifty-three patients, which was coordinated by the AllTrials team and sent on 18 January 2013 to the EMA (Chalmers et al., 2013). The letter demanded that the protocols and results for all clinical trials published since the 1980s should be posted on a public register. Then, in June 2013, the editors of the *BMJ* and *PLoS Medicine* announced the launch of RIAT,[4] an initiative to restore invisible and abandoned trials, and officially endorsed the initiative (Doshi & Jefferson, 2013; Loder, Godlee, Barbour, & Winker, 2013; Winker & Barbour, 2013).

Although the AllTrials campaign was not concerned solely with the EMA's transparency policy, it highlighted the role of regulators in blocking or facilitating access to data and, at the political level, focused attention on opportunities offered by the new Clinical Trials Regulation to strengthen citizens' right of access (see later discussion; Mansell, 2013a). At a more general level, the initiatives just outlined were both a sign and a driver of increased awareness around, and changing attitudes towards, the broader issue of data publication bias and selective reporting by companies. In 2012, one of the most popular videos on TED.com was the talk by Ben Goldacre titled "What doctors don't know about the drugs they prescribe" (Jackson, 2012); Goldacre's book *Bad Pharma*, published in February 2013, received widespread publicity. Evidence that these concerns had permeated politicians' consciousness – at least in the United Kingdom – can be found in the fact that two UK House of Commons committees, the Committee of Public Accounts and the Science and Technology Committee, made inquiries in 2013 concerning the issue of data transparency. The practice of withholding trial data from the public was described as a "longstanding regulatory and cultural failure" by one committee (UK House of Commons, Committee of Public Accounts, 2014, p. 4), while the other committee recommended that CSRs produced for regulatory purposes should be placed in the public domain with identifiable patient data redacted (UK House of Commons, Science and Technology Committee, 2013, p. 4). That committee also specifically requested that the UK government consider the committee's recommendations in preparing its response to the EMA's ongoing consultation on access to clinical trial data, suggesting that growing awareness and political attention in the United Kingdom may have had some impact at the European Union level. Further evidence of a changing culture comes from the EMA itself. In its early exchanges with the EU Ombudsman, the EMA had claimed there was no value in external researchers scrutinizing the data submitted in support of marketing authorizations since the EMA had already carried out this examination on behalf of the medical community, patients, and the public. However, by 2012, in apparent recognition that it was no longer acceptable to make such claims, senior EMA scientists declared:

> The potential benefits for public health of independent (re)-analysis of data are not disputed and, in an open society, trial sponsors and regulators do

not have a monopoly on analysing and assessing drug trial results. (Eichler, Abadie, Breckenridge, Leufkens, & Rasi, 2012, p. 1)

Equally important has been the close engagement of these actors with the European regulatory body during subsequent stages in the formulation of EMA's transparency initiatives. On the 22 November 2012, following the announcement of its new policy initiatives, the EMA organized a public workshop to further discuss how the policies should be developed (EMA, 2012). This workshop involved participation by a large number and wide range of interested stakeholders, including representatives from industry, other regulatory bodies such as the FDA, and various health technology assessment bodies, academia, and patient and consumer advocates. Critically, many of the pivotal actors discussed earlier attended this workshop and were among the event's key speakers, including Peter Gøtzsche from the Nordic Cochrane Collaboration, Fiona Godlee from the *BMJ*, Virginia Barbour, chief editor of *PLoS Medicine*, Ben Goldacre, and a representative of the European Ombudsman. At the end of the workshop, the EMA proposed a series of working groups to develop more detailed policy recommendations. Again, a number of the individuals associated with the loose networks discussed earlier participated in these advisory groups. For example, in addition to Peter Gøtzsche and Ben Goldacre, workshop participants who joined one or more of the various Clinical Trials Advisory groups included Jörg Schaaber and Teresa Alves from ISDB; Pierre Chirac from *Prescrire* and the MiEF; Barbara Mintzes from HAI; Ilaria Passarani from BEUC; and Carl Heneghan, Tom Jefferson, and Peter Doshi, who had worked on the Cochrane reviews of the NIs (EMA, 2013).

We have suggested that some of the events previously outlined provide evidence of a "mainstreaming" of arguments around data transparency, publication bias, and the suppression of negative findings by companies. Within this broader context, in July 2012 the European Commission announced draft proposals for a new regulation aiming to streamline the process for authorizing clinical trials in order to reverse a decline in medical research in Europe (European Commission, 2012; Cressey, 2014). The draft regulation was intended to replace a widely criticized directive on clinical trials in existence since 2001. The Commission's proposals on transparency were fairly limited, and were justified only in terms of preventing redundancy and duplication of research. In an analysis piece published by the *BMJ*, Peter Gøtzsche pointed to deficiencies in the Commission's proposals with respect to providing access to data, including the fact that the regulation only required sponsors to submit a summary of results to the new EU portal (Gøtzsche, 2012). It was clear, then, that the Commission had drafted its proposals without regard for wider initiatives at the EU level – specifically, the EMA's plans for greater data transparency. This omission is not surprising, since securing data transparency was not the primary purpose of the legislation for the Commission. But what began as an initiative to streamline and accelerate the process for authorizing clinical trials across the EU member states became a vehicle, under the rapporteurship of Glenis Willmott, for strengthening transparency and citizens' right to access clinical trial data. These events represent the fourth and final stream in our analysis.

In October 2012, it was reported that the European Parliament had decided to appoint Willmott, a UK member of the European Parliament (MEP) and leader of the European Parliamentary Labour Party, as the rapporteur for the new Clinical Trials Regulation. "Rapporteurs" are responsible for steering new legislation through the European Parliament – including through the parliamentary committee responsible for reviewing the Commission's draft proposal in the initial stages – and for liaising with the Council and the Commission throughout the legislative process. Consequently, rapporteurs are also in a key position to shape the outcomes of that process. Industry reaction to the news of Willmott's appointment was initially positive, and she was described by the UK BioIndustry Association (BIA) as someone who understood "the concerns of the UK life science sector" (Mansell, 2012). Willmott's initial rapporteur's report, released in January 2013, proposed key revisions to the Clinical Trials Directive, introducing important transparency requirements and penalties for non-compliance. As touched on earlier, text published by the Commission only required sponsors to submit a summary of the trial's results to the EU clinical trial database within one year of a study ending. Willmott amended the provision to read: "Within one year from the end of a clinical trial, the sponsor shall submit to the EU database *the clinical study report, including a lay summary* of the clinical trial" (Amendment 51; European Parliament, Committee on Environment, Public Health and Food Safety, 2013, p. 35, emphasis in original). She also introduced an amendment specifying that financial penalties would be imposed in the event of a sponsor failing to comply with this obligation (Amendment 52; p. 36).

Industry representatives were quick to express concerns that these transparency provisions might threaten investment in clinical trials (Mansell, 2013b). Nevertheless, in May 2013, the Committee on Environment, Public Health and Food Safety unanimously adopted Willmott's amendments, including the provisions requiring sponsors to publish CSRs (Mansell, 2013c). Between June 2013 and April 2014, Willmott steered the draft legislation through the European Union's complex co-decision procedure. And, despite initially wide divergence between the views of MEPs on data transparency (Adams, 2015, p. 18), on 16 April 2014 the European Parliament voted overwhelmingly to introduce the Clinical Trials Regulation (Regulation [EU] No 536/2014). The new regulation included a requirement that, as of May 2016 (when the law came into force), all trials have to be registered on a publicly accessible EU clinical trials register before they can begin, with a summary of the trial results to be posted within twelve months of the end of the trial. In addition, where the purpose of a trial is to obtain a marketing authorization, sponsors are required to file a clinical study report to the EU database thirty days after the marketing authorization has been granted, or after the decision-making process on the marketing authorization application is completed or the application is withdrawn by the sponsor. Critically, the regulation confirmed a general presumption in favour of transparency, stipulating: "For the purposes of this Regulation, in general the data included in a clinical study report should not be considered commercially confidential once a marketing authorization has been granted, the procedure for granting the marketing authorization has been completed, [or] the application for marketing has been withdrawn" (Regulation [EU] No 536/2014, para. 68).

According to Ben Goldacre and Síle Lane from the AllTrials campaign, the UK campaigners worked with Willmott's office during the legislative process and helped to organize mass letter-writing campaigns from AllTrials supporters to their MEPs, asking them to support Willmott's transparency provisions in the draft regulation. These letters may have acted as something of a counterforce to arguments to limit data transparency made by the pharmaceutical industry's 300 lobbyists in Brussels (Butterworth, 2015). At the same time, the coalition of actors discussed in the first stream, including HAI and the MiEF, worked hard in Brussels to advocate for the amendment granting public access to CSRs. The early activities of the MiEF in the context of the first major overhaul of EU pharmaceutical legislation between 2000 and 2004, and its later efforts to oppose the introduction of direct-to-consumer advertising in the European Union (Geyer, 2011; Brooks, 2018), showed that civil society groups could influence and secure improvements in regulation at the European level in the face of daunting industry influence (Mulinari, 2013; Prescrire, 2004). These groups also gained critical experience – particularly in how to engage with members of the European Parliament and government ministers – that would later come in useful in the context of the Clinical Trials Regulation. Briefing papers and letters, signed by several European or international organizations, were sent to ministers of health, MEPs, and member states' permanent representatives to the European Union throughout 2013, explaining the importance of the transparency provisions.[5]

The combined and cumulative effect of the unfolding events in these four streams was to strengthen the pressure on European politicians, bureaucrats, and regulators to take steps to greatly increase data transparency in the European Union. Moreover, the core actors within each of the groupings described joined together into a policy network, acting as a loose coalition committed to closely monitor, report on, and shape events as they unfolded.

The Devil's in the Detail: Industry Fights Back and EMA Backtracks

Following the EMA's initial announcement in 2010, the pharmaceutical industry has engaged in a concerted campaign to undermine and reverse moves towards greater transparency in the European Union. It was apparent during the EMA's November 2012 workshop that industry was opposed to proposals for proactive release of CSRs, with the European Federation of Pharmaceutical Industries and Associations (EFPIA) arguing that requests for data access should be reviewed on a case-by-case basis (Mansell, 2012). Predictably, industry lobbied hard against the most radical elements of the EMA's new policy. A joint letter from two trade associations, EFPIA and the Pharmaceutical Research and Manufacturers of America (PhRMA), to a group of companies, which was leaked to the press in July 2013, revealed a "four-pronged" strategy that would start with "mobilizing patient groups to express concerns about the risks to public health by non-scientific re-use of data." The strategy also outlined plans to persuade researchers of the risks of data sharing, to work with other businesses concerned with the release of trade secrets and confidential data, and to create a network of academics that could be called upon to challenge re-analyses of the data that threatened companies' interests. A source at the European Parliament confirmed MEPs were being lobbied by particular patient groups, attempting to weaken some of the transparency measures (Sample, 2013).

Through constant vigilance, the "coalition" was, however, able to counter some of industry's (and possibly the Commission's) attempts to halt the expansion and deepening of data transparency. In late April and early May 2014, background documents sent to academic researchers who had actively participated in the transparency policy working groups raised a red flag that EMA was beginning to backtrack on its previous commitments. The documents included new proposals that would significantly restrict public access to clinical trial data contained in the new clinical trials database, including screen-only viewing without screen capture; and terms of use (ToU) provisions that required users to "acknowledge ... that the information is protected by copyright and proprietary rights ... and can be considered commercially valuable" and to contractually agree to being sued under UK law for violating the ToU. Rather than proactively disclose complete CSRs, new redaction provisions described a process whereby companies would be responsible in the first instance for redacting material (these would have to be agreed to by EMA) and envisioned that "novel statistical or other analytical methods and exploratory endpoint results about potential new uses of medicine" could be deemed commercially confidential. As Tom Jefferson and colleagues pointed out, safety and efficacy data about off-label use – the kind of use that had sparked concerns about data suppression, misrepresentation, and illegal promotion following US court cases – could be withheld from public view (Jefferson, Doshi, & Lemmens, 2014).

These new proposals were due to be discussed at an EMA Management Board meeting scheduled for June 2014. All the key actors who had fought to secure data transparency, including the Ombudsman and MEP Glenis Willmott, wrote letters to the EMA and issued press releases expressing their dismay at the EMA's severely compromised new "transparency" policy. It appears from documents released to the Ombudsman following her inquiries to the EMA and the European Commission that the Commission may have put pressure on the EMA to backtrack. Minutes from a previous EMA Management Board meeting note:

> A representative of the European Commission stated that they consider this topic to be complex and multi-faceted; therefore, some other parameters should be evaluated before proceeding to any final decisions, such as interaction with the TRIPS Agreement and the European patent system. (European Commission, 2014)

Following the campaign's interventions, the EMA Management Board asked for removal of screen-only restrictions. However, the onerous ToU provisions remained. The agency's final guidelines on redactions are unfortunately vague. The EMA notes that sections of the CSRs may contain commercially confidential information, including those covering the introduction and study objectives (sections 7 and 8); all efficacy and safety measurements assessed (but not the primary efficacy variables); drug concentration measurements (sections 9.5.1, 9.5.2, and 9.5.4); and determination of sample size (section 9.7.2) (EMA, 2015, Annex 1). These are all data that would be critical to evaluating the safety and efficacy of the drugs, and questions remain as to how broadly EMA will interpret the definition of "commercially confidential information."

The industry also launched legal challenges to the EMA's disclosure decisions under its new policy in the European courts. While the new Clinical Trials Regulation was working its way through a complex legislative process, InterMune and AbbVie brought cases challenging the EMA decision to allow third party access to CSRs and requested that the Court of Justice of the European Union (ECJ) issue interim orders to prevent the EMA from releasing the reports prior to trial. These cases were withdrawn by the companies before the EU courts were able to rule on the relevant legal issues. However, in February 2018, the ECJ ruled on three similar cases (brought by PARI Pharma, PTC Therapeutics International, MSD Animal Health Innovation, and Intervet International), upholding the EMA's decision to release documents requested in accordance with Regulation 1049/2001. Importantly, the ECJ confirmed a presumption in favour of openness and ruled that companies would have to give concrete evidence as to how release of clinical trial data would undermine their commercial interests (EMA, 2018).

Discussion

El Emam, Jefferson, and Doshi (2015, para. 1) observe that "in 2010, the European Medicines Agency … became the first regulator in history to promulgate a freedom of information policy that covered the release of manufacturer submitted clinical trial data." The political significance of this development should not be underestimated since it shows that – with enormous determination, persistence, and vigilance – a coalition of civil society organizations, researchers, and political actors can achieve major gains despite the enormous power and influence of the pharmaceutical industry. Nor should the scientific and public health significance of these gains be underestimated. The value of full data transparency for public health was confirmed by the Cochrane Collaboration's updated 2014 reviews of oseltamivir and zanamivir, for which they obtained all relevant clinical study reports (Heneghan et al., 2014; Jefferson, Jones, et al., 2014). The revised reviews, based on the full clinical trial data set, concluded that evidence from the studies did not support the drugs' use to reduce hospitalizations or the risks of serious complications. Against the drugs' minimal efficacy, the researchers pointed to an increased risk of psychiatric events, renal complications, headaches, and nausea and vomiting in patients taking oseltamivir, and they called on the WHO to review its guidance on the use of NIs and inclusion of oseltamivir in its Essential Medicines List (Torjensen, 2014).

Nevertheless, there are continuing concerns. At the political level, commentators suggest that industry and the Commission may attempt to block data transparency through other regulatory routes – for example, through initiatives to strengthen trade secret protection as part of trade negotiations with the United States and Canada (Association Internationale de la Mutualité et al., 2014; Lemmens & Gibson, 2014). At the regulatory level, there are concerns relating to the scope and implementation of the EMA's policies (which, at the time of writing, had been scaled back or suspended due to the EMA's preparations for Brexit and its relocation from London to Amsterdam). First are the unreasonable ToU restrictions imposed by the EMA. Second, some of the most commonly used drugs were not licensed by the EMA under the centralized procedure; rather, they were licensed by the different national competent authorities (NCAs) at the national level. However, the extent to which national regulatory agencies within Europe are willing to grant the public access to documents is highly variable. For example, following the recent controversy over the possible harms of statins in primary prevention of cardiovascular events, one of us (Jefferson) sought access to trial data for the eight original statins from four NCAs within Europe, as well as from Health Canada. While some European regulators, like the Finnish FIMEA, refused to release any reports of statin trials, the British MHRA and the Dutch MEB did so without any restrictions.[6] The divergent approach of different NCAs is not justifiable in light of the EMA's new transparency policies. Third, it is unclear whether sufficient resources and priority will be accorded to the EMA's policy, and the recent experience of one of the authors (Jefferson) points to the potential risks of delay in the release of information when public health is at stake. Following a request for data underlying a conclusion by the EMA's Pharmacovigilance Risk Assessment Committee that available evidence did not support an association between three currently registered HPV vaccines and an increased incidence of complex regional pain syndrome (CRPS) or postural orthostatic tachycardia syndrome (POTS), Jefferson was informed that a response would be forthcoming in two months. An important inference to be drawn from this episode is that the EMA continues to believe that important decisions on public health can be made and publicized without at the same time providing the public or medical community with access to the underlying evidence for these decisions (Jefferson, 2015).

Beyond these concerns about the future scope and implementation of the EMA's policies, there are further ways in which the value of full data transparency may be diminished. The first is where regulators, governments, or public health bodies fail to act on the knowledge generated. For example, although the status of oseltamivir has been downgraded, it remains on the WHO Model List of Essential Medicines (Ebell, 2017).[7]

The second relates to the fact that forensic re-analysis of primary trial data is enormously time consuming and resource intensive (Jefferson, Jones et al., 2014; Le Noury et al., 2015), which may explain why researchers are not making more use of increased data transparency in Europe (Hodkinson et al., 2018). Despite its intense resistance, industry has been the chief beneficiary so far of increased regulatory openness. Doshi and Jefferson (2013) report that, between November 2010 and November 2012, the EMA handled 457 requests for information under its new "reactive" disclosure policy. Of these, industry made the most requests – accounting for 33 per cent of the total – while requests from academic researchers accounted for only 8 per cent. Given the intrinsic difficulties of the sort of review that was undertaken by the Cochrane Acute Respiratory Infections group, it is probably reasonable to assume that, in most cases, assessments of company data by medicines regulators will remain the only "independent" evaluation available to the public. The rigour of these regulatory assessments will therefore continue to be hugely important, and the fact that researchers and citizens feel the need for further independent (re)analysis of data points to a failure on the part of drug regulatory agencies to make decisions the public can trust.

A third potential limit to the value of data transparency relates to the fact that regulatory standards do not always ensure the evidence generated in clinical studies is informative. For example, clinical studies are not always conducted in a relevant population, against a relevant comparator, at the right dose, or for a sufficient period of time to determine the longer-term health impacts (both beneficial and harmful) of treatment (see Persaud, chapter six, this volume). Data transparency is meaningless if those data don't tell clinicians, patients, health technology assessment bodies, or health policy-makers what they need to know. Moreover, broader regulatory trends towards lowering standards for an increasingly wide category of drugs – particularly through the use of surrogate end points that do not reliably predict improvements in the health outcomes that matter to patients (Kesselheim, Wang, Franklin, & Darrow, 2015) – may mean that, in the future, we will be able to "see" the data, but that data will be less and less informative.

Thus, broader problems with the priorities, activities of, and standards promulgated by medicines regulators are as profound as, and cannot be separated from, the problem of data transparency. Regulators need sufficient time and resources to undertake rigorous, in-depth reviews – including, where necessary, re-analysis of patient-level data – and should insist on clinical study designs that produce relevant information on treatment outcomes that matter to patients. Recent gains achieved by transparency campaigners in Europe suggest that further, wide-reaching changes may be possible, but success would depend on the formation of broad coalitions, a compelling framing of the issue, a very high degree of vigilance and engagement, and the support of key political players.

NOTES

1 The one respect in which the EMA outperformed the FDA was in relation to release of information about non-approved or withdrawn applications. Typically, the FDA, citing exemption 4 of the Freedom of Information Act, refuses to release any information about non-approved indications on grounds that it is commercially confidential (Lenzer & Brownlee, 2008).
2 Regulation (EU) No 536/2014 of the European Parliament and of the Council of 16 April 2014 on clinical trials on medicinal products for human use, and repealing Directive 2001/20/EC.
3 For details about the forum and the organizations it comprises, see the description on the *Prescrire* (in English) website: "About the Medicines in Europe Forum." Retrieved from https://english.prescrire.org/en/79/549 /49237/3374/ReportDetails.aspx.
4 For details about the work and programs of the Restoring Invisible and Abandoned Trials (RIAT) Support Center, see the description on its website: "What is RIAT?" Retrieved from https://restoringtrials.org/whatisriat/.
5 For information about the actions that took place in Europe over this period, see the list on the *Prescrire* (in English) website: "Clinical trials and Europe: Actions." Retrieved from http://english.prescrire.org/en/79/549/49220 /3472/SubReportList.aspx.
6 For details of the controversy over statins, see the *BMJ*'s article "Statins – A call for transparent data." Retrieved from https://www.bmj.com/campaign /statins-open-data.
7 See Persaud, chapter six of this volume, for further examples.

REFERENCES

Abbasi, K. (2004). Compulsory registration of clinical trials. *BMJ, 329*(7467), 637–8. https://doi.org/10.1136/bmj.329.7467.637

Abraham, J. (1995). *Science, politics and the pharmaceutical industry: Controversy and bias in drug regulation.* London, UK: UCL Press.

Abraham, J., & Lewis, G. (1998). Secrecy and transparency of medicines licensing in the EU. *Lancet, 352*(9126), 480–2. https://doi.org/10.1016/S0140 -6736(97)11282-X

Abraham, J., & Lewis, G. (2000). *Regulating medicines in Europe: Competition, expertise and public health.* London, UK: Routledge.

Adams, B. (2015). The pioneers of transparency. *BMJ, 350*, 16–19. https://doi
.org/10.1136/bmj.g7717

Armstrong, D. (2006, 15 May). How the New England Journal missed warning
signs on Vioxx. *Wall Street Journal*. Retrieved from https://www.wsj.com
/articles/SB114765430315252591

Association Internationale de la Mutualité (AIM), Health Action International
(HAI) Europe, International Society of Drug Bulletins (ISDB), Medicines
in Europe Forum (MiEF), Nordic Cochrane Collaboration, TransAtlantic
Consumer Dialogue (TACD), & WEMOS. (2014, 17 March). EU Regulation
on clinical trials: Close to the finish line. Press release. Retrieved from
http://haiweb.org/wp-content/uploads/2015/07/EU-Regulation-on-Clinical
-Trials-Close-to-the-Finish-Line-2014.pdf

Barbui, C., Baschirotto, C., & Cipriani, A. (2011). EMA must improve the
quality of its clinical trial reports. *BMJ, 342*, d2291. https://doi.org/10.1136
/bmj.d2291

Bardelay, D., & Kopp, C. (2002). Commentary: Concern over drug industry's
influence on regulatory policy in Europe. *BMJ, 325*(7373), 1167–8. https://
doi.org/10.1136/bmj.325.7373.1164

Boseley, S. (2009, 8 December). Doctors query ability of Tamiflu to stop severe
illness. *The Guardian*. Retrieved from https://www.theguardian.com/world
/2009/dec/08/tamiflu-swine-flu-roche

Brooks, E. (2018). Using the Advocacy Coalition Framework to understand EU
pharmaceutical policy. *European Journal of Public Health, 28*(Suppl. 3), 11–14.
https://doi.org/10.1093/eurpub/cky153

Butterworth, T. (2015, 13 July). The story of AllTrials: Interview with Ben
Goldacre and Síle Lane. Retrieved from http://www.alltrials.net/news/the
-story-of-the-campaign-thats-changing-the-world/

Chalmers, I. (1990). Underreporting research is scientific misconduct. *JAMA,
263*(10), 1405–8. https://doi.org/10.1001/jama.1990.03440100121018

Chalmers, I. (2006). From optimism to disillusion about commitment to
transparency in the medico-industrial complex. *Journal of the Royal Society of
Medicine, 99*(7), 33741. https://doi.org/10.1177/014107680609900715

Chalmers, I., Stephens, R., Gore, L., Smith, R., Stevens, S., Haigh, D., … Fraser,
M. (2013, 18 January). Letter to Guido Rasi, Executive Director, European
Medicines Agency, 18 January 2013. Retrieved from https://www.alltrials
.net/wp-content/uploads/2013/01/letter-to-EMA-from-clinical-trial
-participants-2013-Jan-18.pdf

Cohen, D. (2009). Complications: Tracking down the data on oseltamivir. *BMJ,
339*, b5387. https://doi.org/10.1136/bmj.b5387

Cohen, D. (2012). Search for evidence goes on. *BMJ, 344*, e458. https://doi.org
/10.1136/bmj.e458

Cressey, D. (2014, 4 June). Overhaul complete for EU clinical trials. *Nature.* Retrieved from https://www.nature.com/news/overhaul-complete-for-eu -clinical-trials-1.15339

Davis, C., & Abraham, J. (2013), *Unhealthy pharmaceutical regulation: Innovation, politics and promissory science.* Basingstoke, UK: Palgrave Macmillan.

Davis, C., Naci, H., Gurpinar, E., Poplavska, E., Pinto, A., & Aggarwal, A. (2017). Availability of evidence of benefits on overall survival and quality of life of cancer drugs approved by European Medicines Agency: A retrospective cohort study of drug approvals 2009–13. *BMJ, 359,* j4530. https://doi.org/10.1136 /bmj.j4530

De Angelis, C.D., Drazen, J.M., Frizelle, F.A., Haug, C., Hoey, J., Horton, R., ... Sox, H.C. (2005). Is this clinical trial fully registered? – A statement from the International Committee of Medical Journal Editors. *New England Journal of Medicine, 352*(23), 2436–8. https://doi.org/10.1056/NEJMe058127

Dickersin, K., Chan, S., Chalmers, T.C., Sacks, H.S., & Smith H. (1987). Publication bias and clinical trials. *Controlled Clinical Trials, 8*(4), 343–53. https://doi.org/10.1016/0197-2456(87)90155-3

Dickersin, K., & Rennie, D. (2003). Registering clinical trials. *JAMA, 290*(4), 516–23. https://doi.org/10.1001/jama.290.4.516

Doshi, P. (2009). Neuraminidase inhibitors – The story behind the Cochrane review. *BMJ, 339,* b5164. https://doi.org/10.1136/bmj.b5164

Doshi, P., Dickersin, K., Healy, D., Vedula, S.S., & Jefferson, T. (2013). Restoring invisible and abandoned trials: A call for people to publish the findings. *BMJ, 346,* f2865. https://doi.org/10.1136/bmj.f2865

Doshi, P., & Jefferson, T. (2013). The first 2 years of the European Medicines Agency's policy on access to documents: Secret no longer. *JAMA Internal Medicine, 173*(5), 380–2. https://doi.org/10.1001/jamainternmed.2013.3838

Doshi, P., Jefferson, T., & Del Mar, C. (2012). The imperative to share clinical study reports: Recommendations from the Tamiflu experience. *PloS Medicine, 9*(4), e1001201. https://doi.org/10.1371/journal.pmed.1001201

Easterbrook, P.J., Gopalan, R., Berlin, J.A., & Matthews, D.R. (1991). Publication bias in clinical research. *Lancet, 337*(8746), 867–72. https://doi.org/10.1016 /0140-6736(91)90201-Y

Ebell, M.H. (2017). WHO downgrades status of oseltamivir. *BMJ, 358,* j3266. https://doi.org/10.1136/bmj.j3266

Egilman, D.S., & Presler, A.H. (2006). Report of specific cardiovascular outcomes of the ADVANTAGE Trial. *Annals of Internal Medicine, 144*(10), 781. https://doi.org/10.7326/0003-4819-144-10-200605160-00016

Eichler, H.-G., Abadie, E., Breckenridge, A., Leufkens, H., & Rasi, G. (2012). Open clinical trial data for all? A view from regulators. *PLoS Medicine, 9*(4), e1001202. https://doi.org/10.1371/journal.pmed.1001202

El Emam, K., Jefferson, T., & Doshi, P. (2015, 27 August). Maximizing the value of clinical study reports. *BMJopinion.* Retrieved from https://blogs.bmj.com/bmj/2015/08/27/maximizing-the-value-of-clinical-study-reports/

European Commission. (2012, 17 July). Proposal for a regulation of the European Parliament and of the Council on clinical trials on medicinal products for human use, and repealing Directive 2001/20/EC. Retrieved from https://ec.europa.eu/health//sites/health/files/files/clinicaltrials/2012_07/proposal/2012_07_proposal_en.pdf

European Commission. (2014, 13 July). Reply from the European Commission to the letter from the European Ombudsman concerning the transparency of clinical trials data. Retrieved from https://www.ombudsman.europa.eu/en/resources/otherdocument.faces/en/54672/html.bookmark

European Medicines Agency (EMA). (2010a, 30 November; updated 2018). European Medicines Agency policy on access to documents. Policy/0043. EMA/110196/2006. Retrieved from https://www.ema.europa.eu/en/documents/other/policy/0043-european-medicines-agency-policy-access-documents_en.pdf

European Medicines Agency (EMA). (2010b, 30 November). European Medicines Agency widens public access to documents. Press release. EMA/718259/2010. Retrieved from https://www.ema.europa.eu/documents/press-release/european-medicines-agency-widens-public-access-documents_en.pdf

European Medicines Agency (EMA). (2010c, 30 November; updated 2018). Output of the European Medicines Agency policy on access to documents related to medicinal products for human and veterinary use. EMA/127362/2006. Retrieved from https://www.ema.europa.eu/en/documents/regulatory-procedural-guideline/output-european-medicines-agency-policy-access-documents-related-medicinal-products-human-veterinary_en.pdf

European Medicines Agency (EMA). (2012). Access to clinical-trial data and transparency: Workshop report. Retrieved from https://www.ema.europa.eu/documents/report/access-clinical-trial-data-transparency-workshop-report_en.pdf

European Medicines Agency (EMA). (2013). Clinical trial advisory groups: Membership overview – 20 February 2013. EMA/33488/2013. Retrieved from https://www.ema.europa.eu/en/documents/other/clinical-trial-advisory-groups-membership-overview_en.pdf

European Medicines Agency (EMA). (2015). Questions and answers on the European Medicines Agency policy on publication of clinical data for medicinal products for human use. EMA/357536/2014 Rev. 2. Retrieved from https://www.ema.europa.eu/en/documents/report/questions-answers-european-medicines-agency-policy-publication-clinical-data-medicinal-products_en.pdf

European Medicines Agency (EMA). (2018, 6 February). General Court confirms EMA approach to transparency. Press release. EMA/73690/2018. Retrieved from https://www.ema.europa.eu/en/news/general-court-confirms -ema-approach-transparency

European Medicines Agency (EMA). (2019, 21 March). European Medicines Agency policy on publication of clinical data for medicinal products for human use. Policy 0070. Retrieved from https://www.ema.europa.eu/en /documents/other/european-medicines-agency-policy-publication-clinical -data-medicinal-products-human-use_en.pdf

European Ombudsman. (2010, 24 November). Decision of the European Ombudsman closing his inquiry into complaint 2560/2007/BEH against the European Medicines Agency. Retrieved from https://www.ombudsman .europa.eu/cases/decision.faces/en/5459/html.bookmark

European Parliament, Committee on Environment, Public Health and Food Safety. (2013). Draft report on the proposal for a regulation of the European Parliament and of the Council on clinical trials on medicinal products for human use, and repealing Directive 2001/20/EC. Retrieved from https:// www.europarl.europa.eu/doceo/document/ENVI-PR-504236_EN.pdf

Eyding, D., Lelgemann, M., Grouven, U., Härter, M., Kromp, M., Kaiser, T., ... Wieseler, B. (2010). Reboxetine for acute treatment of major depression: Systematic review and meta-analysis of published and unpublished placebo and selective serotonin reuptake inhibitor controlled trials. *BMJ, 341*, c4737. https://doi.org/10.1136/bmj.c4737

Garattini, S. (2005). EMEA: For patient or for industry? *Pharmacoeconomics, 23*(3), 207–8. https://doi.org/10.2165/00019053-200523030-00001

Garattini, S., & Bertele', V. (2001). Adjusting Europe's drug regulation to public health needs. *Lancet, 358*(9275), 64–7. https://doi.org/10.1016/S0140 -6736(00)05258-2

Garattini, S., & Bertele', V. (2007). How can we regulate medicines better? *BMJ, 335*(7624), 803–5. https://doi.org/10.1136/bmj.39281.615706.94

Geyer, R. (2011). The politics of EU health policy and the case of direct-to -consumer advertising for prescription drugs. *The British Journal of Politics and International Relations, 13*(4), 586–602. https://doi.org/10.1111/j.1467-856X .2011.00460.x

Godlee, F. (2009). We want raw data, now. *BMJ, 339*, b5405. https://doi.org /10.1136/bmj.b5405

Godlee, F. (2012). Clinical trial data for all drugs in current use. *BMJ, 345*, e7304. https://doi.org/10.1136/bmj.e7304

Godlee, F., & Clarke, M. (2009). Why don't we have all the evidence on oseltamivir? *BMJ, 339*, b5351. https://doi.org/10.1136/bmj.b5351

Godlee, F., & Loder, E. (2010). Missing clinical trial data: Setting the record straight. *BMJ, 341*, c5641. https://doi.org/10.1136/bmj.c5641

Gøtzsche, P.C. (2012). Deficiencies in proposed new EU regulation of clinical trials. *BMJ, 345*, e8522. https://doi.org/10.1136/bmj.e8522

Gøtzsche, P.C., & Jørgensen, A.W. (2011). Opening up data at the European Medicines Agency. *BMJ, 342*, d2686. https://doi.org/10.1136/bmj.d26861

Groves, T. (2008). Mandatory disclosure of trial results for drugs and devices. *BMJ, 336*(7637), 170. https://doi.org/10.1136/bmj.39469.465139.80

Health Action International (HAI) Europe, International Society of Drug Bulletins (ISDB), & Medicines in Europe Forum (MiEF). (2009, 23 September). EMA transparency policy falls short: A weak and irresponsible project. Retrieved from https://english.prescrire.org/Docu/Archive/docus/JointAnswerEMEATranspPolicy_Sept2009.pdf

Hemminki, E. (1980). Study of information submitted by drug companies to licensing authorities. *BMJ, 280*, 833–6. https://doi.org/10.1136/bmj.280.6217.833

Heneghan, C.J., Onakpoya, I., Thompson, M., Cohen, H.D., Spencer, E.A., Jones, M., & Jefferson T. (2014). Zanamivir for influenza in adults and children: Systematic review of clinical study reports and summary of regulatory comments. *BMJ, 348*, g2547. https://doi.org/10.1136/bmj.g2547

Hill, K.P., Ross, J.S., Egilman, D.S., & Krumholz, H.M. (2008). The ADVANTAGE seeding trial: A review of internal documents. *Annals of Internal Medicine, 149*(4), 251–8. https://doi.org/10.7326/0003-4819-149-4-200808190-00006

Hodkinson, A., Dietz, K.C., Lefebvre, C., Golder, S., Jones, M., Doshi, P., ... Stewart, L. (2018). The use of clinical study reports to enhance the quality of systematic reviews: A survey of systematic review authors. *Systematic Reviews, 7*, 117. https://doi.org/10.1186/s13643-018-0766-x

Horton, R., & Smith, R. (1999). Time to register randomized trials. *BMJ, 319*(7214), 865–6. https://doi.org/10.1136/bmj.319.7214.865

Hrachovec, J.B., & Mora, M. (2001). Comment: Reporting of 6-month vs 12-month data in a clinical trial of celecoxib. *JAMA, 286*(19), 2398–400. https://doi.org/10.1001/jama.286.19.2398

International Society for Drug Bulletins (ISDB). (2001). The failings of the European Medicines Evaluation Agency. *ISDB Newsletter, 115*(1), 11–13.

Ioannidis, J.P.A. (1998). Effect of the statistical significance of results on the time to completion and publication of randomized efficacy trials. *JAMA, 279*(4), 281–6. https://doi.org/10.1001/jama.279.4.281

Jackson, T. (2012). Open data: Seize the moment. *BMJ, 345*, e7332. https://doi.org/10.1136/bmj.e7332

Jefferson, T. (2015, November 13). Happy birthday Ombudsman. *BMJopinion*. Retrieved from https://blogs.bmj.com/bmj/2015/11/13/tom-jefferson-happy-birthday-ombudsman/

Jefferson, T., & Doshi, P. (2014). Multisystem failure: The story of anti-influenza drugs. *BMJ, 348*, g2263. https://doi.org/10.1136/bmj.g2263

Jefferson, T., Doshi, P., & Lemmens, T. (2014, 22 May). EMA's data sharing policy – Towards peeping tom based medicine? *BMJopinion.* Retrieved from https://blogs.bmj.com/bmj/2014/05/22/tom-jefferson-et-al-emas-data -sharing-policy-towards-peeping-tom-based-medicine/

Jefferson, T., Doshi, P., Thompson, M., & Heneghan, C. (2011). Ensuring safe and effective drugs: Who can do what it takes? *BMJ, 342,* c7258. https://doi .org/10.1136/bmj.c7258

Jefferson, T., Jones, M., Doshi, P., & Del Mar, C. (2009). Neuraminidase inhibitors for preventing and treating influenza in health adults: Systematic review and meta-analysis. *BMJ, 339,* b5106. https://doi.org/10.1136/bmj.b5106

Jefferson, T., Jones, M., Doshi, P., Spencer, E.A., Onakpoya, I., & Heneghan, C. (2014). Oseltamivir for influenza in adults and children: Systematic review of clinical study reports and summary of regulatory comments. *BMJ, 348,* g2545. https://doi.org/10.1136/bmj.g2545

Jones, C.W., Handler, L., Crowell, K.E., Keil, L.G., Weaver, M.A., & Platts-Mills, T.F. (2013). Non-publication of large randomized clinical trials: Cross sectional analysis. *BMJ, 347,* f6104. https://doi.org/10.1136/bmj.f6104

Jørgensen, L., Gøtzsche, P.C., & Jefferson, T. (2018). Index of the human papillomavirus (HPV) vaccine industry clinical study programmes and non-industry funded studies: A necessary basis to address reporting bias in a systematic review. *Systematic Reviews, 7,* 8. https://doi.org/10.1186 /s13643-018-0675-z

Kesselheim, A.S., Wang, B., Franklin, J.M., & Darrow, J.J. (2015). Trends in utilization of FDA expedited drug development and approval programs, 1987–2014: Cohort study. *BMJ, 351,* h4633. https://doi.org/10.1136/bmj .h4633

Kondro, W. (2004). Drug company experts advised staff to withhold data about SSRI use in children. *CMAJ, 170*(5), 783. https://doi.org/10.1503/cmaj.1040213

Krleža-Jerić, K., Chan, A.-W., Dickersin, K., Sim, I., Grimshaw, J., & Gluud, C. (2005). Principles for international registration of protocol information and results from human trials of health related interventions: Ottawa statement (part 1). *BMJ, 330,* 956–8. https://doi.org/10.1136/bmj.330.7497.956

Krleža-Jerić, K., Lemmens, T., Reveiz, L., Cuervo, L.G., & Bero, L.A. (2011). Prospective registration and results disclosure of clinical trials in the Americas: A roadmap towards transparency. *Revista Panamericana de Salud Publica, 30*(1), 87–96.

Krumholz, H.M., Hines, H.H., Ross, J.S., Presler, A.H., & Egilman, D.S. (2007). What have we learnt from Vioxx? *BMJ, 334,* 120–3. https://doi.org/10.1136 /bmj.39024.487720.68

Lee, K., Bacchetti, P., & Sim, I. (2008). Publication of clinical trials supporting successful new drug applications: A literature analysis. *PLoS Medicine, 5*(9), e191. https://doi.org/10.1371/journal.pmed.0050191

Lehman, R., & Loder, E. (2012). Missing clinical trial data: A threat to the integrity of evidence based medicine. *BMJ, 344*, d8158. https://doi.org/10.1136/bmj.d8158

Lemmens, T., & Gibson, S. (2014). Decreasing the data deficit: Improving post-market surveillance in pharmaceutical regulation. *McGill Law Journal, 59*(4), 943–88. https://doi.org/10.7202/1026134ar

Le Noury, J., Nardo, J.M., Healy, D., Jureidini, J., Raven, M., Tufanaru, C., & Abi-Jaoude, E. (2015). Restoring Study 329: Efficacy and harms of paroxetine and imipramine in treatment of major depression in adolescence. *BMJ, 351*, h4320. https://doi.org/10.1136/bmj.h4320

Lenzer, J., & Brownlee, S. (2008). An untold story? *BMJ, 336*, 532–4. https://doi.org/10.1136/bmj.39504.662685.0F

Lexchin, J., & Mintzes, B. (2004). Transparency in drug regulation: Mirage or oasis? *CMAJ, 171*(11), 1363–5. https://doi.org/10.1503/cmaj.1041446

Loder, E., Godlee, F., Barbour, V., & Winker, M. (2013). Restoring the integrity of the clinical trial evidence base. *BMJ, 346*, f3601. https://doi.org/10.1136/bmj.f3601

Loder, E., Tovey, D., & Godlee, F. (2014). The Tamiflu trials: Progress towards data sharing but many battles still to fight. *BMJ, 348*, g2630. https://doi.org/10.1136/bmj.g2630

MacLean, C.H., Morton, S.C., Ofman, J.J., Roth, E.A., & Shekelle, P.G. (2003). How useful are unpublished data from the Food and Drug Administration in meta-analysis? *Journal of Clinical Epidemiology, 56*(1), 44–51. https://doi.org/10.1016/s0895-4356(02)00520-6

Mansell, P. (2012, 6 December). Deep divisions remain at EMA transparency workshop. *PharmaTimes*. Retrieved from http://www.pharmatimes.com/news/deep_divisions_remain_at_ema_transparency_workshop_976083

Mansell, P. (2013a, 10 January). AllTrials campaign raises the game on clinical trial transparency. *PharmaTimes*. Retrieved from http://www.pharmatimes.com/news/alltrials_campaign_raises_the_game_on_clinical-trial_transparency_1004196

Mansell, P. (2013b, 26 February). Transparency demands could threaten early trial investment. *PharmaTimes*. Retrieved from http://www.pharmatimes.com/news/transparency_demands_could_threaten_early_trial_investment_1004528

Mansell, P. (2013c, 30 May). Environment Committee adopts Willmott amendments to CT regulation. *PharmaTimes*. Retrieved from http://www.pharmatimes.com/news/environment_committee_adopts_willmott_amendments_to_ct_regulation_1005103

McGauran, N., Wieseler, B., Kreis, J., Schüler, Y.-B., Kölosch, H., & Kaiser, T. (2010). Reporting bias in medical research – A narrative review. *Trials, 11*(37), 1–15. https://doi.org/10.1186/1745-6215-11-37

Medicines in Europe Forum (MiEF). (n.d.). Petition to the president of the
European Parliament: Putting European drugs policy back on tracks. Retrieved
from http://english.prescrire.org/Docu/Archive/docus/petition1En.pdf

Melander, H., Ahlqvist-Rastad, J., Meijer, G., & Beermann, B. (2003). Evidence
b(i)ased medicine – Selective reporting from studies sponsored by
pharmaceutical industry: Review of studies in new drug applications. *BMJ*,
326(1171), 1–5. https://doi.org/10.1136/bmj.326.7400.1171

Mintzes, B., Lexchin, J., & Quintano, A.S. (2015). Clinical trial transparency:
Many gains but access to evidence for new medicines remains imperfect.
British Medical Bulletin, *116*, 43–53. https://doi.org/10.1093/bmb/ldv042

Moscicki, R. (2013). Responsible sharing of clinical trial data: An FDA
perspective. Retrieved from https://www.fdanews.com/ext/resources/files
/Conference/CTDTPresentations/archives/10113-01/Moscicki-Clinical
%20Trial%20and%20Transparency%20Summit%207-23-13.pdf

Mukherjee, D., Nissen, S.E., & Topol, E.J. (2001). Risk of cardiovascular events
associated with selective COX-2 inhibitors. *JAMA*, *286*(8), 954–9. https://doi
.org/10.1001/jama.286.8.954

Mulinari, S. (2013). Regulating drug information in Europe: A pyrrhic victory
for pharmaceutical industry critics? *Sociology of Health & Illness*, *35*(5), 761–77.
https://doi.org/10.1111/j.1467-9566.2012.01528.x

Mulinari, S., & Davis, C. (2017). Why European and United States drug
regulators are not speaking with one voice on anti-influenza drugs: Regulatory
review methodologies and the importance of "deep" product review. *Health
Research Policy and Systems*, *15*, 93. https://doi.org/10.1186/s12961-017-0259-8

Naci, H., Cooper, J., & Mossialos, E. (2015). Timely publication and sharing
of trial data: Opportunities and challenges for comparative effectiveness
research in cardiovascular disease. *European Heart Journal – Quality of Care and
Clinical Outcomes*, *1*(2), 58–65. https://doi.org/10.1093/ehjqcco/qcv012

New York State Court. (2004, 2 June). *Spitzer v GlaxoSmithKline PLC New York*,
Supreme Court, No 04/401707.

Nissen, S.E., & Wolski, K. (2007). Effect of rosiglitazone on the risk of
myocardial infarction and death from cardiovascular causes. *NEJM*, *356*(24),
2457–71. https://doi.org/10.1056/NEJMoa072761

Nissen, S.E., Wolski, K., & Topol, E.J. (2005). Effect of muraglitazar on death and
major adverse cardiovascular events in patients with type 2 diabetes mellitus.
JAMA, *294*(20), 2581–6. https://doi.org/10.1001/jama.294.20.joc50147

Payne, D. (2012). Tamiflu: The battle for secret drug data. *BMJ*, *345*, e7303.
https://doi.org/10.1136/bmj.e7303

PharmaTimes. (2012, 16 October). BIA welcomes UK MEP's inclusion on
clinical trials rethink. *PharmaTimes*. Retrieved from http://www.pharmatimes
.com/appointments/bia_welcomes_uk_meps_inclusion_on_clinical_trials
_rethink_1008662

Prescrire. (2002). European Medicines Policy. *Prescrire International*. Retrieved from https://www.prescrire.org/docus/euMedPolEn.pdf

Prescrire. (2004, August). Medicines in Europe: The most important changes in the new legislation. *Prescrire International*. Translated from *La Revue Prescrire* (2004, July–August), *24*(252), 481. Retrieved from https://english.prescrire.org/Docu/DOCSEUROPE/europeSyntheseEn.pdf

Prescrire. (2009). Caviardage en guise de "transparence": la censure d'un rapport d'évaluation du rimonabant (ex-Acomplia) par l'Agence européanne du médicament. *La Revue Prescrire*, *29*(309), 537. Retrieved from https://www.prescrire.org/editoriaux/EDI33693.pdf

Prescrire. (2010, 20 August). Letter to P. Nikiforos Diamandouros, the European Ombudsman. Retrieved from https://english.prescrire.org/Docu/Archive/docus/Prescrire%20to%20European%20Ombudsman%20five%20complaints%20against%20EMA%2030%20August%202010.pdf

Prescrire. (2012, April). In the wake of the Mediator scandal: Some progress in France, but apathy at the European level. *Prescrire International*, *21*(126), 110.

Psaty, B.M., & Kronmal, R.A. (2008). Reporting mortality findings in trials of rofecoxib for Alzheimer disease or cognitive impairment: A case study based on documents from rofecoxib litigation. *JAMA*, *299*(15), 1813–17. https://doi.org/10.1001/jama.299.15.1813

Regulation (EU) No. 536/2014 of the European Parliament and of the Council of 16 April 2014 on clinical trials on medicinal products for human use, and repealing Directive 2001/20/EC. Retrieved from https://ec.europa.eu/health/sites/health/files/files/eudralex/vol-1/reg_2014_536/reg_2014_536_en.pdf

Rennie, D. (2004). Trial registration: A great idea switches from ignored to irresistible. *JAMA*, *292*(11), 1359–62. https://doi.org/10.1001/jama.292.11.1359

Rising, K., Bacchetti, P., & Bero, L. (2009). Reporting bias in drug trials submitted to the Food and Drug Administration: Review of publication and presentation. *PLoS Medicine*, *5*(11), e217. https://doi.org/10.1371/journal.pmed.0050217

Sample, I. (2013, 21 July). Big pharma mobilizing patients in battle over drugs trial data. *The Guardian*. Retrieved from https://www.theguardian.com/business/2013/jul/21/big-pharma-secret-drugs-trials

Simes, R.J. (1986). Publication bias: The case for an international registry of clinical trials. *Journal of Clinical Oncology*, *4*(10), 1529–4. https://doi.org/10.1200/jco.1986.4.10.1529

Simmonds, M.C., Brown, J.V.E., Heirs, M.K., Higgins, J.P.T., Mannion, R.J., Rodgers M.A., & Stewart L.A. (2013). Safety and effectiveness of recombinant human bone morphogenetic protein-2 for spinal fusion. *Annals of Internal Medicine*, *158*(12), 877–89. https://doi.org/10.7326/0003-4819-158-12-201306180-00005

Song, F., Parekh, S., Hooper, L., Loke, Y.K., Ryder, J., Sutton, A.J., ... Harvey, I. (2010). Dissemination and publication of research findings: An updated review of related biases. *Health Technology Assessment, 14*(8). https://doi.org/10.3310/hta14080

Teather, D., & Boseley, S. (2004, 3 June). Glaxo faces drug fraud lawsuit: Firm accused of keeping back negative trial results. *The Guardian.* Retrieved from https://www.theguardian.com/business/2004/jun/03/mentalhealth.medicineandhealth

Torjensen, I. (2014). Cochrane review questions effectiveness of neuraminidase inhibitor. *BMJ, 348,* g2675. https://doi.org/10.1136/bmj.g2675

Turner, E.H. (2004). A taxpayer-funded clinical trials registry and results database. *PLoS Medicine, 1*(3), e60. https://doi.org/10.1371/journal.pmed.0010060

Turner, E.H., Matthews, A.M., Linardatos, E., Tell, R.A., & Rosenthal, R. (2008). Selective publication of antidepressant trials and its influence on apparent efficacy. *NEJM, 358*(3), 252–60. https://doi.org/10.1056/nejmsa065779

UK House of Commons, Committee of Public Accounts. (2014). *Access to clinical trial information and the stockpiling of Tamiflu.* Thirty-fifth report of Session 2013–14. London, UK: The Stationary Office. Retrieved from https://publications.parliament.uk/pa/cm201314/cmselect/cmpubacc/295/295.pdf

UK House of Commons, Science and Technology Committee. (2013). *Clinical trials.* Third report of Session 2013–14. London, UK: The Stationary Office. Retrieved from https://publications.parliament.uk/pa/cm201314/cmselect/cmsctech/104/104.pdf

US Congress, House Committee on Government Reform. (2005a, 5 May). Memorandum: The marketing of Vioxx to physicians. Retrieved from https://democrats-oversight.house.gov/sites/democrats.oversight.house.gov/files/documents/20050505114932-41272.pdf

US Congress, House Committee on Government Reform. (2005b, 5 May). Statement of Rep. Henry A. Waxman for the hearing, "The roles of FDA and pharmaceutical companies in ensuring the safety of approved drugs, like Vioxx." Retrieved from https://democrats-oversight.house.gov/sites/democrats.oversight.house.gov/files/documents/20050505113149-41995.pdf

US Senate, Committee on Finance. (2004, 18 November). *FDA, Merck and Vioxx: Putting patient safety first?* S. HRG 108-791. Washington DC: US Government Printing Office. Retrieved from https://www.finance.senate.gov/imo/media/doc/99575.pdf

US Senate, Committee on Finance. (2010, January). Staff report on GlaxoSmithKline and the diabetes drug Avandia. Retrieved from https://www.finance.senate.gov/imo/media/doc/prg022010a.pdf

Vedula, S.S., Bero, L., Scherer, R.W., & Dickersin, K. (2009). Outcome reporting in industry-sponsored trials of gabapentin for off-label use. *NEJM, 361,* 1963–71. https://doi.org/10.1056/nejmsa0906126

Vitry, A., Lexchin, J., Sasich, L., Dupin-Spriet, T., Reed, T., Bertele', V., ...
Hurley, E. (2008). Provision of information on regulatory authorities'
websites. *Internal Medicine Journal, 38*(7), 559–67. https://doi.org/10.1111
/j.1445-5994.2007.01588.x

Whittington, C.J., Kendall, T., Fonagy, P., Cottrell, D., Cotgrove, A., &
Boddington, E. (2004). Selective serotonin reuptake inhibitors in childhood
depression: Systematic review of published versus unpublished data. *Lancet,
363*(9418), 1341–5. https://doi.org/10.1016/s0140-6736(04)16043-1

Wieseler, B., Kerekes, M.F., Vervoelgyi, V., McGauran, N., & Kaiser, T. (2012).
Impact of document type on reporting quality of clinical drug trials: A
comparison of registry reports, clinical study reports, and journal publications.
BMJ, 344, d8141. https://doi.org/10.1136/bmj.d8141

Wieseler, B., McGauran, N., & Kaiser, T. (2010). Finding studies on reboxetine:
A tale of hide and seek. *BMJ, 341*, c4962. https://doi.org/10.1136/bmj.c4942

Wieseler, B., Wolfram, N., McGauran, N., Kerekes, M.F., Vervölgyi, V., Kohlepp,
P., ... Grouven, U. (2013). Completeness of reporting of patient-relevant
clinical trial outcomes: Comparison of unpublished clinical study reports
with publicly available data. *PLoS Medicine, 10*(10), e1001526. https://doi.org
/10.1371/journal.pmed.1001526

Wilde Mathews, A., & Martinez, B. (2004, 1 November). Emails suggest Merck
knew Vioxx's dangers at early stage. *Wall Street Journal.* Retrieved from https://
www.wsj.com/articles/SB109926864290160719

Winker, M.A., & Barbour, V. (2013, 13 June). Restoring invisible and abandoned
trials: A creative approach to a public good; Now a creative approach to
implementation is needed. *PLoS Blogs.* Retrieved from https://blogs.plos.org
/speakingofmedicine/2013/06/13/restoring-invisible-and-abandoned-trials-a
-creative-approach-to-a-public-good-now-a-creative-approach-to-implementation
-is-needed/

World Health Organization (WHO). (n.d.). International Clinical Trials Registry
Platform (ICTRP). Organisations with policies. Retrieved from https://www
.who.int/ictrp/trial_reg/en/index2.html

4 The FDA and Health Canada: Similar Origins, yet Divergent Paths and Approaches to Transparency

MARGARET E. McCARTHY AND JOSEPH S. ROSS

Early History of US and Canadian Drug Regulation

The US Food and Drug Administration (FDA) and Health Canada differ widely in their degree of transparency to the public, although both agencies arose from similar foundations. The origins of transparency in both the FDA and Health Canada lie in efforts to regulate the safety of food and drugs in the late nineteenth and early twentieth centuries, when a primary focus was the adulteration of consumer products. Regulatory agencies gained power by mobilizing public support and building on the outrage from widely publicized deaths due to unsafe drugs.

In both the United States and Canada, government chemists began to publish bulletins reporting on adulterants in food and drugs in 1887 (Herder, 2015; Young, 1990). These bulletins provided details of the contents of food and drug products, as well as the health effects of additives. The contents of bulletins were the subject of controversy and censorship: from 1907 to 1911, the US government censored many manuscripts, based on the objections of those from affected industries, while in Canada, the publication of names of manufacturers and vendors of suspected adulterated products faced some criticism from members of Parliament (Herder, 2015; Lewis, 2002).

In the United States, the need to develop public support for legislation around food and drug safety meant that scientists involved the press and the public. Beginning in 1902, the Agriculture Department's Bureau of Chemistry began a five-year experiment, feeding food laced with common additives to a dozen young male volunteers, nicknamed the "poison squad." The experiments were heavily publicized and reported in the national press, and at the same time, the head of the Bureau of Chemistry made speeches around the country at women's clubs and civic organizations in support of the campaign for greater regulation (Lewis,

2002). The US Bureau of Chemistry continued to publish bulletins regarding the deleterious effects of common food and drug additives. These combined efforts were successful, and with the enactment of the Pure Food and Drug Act of 1906, the US federal government gained the power to regulate drugs for the first time. Yet, patent medicine manufacturers were largely able to successfully evade government control: under a 1912 amendment to the law, successful prosecution for making false therapeutic claims required proof that the promoter intended to defraud the public (Janssen, 1981).

Early legislation in Canada similarly allowed patent medicine to escape government regulation. The Adulteration Act, passed in 1884, did not apply to patent or proprietary medicines (Herder, 2015). The same investigative journalism pieces that helped sway sentiment in favour of additional legislation in the United States were also influential in the passage of additional protections in Canada. Under the 1908 Canadian Proprietary Medicine Act, preregistration of proprietary medicines was required for the first time. Proprietary medicine manufacturers had to make limited disclosure of the ingredients in products to the government – but not the precise formulas. Drug labels contained even less information than that disclosed to the government (Herder, 2015).

Public disclosure of drug information by regulatory agencies ceased after passage of new laws. The last Canadian bulletins were published in 1920 (Herder, 2015). With Canadian requirements for labelling enacted in 1919, as well as the passage of the Food and Drugs Act in 1920, information regarding adulteration was no longer publicly available. In the United States, the Bureau of Chemistry ceased publication of bulletins in 1913 (Lewis, 2002). Herder (2015) suggests that, at least in the Canadian context, the power to regulate came with a price: lack of information for the public.

In the United States, the FDA continued to selectively release information to the public when it needed public support to obtain new regulatory power. Beginning in 1933, the FDA began to drum up support within the government as well as from the public for greater authority. FDA staff assembled an exhibit of food, drugs, and cosmetics that fell outside the provisions of the law, the "Chamber of Horrors," which was displayed to Congress and to the public, including at the 1933 World's Fair (US Food and Drug Administration, 2018). The FDA's chief education officer published a book detailing the loopholes in the existing law, which was dedicated to the heads of the women's organizations supporting passage of a bill (Lamb, 1936). Eventually, after at least 100 deaths due to elixir of sulfanilamide (which contained extremely toxic diethylene glycol), the 1938 US Federal Food, Drug, and Cosmetic Act was passed, which required manufacturers to submit proof of safety to the FDA prior to introduction of drugs to the US market.

In 1951, Canada instituted similar safety requirements for pre-market evaluation of new drugs. However, that requirement did not keep thalidomide from the Canadian market, both as samples of an unapproved drug sent to physicians and after approval by Canadian authorities. By the time thalidomide was pulled from the market in Canada in 1962, more than 100 Canadian children had been born with serious birth defects as a result of thalidomide use during pregnancy. Although thalidomide was never approved by the FDA, it had been provided to physicians by the US manufacturer, and at least 17 children were born with thalidomide-related birth defects (Bren, 2001).

Despite the important role that a Canadian FDA scientist, Frances Kelsey, played in keeping thalidomide off the US market, the key US news story regarding thalidomide was the result of leaks from congressional staff, not the FDA (Carpenter, 2014). The thalidomide tragedy served as an impetus for passage of the 1962 Kefauver amendments to the US Federal Food, Drug, and Cosmetic Act. For the first time, drug sponsors were required by statute to show proof of safety and efficacy through conducting adequate and well-controlled studies in order to have a drug approved, although FDA regulations had already required proof of efficacy since 1956 (Carpenter, 2014). Canada enacted similar provisions in 1962, requiring that substantial evidence of safety and efficacy for the indicated use be provided in connection with an application for marketing authorization.

Despite the great public interest in deaths and disability due to unsafe medical products, from elixir of sulfanilamide to thalidomide, government regulation of drugs occurred outside the public view, absent voluntary release of information by Canadian and US regulatory authorities. That situation did not change until the passage of general access to information laws provided a way for the public to obtain information from governmental agencies.

Access to Information Legislation

The US Freedom of Information Act

In proclaiming the Freedom of Information Act (FOIA), the United States became the third country in the world to enact an access to information law, following Sweden in 1766 and Finland in 1951 (freedominfo.org, 2017). The 1966 FOIA and its 1974 amendment ushered in a new era of government accountability in the United States. A wave of open government laws followed, including the Advisory Committee Act in 1972 and the Government in the Sunshine Act in 1976, which require that public notice be given for meetings; that meeting agendas, minutes, and most materials prepared for committee review be made available to the public; and that meetings of most adjudicative bodies or committees be open to the public.

Although the United States was an early leader in access to information, these laws were enacted despite tremendous opposition. The weaknesses in the original 1966 Freedom of Information Act allowed federal agencies to delay or obstruct provision of requested documents and to charge excessive fees. Initially, the FDA interpreted the FOIA narrowly, and broadly construed the exceptions for trade secrets or confidential commercial information, opposing disclosure of health and safety information that was provided to the FDA as part of an approved new drug application (Halperin, 1979; Rodwin, 1973).

For example, in 1970 the FDA denied an FOIA request filed by a woman who sought to examine the underlying clinical test information that led to approval of birth control pills; the FDA indicated in court filings that it always considered this information to be confidential (*Carolyn D.M. Morgan v. Food and Drug Administration, et al.*, 1974; Rodwin, 1973). This case was concurrent with congressional hearings regarding the safety of oral contraceptives, during which doctors testified that the FDA was giving women inadequate information and feminist organizations criticized the FDA (Carpenter, 2014). The FDA also refused to release transcripts of closed committee meetings of the Drug Efficacy Study Implementation (DESI) program, resulting in litigation leading to their release under the FOIA (*Wolfe v. Weinberger*, 1975). The assistant secretary of the Department of Health, Education and Welfare, testifying in Congress in 1972, singled out the FDA as particularly poor at meeting the requirements of the FOIA in a timely fashion (US Committee on Government Operations, 1972). Only when congressional hearings were scheduled in 1972 did agencies, including the FDA, issue revised regulations with broader provisions favouring information release (US Committee on Government Operations & US House of Representatives, 1972).

The Watergate scandal provided enough political momentum for the 1974 FOIA amendments (passed over presidential veto) and the Government in the Sunshine Act to be enacted. The FDA issued final regulations under the FOIA in 1974. According to the FDA, prior to the 1972 draft regulations, only 10 per cent of records were available for disclosure, while 90 per cent of agency records were available for disclosure from 1972 to 1974 (39 Fed. Reg. 44602, 1974). The new regulations allowed

Table 4.1. Processing Time for Simple and Complex Requests, US Food and Drug Administration, Fiscal Year 2017

FDA fiscal year 2017	Simple requests	Complex requests
Median processing time (days)	3	50
Lowest (days)	1	1
Highest (days)	1,064	1,536

Source: US Department of Health and Human Services, 2017.

the FDA to release summary-level information regarding approved drugs and also regarding abandoned, rejected, or withdrawn new drug applications (39 Fed. Reg. 44602, 1974; Herder, 2018). In at least one case, FDA scientists published an article in a peer-reviewed journal explaining the reasons why a new drug application (NDA) was denied approval (Herder, 2018; Temple & Pledger, 1980).

Unfortunately, by 1984 the FDA had retreated from its expansive interpretation of its obligations under the FOIA. After the FOIA statute was amended, the FDA's regulations were more narrowly drawn, restricting access to information (Herder, 2015). Successive amendments to the FOIA have required electronic or virtual reading rooms for the public to access documents via the internet, created a mediation service for FOIA disputes, and required agencies to identify records for proactive disclosure to the public (Electronic Freedom of Information Act Amendments of 1996; FOIA Improvement Act of 2016; Open Government Act of 2007). Information obtained under the FOIA is considered in the public domain, and once released, there are no limitations on its use.

The FOIA allows requestors to the FDA to seek information created by the agency or submitted to the agency. FOIA exemptions for trade secrets and confidential commercial information pose the greatest barrier to obtaining information provided to the FDA by medical product manufacturers. The FOIA requires the FDA to notify a company if material it submitted to the FDA is sought under the FOIA so that the company can raise a trade secret and/or confidential commercial information objection. Another barrier to obtaining documents under the FOIA is processing time. The FDA assigns requests to either a simple or complex track, depending on the likely staff time involved; as depicted in Table 4.1, it can take years to reach the front of the complex track queue, absent litigation. FOIA litigation most frequently involves disputes over interpretation of the exception for confidential commercial information (Lurie & Zieve, 2006).

Table 4.2. FDA and Health Canada Access to Information Statistics

FOIA and ATIA requests	FDA	Health Canada
Year	1 Oct. 2016– 30 Sept. 2017	1 April 2017– 30 March 2018
Backlog at beginning of year	2,489	1,612
Requests received	11,062	1,806
Requests processed	10,881	1,808
Backlog at end of year	2,670	1,610
Full disclosure of information requested	8,318	286
Partial disclosure of information requested	83	848
Informal request for previously disclosed information	n/a	627
Full-time equivalent employees	147.5	68.39
Agency money expended (in US dollars)	$34,345,566.00	$4,724,232.26

Sources: Health Canada, 2018b; US Department of Health and Human Services, 2017.
Notes: ATIA = Access to Information Act (Canada); FDA = (US) Food and Drug
Administration; FOIA = Freedom of Information Act (United States)

Canada's Access to Information Act

With the enactment of the Access to Information Act (ATIA) in 1982, Canada was the seventh country in the world to pass an access to information law (freedominfo.org, 2017). However, the level of access to information in Canada still remains significantly less than in other Commonwealth countries and the United States (Tromp, 2019). Until recent 2019 amendments, the ATIA had not been significantly updated since its passage, and these amendments are anticipated to bring only minimal improvements in access to information (Tromp, 2019). Comprehensive recommendations to expand access to information recommended by the Information Commissioner of Canada were not included in the final legislation (Information Commissioner of Canada, 2017). Canada limits its ATIA process to residents, unlike the United States and many other countries (Access to Information Act, 1985; Access to Information Act Extension Order, No. 1, 1989; Tromp, 2019). As detailed in Table 4.2, Health Canada receives significantly fewer information requests than the FDA.

The overall openness of the federal government differs substantially between the United States and Canada. The FDA advisory committee meetings are open to the public, with the agenda and materials for review provided to the public ahead of time and transcripts available after the meeting; in Canada, however, many government committee meetings, including Health Canada consultation meetings, are not open to the public, and meeting materials are not routinely provided to the public. In the United States, due to pressure from patient groups beginning with AIDS activists in the late 1980s, patients and patient advocacy groups have become involved in many FDA committees and are frequently consulted (US Food and Drug Administration, 2019). By contrast, Health Canada has only recently begun to create mechanisms for patient involvement in therapeutic product evaluation (Klein, Hardy, Lim, & Marshall, 2016).

Other limits to federal transparency in Canada are the result of devolution of responsibilities to provinces and territories, which have their own access to information procedures (Abelson & Eyles, 2002). For example, after a drug is approved by Health Canada, decisions on whether it will be included on public drug formulary listings are made at the provincial or territorial level, and thus are not subject to the ATIA (Rosenberg-Yunger & Bayoumi, 2017).

The ability to obtain information from the Canadian government under the ATIA differs substantially from obtaining information in the United States under the FOIA. First, the ATIA exempts many government subdivisions, although it applies to Health Canada. Second, the ATIA contains additional exceptions, including an exception for information that would harm the economic position of Canada and exceptions for information provided by third parties, such as trade secrets and confidential business information, which have been interpreted very expansively (Access to Information Act, 1985).

One deliberate attempt to evade the ATIA involving Health Canada was the 1989 destruction of all the Canadian Blood Committee's audiotapes and transcripts of meetings from its inception. The destruction occurred in an attempt to thwart a request for information made less than a week before, in the context of knowledge concerning contamination of donated blood in Canada with HIV and hepatitis C (Information Commissioner of Canada, 1997). As a result of this deliberate destruction of records, the ATIA was amended to include penalties, including fines and imprisonment, for intentional evasion of ATIA responsibilities (Access to Information Act, §67.1, 1999).

Responses to ATIA requests have been criticized as overly tied to political considerations. Some of the inappropriate practices include the identification of requests from the media or members of Parliament as "sensitive," which then have resulted in delayed response time while the relevant government agencies prepared a media response; disclosure of the names of journalists who have filed requests to ministerial staff; pressure placed on ATIA officials to interpret the statute restrictively; and failure to keep official records in order to evade the requirements of the ATIA (Gilbert, 2000; Roberts, 2006). Although these overall system faults were identified in 2006, Health Canada in 2008 continued to identify requests as "sensitive" and delayed response (Information Commissioner of Canada, 2009). An official investigation in 2014 led to a finding that Health Canada's response to one request for information regarding membership in an advisory panel on asbestos in 2009 had been inappropriately influenced by ministerial staff (Information Commissioner of Canada, 2014).

The Protecting Canadians from Unsafe Drugs Act (Vanessa's Law)

Prior to 2014, the broad exclusions for confidential business information under the ATIA meant that requests to Health Canada for clinical information submitted by drug companies were largely denied. The death in 2000 of his daughter, Vanessa Young, from a heart attack related to cisapride (Prepulsid), a drug that was withdrawn from the market in both the United States and Canada later that year due to serious cardiac adverse events, led her father, Terence Hart Young, to run for Parliament. Once there, he successfully campaigned to change the law to provide Health Canada with greater powers, including mandatory reporting of adverse events, recall powers, and changes to access to information.

Vanessa's Law, enacted in 2014, amended the Food and Drugs Act to provide a definition of confidential business information and empowered the health minister to disclose confidential business information about therapeutic products, without notice to or consent from the company, related to "protection or promotion of human health or the safety of the public." Confidential business information could be released to the following:

a. government;
b. a person from whom the Minister seeks advice; or
c. a person who carries out functions relating to the protection or promotion of human health or the safety of the public. (Food and Drugs Act [R.S.C., 1985, c. F-27], §2, §21[1][c]; 2014, c. 24, s. 3)

Notably, Vanessa's Law did not provide a public right of access to information regarding therapeutic products, although it did create a power to remove some data from the category of confidential business information through regulations (see later discussion). With regard to access by requestors under subsection (c), the implementing guidance, finalized in 2016, significantly narrowed the stated purpose of the law and required entry into a confidentiality agreement prohibiting re-disclosure as a condition of information receipt, in addition to requiring a detailed proposal (Health Canada, 2017a). The procedure was widely criticized (Herder, Lemmens, Lexchin, Mintzes, & Jefferson, 2016) and resulted in one researcher suing the government to invalidate the restrictions in the confidentiality agreement. In 2018, the court struck down the restrictions in the confidentiality agreement as a violation of the right to freedom of expression under the Canadian Charter of Rights and Freedoms, and ordered Health Canada to supply the researcher with the requested data (*Doshi v. Attorney General of Canada*, 2018).

Transparency and Proactive Disclosure

Under the 2007 Food and Drug Administration Amendments Act (FDAAA), the FDA is required to release agency decision-making documents for approved drugs going back to 1997 and to forward these documents within thirty days of initial approval of approved drugs (new molecular entities) (Food and Drug Administration Amendments Act, 2007). The release consists of an "action package" containing FDA scientists' original medical and statistical analyses and evaluations of information provided by the company, as well as correspondence. Action packages, which are downloadable on the agency website, can exceed two thousand pages in length. The FDA also proactively discloses product labels and approval letters on its website. No registration is needed to download documents from the FDA website, and there are no limitations on its use.

Since 2005, Health Canada has released a Summary Basis of Decision on all drugs newly granted marketing authorization. However, these extremely brief descriptions fail to contain key information important to patients and providers (Habibi & Lexchin, 2014). Since 2015, a Regulatory Decision Summary is released when a regulatory decision is made granting or denying marketing authorization for a new drug submission (NDS). Since 2014, a Safety Summary is released after a post-market safety review is conducted. These documents are quite short – a few pages in length – and provide far less information than those available from the FDA.

Information submitted by pharmaceutical companies to the FDA and Health Canada follows a standardized format. Both the FDA and Health Canada use the electric common technical document (eCTD) format, developed by the International Committee on Harmonization (ICH), for applications for new drug approval. In addition, the FDA routinely requests patient-level analysable data sets from industry and conducts independent statistical analyses as part of its review of materials submitted for approval.

Recent Transparency Initiatives

The adoption of the eCTD for pharmaceutical company submissions to regulatory agencies has allowed companies to submit nearly identical applications to multiple regulatory agencies, across continents, for the same product. This standardization means that proactive transparency measures regarding manufacturer submissions adopted by one jurisdiction may effectively result in proactive disclosure of submissions made to regulatory agencies in less transparent jurisdictions.

As noted in chapter three, the European Medicines Agency (EMA) began in 2016 to proactively disclose portions of the eCTD and clinical study reports submitted to the agency for marketing authorization. EMA Policy 0070 applies to applications made from 1 January 2015 onward and to supplemental or modification applications made from 1 July 2015 onward. Disclosure is made for approved applications, withdrawn applications, and applications refused marketing authorization. In phase I, no individual patient-level data are disclosed. In phase II, which has not commenced, the agency plans to release anonymized patient-level data. Notably, the EMA policy has been suspended as of 1 August 2018 due to the EMA's relocation from the United Kingdom as a result of the UK withdrawal from the European Union (European Medicines Agency, 2018).

Both the Canadian and US governments have similarly embarked on new transparency initiatives in the past decade. Beginning in 2010, the FDA Transparency Task Force made recommendations to systematically increase transparency at the FDA in three phases: FDA basics; public disclosure; and transparency to regulated industry (US Food and Drug Administration, 2017). As detailed in Table 4.3, none of the specific proposals for proactive release of information regarding the status of medical product applications was adopted (US Food and Drug Administration, 2010, 2015). The recommendations that were implemented resulted in greater disclosure on the FDA website of existing FDA-created documents and data, and creation of user-friendly guides for consumers and industry. The FDA has also created a user-friendly adverse events database that is searchable on its website.

In 2013, the FDA published a proposal to release de-identified pooled patient-level data sets created from data submitted by industry. A broad set of responses were received, with a number of patient and medical groups supporting the proposal. The response from industry was mixed.

Table 4.3. FDA Transparency Initiative, May 2010 Proposals and Status of FDA Action

Category and recommendations	Status
Adverse event reports	
• The FDA should provide online access to searchable adverse event report information that allows users to generate summary reports.	Completed
Docket management process	
• Public comments submitted by individuals on www.regulations.gov should be shared with the public.	Completed
Enforcement priorities and actions	
• Status of enforcement cases should be made public on a weekly basis.	No action
• Enforcement priorities set out in agency work plans should be shared once they are more than 5 years old.	Completed
Import procedures	
• The FDA should make public the outcomes of FDA evaluations of importer filings regarding products being imported to the United States.	Completed
Inspections	
• The FDA should disclose information regarding inspections conducted, including inspection outcomes.	Completed
• The FDA should create and share information regarding most common problems found during inspections.	Completed
Product applications (including investigational applications)	
• The FDA should disclose the existence of investigational applications, including the proposed use of the product, and the application sponsor.	No action
• The FDA should disclose whether an investigational application has been placed on hold, terminated, or withdrawn.	No action
• The FDA should disclose at the time of filing that an application for marketing, including a new drug application (NDA), was submitted or resubmitted.	No action
• The FDA should disclose that an application for approval of a drug, biologic, animal drug, or pre-market authorization of a device was withdrawn or abandoned by the sponsor. The FDA should disclose any significant safety concern.	No action
• When an application for an orphan drug or minor species animal drug has been withdrawn, terminated, or abandoned, the FDA should disclose if the product was not withdrawn for safety reasons and also if the FDA thinks that it could represent a significant therapeutic advance.	No action
• The FDA should disclose when it rejects an application for a drug or biologic (complete response) or refuses to file an application, and should also disclose the rejection letter itself.	No action
• The FDA should disclose when it refuses to approve an animal drug, and should disclose the rejection letter.	No action

(Continued)

Table 4.3. (*Continued*)

Category and recommendations	Status
• The FDA should disclose when it issues a not approvable letter for a device or a letter requesting more information. The letter itself should be disclosed.	No action
• The FDA should disclose safety or efficacy information from an investigational or pending market evaluation when disclosure is needed to correct misleading information about the product.	No action
• The FDA should convene an internal and external stakeholder group to discuss if, when, and how release of non-summary safety and effectiveness data from applications should be released.	Federal Register notice solicited comments; no policy change prior to 2018
Recalls	
• If the FDA can require submission of information about a recall by companies, and the FDA receives information about a recall, the FDA should release that information to the public as soon as practicable.	No action
• Where confusion exists about which food products are implicated in a food outbreak, the FDA can communicate information to the public that is in the interest of public health to alleviate confusion.	Completed
• The FDA should inform the public when a recall is terminated.	No action
Warning and untitled letters	
• The FDA already posts warning letters. The FDA should post untitled letters on its website and also company responses.	Completed

Sources: US Food and Drug Administration, 2010, 2015.

However, after publishing the initial proposal for comment, the FDA took no action (US Food and Drug Administration, 2013).

In a deliberate attempt to revisit the FDA Transparency Task Force report proposals of May 2010 and the lack of action by the FDA, a group of academic researchers published "Blueprint for Transparency at the U.S. Food and Drug Administration" (Sharfstein et al., 2018), detailing eighteen proactive transparency actions regarding medical product regulation in five areas identified in the 2010 Transparency Task Force Report that could be accomplished without new legislation:

1 FDA should disclose more information about key milestones in the application process.
2 FDA should disclose more of its own analysis and decision-making.
3 FDA should disclose more about the application and review process for generic drugs and biosimilars.

4 FDA should correct misleading information in the market.
5 FDA should disclose data from scientific studies to enhance understanding of medical products. (Excerpted from Sharfstein, et al., 2018)

In January 2018, in response to the Blueprint, the FDA announced a pilot project for voluntary release of portions of clinical study reports (Gottlieb, 2018), but did not adopt any of the Blueprint recommendations. Although the FDA intended to include nine drugs in the pilot project, only one manufacturer agreed to participate; only portions of one clinical study report for one drug were posted on the FDA website before the pilot was concluded (US Food and Drug Administration, 2020). The portions of the clinical study report released under the FDA pilot project are fewer than those released under EMA Policy 0070. The United States has not proactively released eCTD new drug applications or clinical study reports, other than through this now-terminated voluntary pilot project.

By contrast, in 2017 Health Canada began a process to amend its policies to allow for proactive disclosure of information currently exempt from disclosure as confidential business information (Health Canada, 2017b, 2018a). In place of the restrictive disclosure provisions in Vanessa's Law, the final regulations introduced a proactive transparency scheme similar to phase I of the EMA's Policy 0070, with portions of the eCTD and clinical study reports to be released. There is no provision for individual patient-level data release (Health Canada, 2019). The regulation provides for proactive disclosure of information from all applications once a final regulatory decision is reached, and the public portal for information disclosure is now live. Largely in response to industry recommendations, Health Canada has mirrored phase I of Policy 0070 as closely as possible.

Researchers have expressed concern that Health Canada's regulations do not go far enough in advancing transparency. Criticisms of the regulations include the proposed granting of two exceptions from disclosure: for clinical study reports submitted by manufacturers but not used to support the application for regulatory approval; and for tests, methods, and assays used exclusively by the manufacturer (Lexchin et al., 2018). In addition, the lack of any plan for release of de-identified patient-level data decreases the ability of independent researchers to make use of proactively disclosed information.

Conclusion

Both the FDA and Health Canada have taken significant steps in the past decade to increase transparency regarding medical product regulation. However, both agencies are far from completely transparent. Key issues to consider in comparing the degree of transparency and proactive disclosure is the authority granted to each agency, the level of staffing committed to information disclosure, and the amount of information generated by the agency itself.

The FDA has had authority for decades to require post-market studies, not only at the time of approval but also as a result of post-market information, including safety surveillance. The FDA can also request drug withdrawal. Only as part of Vanessa's Law in 2014 did Health Canada obtain the authority to mandate post-market adverse event reporting, along with the power to require post-market studies as a result of post-market information, including safety surveillance, and to mandate drug withdrawal.

To our knowledge, the FDA is the only drug regulatory agency in the world to routinely request submission of analysable patient-level data sets from manufacturers when reviewing regulatory applications and to be staffed to the level capable of performing such analyses routinely. The FDA currently releases agency analyses of manufacturer-supplied data for new drug applications, but not for supplemental applications. Notably, although the EMA and Health Canada now release information regarding rejected drug applications, the FDA does not, and it failed to implement the recommendation of its 2010 Transparency Task Force that it release information explaining its decision to reject drug applications or withdraw drugs from the market.

Now that Health Canada has implemented the recently proposed regulatory changes, it stands to become more transparent than the FDA with regard to information supplied to the regulatory agency by industry. This marks a radical change from Health Canada's restrictive policies on access to information. However, Health Canada still lacks transparency in a number of important areas. Since many of Health Canada's consultations are closed to the public, and meeting materials and minutes are not routinely published on its website, its regulatory decision-making is not accessible to the public. Health Canada is still formulating policies for patient involvement in consultations and decision-making. The proposed policy will make information available that will be of primary interest to researchers, rather than the public. Although product monographs are available on its website, Health Canada lacks public-facing, easily comprehensible information regarding drugs.

Why has the FDA historically been more transparent than Health Canada? In large part, it is because the FOIA applies to more agency records than the ATIA and because there are stronger federal open meeting laws in the United States. The right to information under the

FOIA has three principle characteristics. First, the FOIA provides an avenue to obtain information regarding the inner workings of government. Second, information is made available if disclosed on individual request. Finally, once disclosed, the information is considered public. If the information sought does not shed light on the inner workings of government, it is less likely to be disclosed, even as a result of contested litigation, after an FOIA request is denied. These characteristics have largely shaped the FDA approach to transparency, which favours release of information created by government agencies and disfavours release of information provided by industry. Unfortunately, the result of this emphasis on a private right to obtain information that then becomes public on release means that the FDA has not been influenced by the EMA policy for proactive disclosure of information submitted by industry in support of applications for regulatory approval.

REFERENCES

39 Fed. Reg. 44602. (1974).

Abelson, J., & Eyles, J. (2002). Public participation and citizen governance in the Canadian health system. Discussion Paper No. 7. Commission on the Future of Health Care in Canada. Retrieved from http://publications.gc.ca /collections/Collection/CP32-79-7-2002E.pdf

Access to Information Act (R.S.C., 1985, c. A-1).

Access to Information Act (R.S.C., 1985, c. A-1), §67.1 (1999).

Access to Information Act Extension Order, No. 1 (SOR/89-207) (1989).

Bren, L. (2001). Frances Oldham Kelsey: FDA medical reviewer leaves her mark on history. *FDA Consumer, 35*(2), 24–9. Retrieved from https://pdfs .semanticscholar.org/5f81/264165bed665f11ad0f37d6569ce83c98784.pdf

Carolyn D.M. Morgan v. Food and Drug Administration, et al. 41147, 1974 WL 415189 (District Court, District of Columbia, 1974).

Carpenter, D. (2014). *Reputation and power: Organizational image and pharmaceutical regulation at the FDA.* Princeton, NJ: Princeton University Press.

Doshi v. Attorney General of Canada, 2018 710 (Ottawa, 2018, 9 July).

Electronic Freedom of Information Act Amendments of 1996, Pub. L. No. 104–231 (1996, 2 October).

European Medicines Agency. (2018). Clinical data publication. Retrieved from https://www.ema.europa.eu/en/human-regulatory/marketing-authorisation /clinical-data-publication

FOIA Improvement Act of 2016, Pub. L. No. 114–85 (2016, 30 June).

Food and Drug Administration Amendments Act, Pub. L. No. 110–85 (2007).

Food and Drugs Act (R.S.C., 1985, c. F-27), §2, §21(1)(c).

freedominfo.org. (2017, 28 September). Alphabetical and chronological lists of countries with FOIA regimes. Retrieved from http://www.freedominfo .org/2017/09/chronological-and-alphabetical-lists-of-countries-with-foi-regimes/

Gilbert, J. (2000). Access denied: The Access to Information Act and its effect on public records creators. *Archivaria, 49,* 84–123. Retrieved from https:// archivaria.ca/index.php/archivaria/article/view/12740

Gottlieb, S. (2018). FDA Commissioner Scott Gottlieb, M.D., on new steps FDA is taking to enhance transparency of clinical trial information to support innovation and scientific inquiry related to new drugs. FDA news release. Retrieved from https://www.fda.gov/news-events/press-announcements/fda -commissioner-scott-gottlieb-md-new-steps-fda-taking-enhance-transparency -clinical-trial

Habibi, R., & Lexchin, J. (2014). Quality and quantity of information in Summary Basis of Decision documents issued by Health Canada. *PLOS One, 9*(3), e92038. https://doi.org/10.1371/journal.pone.0092038

Halperin, R.M. (1979). FDA disclosure of safety and effectiveness data: A legal and policy analysis. *Duke Law Journal, 28*(1), 286–326. https://doi.org/10.2307 /1372230

Health Canada. (2017a). *Guidance document: Disclosure of confidential business information under paragraph 21.1(3)(c) of the Food and Drugs Act.* Retrieved from https://www.canada.ca/content/dam/hc-sc/documents/services/drug -health-product-review-approval/cbi-gd-ld-ccc-eng.pdf

Health Canada. (2017b, 9 December). Regulations amending the food and drug regulations (public release of clinical information). *Canada Gazette, 151*(49). Retrieved from http://gazette.gc.ca/rp-pr/p1/2017/2017-12-09/html/reg4 -eng.html

Health Canada. (2018a, 10 April). *Draft guidance document: Public release of clinical information.* Retrieved from https://www.canada.ca/content/dam/hc-sc /documents/programs/consultation-public-release-clinical-information-drug -submissions-medical-device-applications/draft-guide-public-release-clinical -information.pdf

Health Canada. (2018b, 26 September 26). *Health Canada Access to Information Act annual report 2017–2018.* Retrieved from https://www.canada.ca/en /health-canada/corporate/about-health-canada/reports-publications/access -information-privacy/health-canada-access-information-act-annual-report -2017-2018.html

Health Canada. (2019, 4 March). Regulations amending the food and drug regulations (public release of clinical information): SOR/2019-62. *Canada Gazette,* Part II, *153*(6). Retrieved from http://www.gazette.gc.ca/rp-pr/p2 /2019/2019-03-20/html/sor-dors62-eng.html

Herder, M. (2015). Denaturalizing transparency in drug regulation. *McGill Journal of Law and Health, 8*(2), S57–S144. Retrieved from https://mjlhmcgill .files.wordpress.com/2017/07/mjlh_8_2_herder.pdf

Herder, M. (2018). Reviving the FDA's authority to publicly explain why new drug applications are approved or rejected. *JAMA Internal Medecine, 178*(8), 1013–14. https://doi.org/10.1001/jamainternmed.2018.3137

Herder, M., Lemmens, T., Lexchin, J., Mintzes, B., & Jefferson, T. (2016, 6 June). Pharmaceutical transparency in Canada: Tired of talk. *BMJopinion*. Retrieved from https://blogs.bmj.com/bmj/2016/06/06/pharmaceutical-transparency-in-canada-tired-of-talk/

Information Commissioner of Canada. (1997). *Annual report of the Canada Blood Committee, 1996–1997*. Ottawa, ON: Office of the Information Commissioner.

Information Commissioner of Canada. (2009). *Report cards 2007–2008: Systemic issues affecting access to information in Canada: A special report to Parliament by Robert Marleau, Information Commissioner of Canada, February 2009*. Retrieved from http://publications.gc.ca/collections/collection_2010/infocom/IP4-4-2009-eng.pdf

Information Commissioner of Canada. (2014). *Interference with access to information: Part 2: Special report to Parliament by Suzanne Legault, Information Commissioner of Canada, April 2014*. Retrieved from http://publications.gc.ca/collections/collection_2015/ci-oic/IP4-9-2-2014-eng.pdf

Information Commissioner of Canada. (2017). *Failing to strike the right balance for transparency: Recommendations to improve Bill C-58: An act to amend the Access to Information Act and the Privacy Act and to make consequential amendments to other acts, September 2017*. Retrieved from https://www.oic-ci.gc.ca/en/resources/reports-publications/failing-strike-right-balance-transparency#1

Janssen, W.F. (1981, June). The story of the laws behind the labels. *FDA Consumer, 15*(June). Retrieved from https://www.fda.gov/media/116890/download

Klein, A.V., Hardy, S., Lim, R., & Marshall, D.A. (2016). Regulatory decision making in Canada – Exploring new frontiers in patient involvement. *Value in Health, 19*(6), 730–3. https://doi.org/10.1016/j.jval.2016.03.1855

Lamb, R.D. (1936). *The American chamber of horrors*. New York, NY: Farrar and Rinehart.

Lewis, C. (2002). The "poison squad" and the advent of food and drug regulation. *FDA Consumer, 36*(6), 12–15. Retrieved from https://foodsafety.wisc.edu/assets/pdf_Files/PoisonSquad.pdf

Lexchin, J., Doshi, P., Gagnon, M.-A., Graham, J.E., Herder, M., Jefferson, T., ... Mintzes, B. (2018). *Re: Regulations amending the Food and Drug Regulations (Public Release of Clinical Information)*. Unpublished comments submitted to Health Canada.

Lurie, P., & Zieve, A. (2006). Sometimes the silence can be like the thunder: Access to pharmaceutical data at the FDA. *Law and Contemporary Problems, 69*(Summer), 85–98. https://www.jstor.org/stable/27592139

Open Government Act of 2007, Pub. L. No. 110–75 (2007, December 31).

Roberts, A. (2006). Two challenges in administration of the Access to Information Act. In J.H. Gomery, Commissioner, *Restoring accountability – Research Studies:*

Vol. 2. The public service and transparency (pp. 115–62). Ottawa, ON: Commission of Inquiry into the Sponsorship Program and Advertising Activities. Retrieved from https://www.humanrightsinitiative.org/programs/ai/rti/international /laws_papers/canada/al_roberts_submission_to_gomery.pdf

Rodwin, R.M. (1973). The Freedom of Information Act: Public probing into (and) private production. *Food, Drug, Cosmetic Law Journal, 28*(8), 533–44. https://www.jstor.org/stable/26656867

Rosenberg-Yunger, Z.R.S., & Bayoumi, A.M. (2017). Evaluation criteria of patient and public involvement in resource allocation decisions: A literature review and qualitative study. *International Journal of Technology Assessment in Health Care, 33*(2), 270–8. https://doi.org/10.1017/S0266462317000307

Sharfstein, J.M., Miller, J.D., Davis, A.L., Ross, J.S., McCarthy, M.E., Smith, B., ... Kesselheim, A.S. (2018). Blueprint for transparency at the U.S. Food and Drug Administration: Recommendations to advance the development of safe and effective medical products. *Journal of Law, Medicine & Ethics, 45*(2 Suppl.), 7–23. https://doi.org/10.1177/1073110517750615

Temple, R., & Pledger, G.W. (1980). The FDA's critique of the Anturane reinfarction trial. *New England Journal of Medicine, 303*(25), 1488–92. https:// doi.org/10.1056/NEJM198012183032534

Tromp, S.L. (2019). *Fallen behind: Canada's Access to Information Act in the world context* (2nd ed.). Vancouver, BC: BC Freedom of Information and Privacy Association. Retrieved from https://fipa.bc.ca/wordpress/wp-content /uploads/2020/05/2020_FallenBehind.pdf

US Committee on Government Operations. (1972). *U.S. Government Information Policies and Practices – Administration and Operation of the Freedom of Information Act: Part 5. Hearings before a subcommittee of the Committee on Government Operations, House of Representatives, March 20, 23, 24, 27 and 28, 1972.* Washington, DC: Committee on Government Operations.

US Committee on Government Operations & US House of Representatives. (1972). *House Report No. 92-1419, Administration of the Freedom of Information Act, September 20, 1972.* Washington, DC: US Government Printing Office.

US Department of Health and Human Services. (2017, 6 March). HHS fiscal year 2017 Freedom of Information annual report. Retrieved from https:// www.hhs.gov/foia/reports/annual-reports/2017/index.html

US Food and Drug Administration. (2010). *FDA Transparency Initiative: Draft proposals for public comment regarding disclosure policies of the U.S. Food and Drug Administration.* Retrieved from http://web.archive.org/web/20100522053732 /http://www.fda.gov/downloads/AboutFDA/WhatWeDo/FDATransparency TaskForce/TransparencyReport/GlossaryofAcronymsandAbbreviations /UCM212110.pdf

US Food and Drug Administration. (2013, 4 June). Availability of masked and de-identified non-summary safety and efficacy data; Request for comments.

Federal Register, 78(107), 33421–3, at 33422. Retrieved from https://www
.federalregister.gov/documents/2013/06/04/2013-13083/availability-of
-masked-and-de-identified-non-summary-safety-and-efficacy-data-request-for
-comments

US Food and Drug Administration. (2015, 24 September). FDA Transparency
Initiative: Phase II progress report. Retrieved from http://web.archive.org
/web/20171114171944/https://www.fda.gov/AboutFDA/Transparency
/TransparencyInitiative/ucm273854.htm

US Food and Drug Administration. (2017, 13 December). FDA Transparency
Initiative: Overview. Retrieved from https://www.fda.gov/about-fda
/transparency/transparency-initiative

US Food and Drug Administration. (2018). 80 years of the Federal Food, Drug,
and Cosmetic Act. Retrieved from https://www.fda.gov/about-fda/virtual
-exhibits-fda-history/80-years-federal-food-drug-and-cosmetic-act

US Food and Drug Administration. (2019). Evolution of patient engagement at
FDA. Retrieved from https://www.fda.gov/patients/learn-about-fda-patient
-engagement/evolution-patient-engagement-fda-text-description

US Food and Drug Administration. (2020). Clinical Data Summary Pilot Program.
Retrieved from https://www.fda.gov/drugs/development-approval-process
-drugs/clinical-data-summary-pilot-program

Wolfe v. Weinberger, 403 238 (District Court, District of Columbia, 1975).

Young, J.H. (1990). Food and Drug Regulation under the USDA, 1906–1940.
Agricultural History Society, 64(2), 134–42. https://www.jstor.org/stable/3743803

5 Clinical Trial Data Transparency in Canada: Mapping the Progress from Laggard to Leader

MARC-ANDRÉ GAGNON, MATTHEW HERDER,
JANICE GRAHAM, KATHERINE FIERLBECK,
AND ANNA DANYLIUK

Introduction

The case for transparency of clinical trial data submitted for drug approval has been gaining momentum over the years in many countries, and national regulatory agencies have taken steps to allow better access. In Canada, the main regulatory authority for pharmaceuticals, Health Canada, dragged its feet on this issue for many years. Health Canada has been criticized for being too slow in responding to drug safety challenges and for putting the interests of drug companies ahead of the interests of patients (Lexchin, 2016; Young, 2009). Following the passing of Vanessa's Law in 2014, Health Canada began disclosing clinical trial data to eligible researchers but with the stipulation that they could only publish an analysis of the data rather than the actual data; the latter were to be kept strictly confidential. In July 2018, however, the Federal Court ruled that Health Canada could not withhold clinical trial data from a researcher refusing to sign a confidentiality agreement (*Doshi v. Attorney General of Canada*, 2018); since April 2019, Health Canada has published clinical data submitted in support of over 100 drug approvals on its website. With this important milestone for transparency, Health Canada became a leader in providing access to pharmaceutical clinical trial data demanded by third-party researchers.

In this chapter, we describe how the debate surrounding disclosure of clinical trial data evolved, emphasizing the importance of the passing of Vanessa's Law in Canada. Steps towards regulatory modernization at Health Canada, beginning in the early 2000s, followed other international regulatory efforts. The Office of Consumer and Public Involvement within the Health Products and Food Branch provided services and guidance, and developed policy (Jones & Graham, 2009). Additionally, a series of instruments, including means to engage wider communities of regulators, pharmaceutical corporations, academics, and other "stakeholders" in invited (if not entirely open) fora for consultation, were used to introduce the principle of progressive licensing and the adaptive pathways lifecycle approach (Graham & Jones, 2010). A key insight gained from this discussion is the progression of policy development: while safety, rather than transparency, was the primary objective of the original changes to the Food and Drugs Act, the process of regulatory change opened a "window of opportunity" that facilitated the introduction of transparency.

Evolution of Pharmaceutical Regulation in Canada

Under section 92(7) of Canada's Constitution Act, 1982, health care in Canada is generally considered to be under provincial jurisdiction. However, prescription drugs are an exception. While the provision of most drugs to patients in hospitals and other health-care facilities is paid for by the provinces, drugs provided at community pharmacies are often purchased through private health plans, a patchwork of public health plans (for example, plans for seniors or low-income individuals), or out of pocket. However, the regulation of prescription drugs is largely a federal matter, as it is based on the patent system and criminal law, both under federal jurisdiction (sections 91[22] and 91[27]; Leeson, 2002). The patent system determines market exclusivity, regulates prices, and forces the disclosure of details about inventions, while criminal law determines which substances are illegal or should have restricted use.

Pharmaceutical regulation in Canada began in 1874 with the Inland Revenue Act, which criminalized the adulteration of drink, food, or drugs and their subsequent sale. Lack of enforcement led to the Adulteration Act in 1884, which codified and specified what was to be deemed an adulterated drug, focusing on harmful adulteration (Herder, 2015). The 1908 Proprietary and Patent Medicine Act required documentation and approval of "secret formulae" drugs issued by physicians. It imposed conditions on the sale of potent drugs, required the printing of the quantities of ingredients used, and forbade exaggerated claims on the product label. While the legislation did not limit public access to these products, it did help consumers avoid taking some ingredients (like opiates) by mistake (Malleck, 2015). By requiring registration before the drug entered the market rather than focusing on adulteration after market entry, the Proprietary and Patent Medicine Act is the first form of pre-market regulation in Canada and remained in force until 1975 (Herder, 2015). The federal Department of Health was created in 1919, and Canada's Food and Drugs Act, which codified the various requirements for licensing drugs, was introduced in 1920. The Food and Drugs Act was modified in 1947 to lay down the foundations of pharmaceutical regulation that remain today. In 1951, it became mandatory under the Food and Drugs Act for information about new drugs to be submitted to the Food and Drugs Division of the Department of Health and Welfare (predecessor to the Health Protection Branch) for approval prior to marketing (Lexchin, 1984).

For the most part, Canada followed the regulatory changes happening in other countries, with the Canadian government maintaining a minimal role in regulating pharmaceuticals (Herder, Gibson, Graham, Lexchin, & Mintzes, 2014). Pharmaceutical regulation was transformed in Canada, along with regulation in most Organisation for Economic Co-operation and Development (OECD) countries, following the thalidomide crisis. Introduced in 1957 as a sleeping pill in West Germany, thalidomide was distributed in almost fifty other countries (Tuffs, 2007), including Canada starting in 1959. Two years later, the link between the pill and serious birth defects in newborns was discovered. Approximately 12,000 children worldwide were affected. While the teratogenic side effects caused by this drug were known and recognized, the federal government had no legal authority to recall this drug from the market. Instead, Health Canada requested a voluntary recall on 2 March 1962; however, physicians continued to distribute samples to their patients (Tuffs, 2007). The Food and Drugs Act was amended on 4 December 1962 to limit the distribution of drug samples to "prescribed conditions" and to prohibit the sale of thalidomide (Herder et al., 2014). Further amendments also defined conditions that had to be satisfied to obtain market authorization (a "Notice of Compliance" [NOC] in Canada). The key provisions were that drug companies had to file a preclinical submission for clinical testing and provide Health Canada with substantial evidence that the new drug was not only safe but effective.

Although the Food and Drugs Act is under federal jurisdiction, provinces also partly regulate pharmaceuticals when it comes to health technology assessment, reimbursement, and pricing, since public drug plans are generally offered at the provincial level. Health Canada's reluctance to be proactive on pharmaceutical regulatory issues is thus partly jurisdictional, but it is also associated with other factors such as networked governance, corporate bias, and reflex regulation. A thorough analysis of Canadian governance in biotechnology shows that governance and regulation are carried out via networks of public-and-private collaborative councils, research institutions and their funders, private industry, and non-governmental advocacy groups (Doern & Prince, 2012). This same networked governance for pharmaceuticals in Canada is also known as clientele pluralism (Lexchin, 2013). Employing networked governance, Health Canada navigates pharmaceutical issues via a close relationship with business stakeholders and advocacy groups (often closely aligned with commercial interests). Many examples of the evolution of pharmaceutical policy in Canada portray Health Canada as having a corporate bias when reacting to problematic events (Lexchin, 2016; Davis & Abraham, 2013). A corporate influence does not indicate regulatory capture per se; it refers, instead, to the broader political context of government policies responsive to industry interests. Furthermore, as the examples discussed later will illustrate, Health Canada's standard reactions, characterized as having corporate bias, often seem to be the product of "reflex regulation" based on a set of reactive institutional habits, routines, and reflexes (Brown & Beynon-Jones, 2012).

For decades after the 1962 amendments, Health Canada avoided tackling controversial issues that could irritate industry stakeholders, such as conflicts of interest in drug reviews or transparency for important pharmaceutical data (Lexchin, 2016). In 1995, Dann Michols, director general of the Health Protection Branch at Health Canada, announced that the organization was considering implementing a Canadian Summary Basis of Approval to provide relevant information concerning why and under what conditions specific drugs were approved. It took until April 1998 for Health Canada to request input on the proposal; in June, Michols stressed the importance of going forward quickly with a Canadian Summary Basis of Decision, but the proposal disappeared from the radar for years.

In the ensuing years, the Health Protection Branch dropped "protection" from its new name, the Health Products and Food Branch. The regulator's resistance to disrupting pharmaceutical industry practices, and seeming disregard for its own deregulation direction (Graham, 2005), was evident from its position on adverse drug reaction (ADR) data transparency. In early 2004, the Canadian Broadcasting Corporation (CBC) ran a series of reports about drug safety, obtaining all ADR reports submitted to Health Canada since 1965. These reports revealed accumulated evidence against COX-2 inhibitors like Vioxx. Nonetheless, Health Canada issued a statement declaring that "Health Canada is concerned that the Canadian public may misinterpret this adverse drug reaction information posted on the CBC website" (Lexchin, 2016, p. 127).

Declared the most secretive of government departments by the Canadian Association of Journalists, Health Canada was awarded a "Code of Silence" award for its "remarkable zeal in suppressing information" and "concealing vital data about dangerous drugs" in 2004 (Kermode-Scott, 2004). Media pressure forced Health Canada to take steps towards greater transparency on drug information; the information on ADRs was made publicly available online in 2005. Health Canada also resurrected Michol's proposal of a Canadian Summary Basis of Decision to be implemented in two phases, starting with phase I in 2005. However, significant omissions in the level of clinical trial information, often presented haphazardly with disputed methods, provided physicians little to no help in determining whether to prescribe specific drugs to patients (Habibi & Lexchin, 2014). (Phase II, focusing on Health Canada's benefit/risk analysis for both drugs and medical devices, was implemented in 2012.)

In the meantime, on 8 April 2008, Bill C-51 (Proposed Amendments to the Food and Drugs Act) and Bill C-52 (Proposed Consumer Product Safety Act) were introduced in the House of Commons. This legislation would have been the first major set of amendments to the Food and Drugs Act since 1962. In particular, Bill C-51 proposed a radical change in drug regulation in favour of progressive licensing, an approach in which drugs can be marketed faster but require ongoing re-evaluation of the risks and benefits of medications through post-marketing studies (Lemmens & Gibson, 2014). While Bill C-51 would have been favourable to commercial interests by allowing faster drug approval (Hébert, 2007), it would have enabled the federal health minister to compel manufacturers to provide more drug information and would also have given the minister the power "to disclose to the public information about the risks or benefits that are associated with a therapeutic product" (Government of Canada, 2008). It is not clear, however, if such disclosure would have been exceptional or standard. An additional concern was the quality of post-marketing studies conducted by drug companies, which often only serve as marketing devices (Spelsberg et al., 2017). In the end, these concerns were moot; an election was called in 2008, and both bills died on the order paper when Parliament was dissolved (Jepson, 2009).

Clinical Trial Data Transparency and the Canadian Institutes of Health Research

While Parliament was relatively inactive regarding pharmaceutical regulatory reform during the early 2000s, considerable activity was taking place in the research community nationally and internationally. In October 2004, an international group of stakeholders met in Ottawa during the Cochrane Colloquium to discuss trial registration (Krleža-Jerić, 2005). Initiated by the Canadian Institutes of Health Research (CIHR), the "Ottawa Group" endeavoured to rethink trial registration in the interests of research, health, and safety in order to reach a global consensus on clinical trial registration. Signed by over 100 individuals and groups internationally, the Ottawa Statement called for the disclosure of clinical trial protocol details up front and amendments along the way, and the release of results upon completion of the trial. It did not receive endorsements from any of the pharmaceutical corporations (Krleža-Jerić, 2005).

The following year, members of the Ottawa Group participated in the World Health Organization (WHO) technical consultation on trial registration standards. The recommendations from this consultation assisted in the creation of the WHO International Clinical Trials Registry Platform (ICTRP) in 2005 (Krleža-Jerić, Lemmens, Reveiz, Cuervo, & Bero, 2011). The ICTRP was the beginning of international standards for clinical trial registration, the reporting of protocol amendments during the trial, and implementation in a publicly accessible registry. The CIHR endorsed the ICTRP's principles of trial registration in 2006 and updated the CIHR policy in 2010 to require all researchers awarded CIHR funding to "register a trial on one of the WHO primary registries or ClinicalTrials.gov, before participant recruitment; regularly update the information during the trial; report and publicly disclose trial results; and retain all trial information for 25 years" (Greyson, 2011). This policy, in conjunction with the WHO International Standards, the International Committee of Medical Journal Editors, and the Declaration of Helsinki, was to be effective by 20 December 2010 and applied to all CIHR competitions with application deadlines after 1 January 2011. However, four months after the policy was posted, it disappeared (Greyson, 2011). What happened to this policy is unknown, and it remains absent from the CIHR website.

Besides decades of inaction by Parliament, Canadian regulatory authorities were also accused of favouring the pharmaceutical industry over the public in areas of pharmaceutical policy (Lexchin, 2013). This accusation, among others, resulted from an imbalance in the money and number of personnel allocated to facilitate the review of new drug applications compared to allocations for monitoring the safety of products already on the market. Only established in 2002, the Marketed Health Products Directorate monitors the safety of medications and other health products following approval; it received three to four times less funding and fewer personnel compared to the Therapeutic Products Directorate responsible for synthetic (small molecule) pharmaceuticals and the Biologics and Genetic Therapies Directorate (biologics), which review new drug applications (Wiktorowicz, Lexchin, Moscou, Silversides, & Eggertson, 2010). In addition, the Therapeutic Products Directorate had a business transformation plan that prioritized "speed[ing] up the regulatory process for drug approvals," despite clear evidence that drugs with shorter approval times have more serious safety problems (Lexchin, 2013; Graham & Nuttall, 2013). It was not until the enactment of the

Protecting Canadians from Unsafe Drugs Act (Vanessa's Law) in 2014 that the federal government began to take on more responsibility in regulating the post-market safety and distribution of pharmaceuticals.

Vanessa's Law and Its Implementation

Terence Young became a member of Parliament (MP) to advocate for the legislative reform of pharmaceutical policy. He embarked on a crusade to change drug safety laws in Canada after the death of his daughter Vanessa in March 2000 (Fierlbeck, 2016). Vanessa Young had been prescribed Prepulsid, a drug against acid reflux. In June 1998, the Food and Drug Administration (FDA) in the United States had sent a letter to American doctors warning about the danger of an irregular heartbeat associated with Prepulsid. In January 2000, the FDA sent out another letter advising patients to have an electrocardiogram before taking Prepulsid and mentioned that the drug should not be prescribed to patients with eating disorders (which was Vanessa's case). In late February 2000, Health Canada also sent a letter to Canadian physicians highlighting the risks associated with the product and announcing that Health Canada would review the drug more thoroughly. In March 2000, the FDA announced that the drug would be withdrawn from the market, and the manufacturer, Janssen Pharmaceutical, voluntarily stopped marketing it in the United States in July 2000. Health Canada withdrew the drug from Canadian shelves one month later, saying that its decision was "founded on the association of the drug with serious cardiac arrhythmias ... and sudden cardiac deaths" (Ogilvie, 2009). Before it was withdrawn in August 2000, there were roughly 1 million prescriptions of Prepulsid each year in this country. At the time of Vanessa's death, the cardiac risks associated with Prepulsid were well known, and in the United States, the contraindication for patients with eating disorders was clearly highlighted on the product label. In Canada, however, patients and prescribing physicians were mostly ignorant of any potential risks and contraindications for this product (McIver & Wyndham, 2013).

In 2009, Young began the process of submitting a private member's bill to create an independent drug safety agency. The bill died on the order paper but was then reintroduced in subsequent parliamentary sessions. Each time, the bill failed to move forward in the House of Commons. In late 2013, however, Young's latest legislative initiative, Bill C-17, an act to amend the Food and Drugs Act – the Protecting Canadians from Unsafe Drugs Act – finally gained some traction. Known as "Vanessa's Law" in honour of Young's deceased daughter, the law appeared to signal a major potential shift in Canadian pharmaceutical regulation. Vanessa's Law promised to finally introduce several critical patient safety measures into Canada's Food and Drugs Act – the power to unilaterally recall drugs from the market, require labelling changes, and compel post-market studies – while also significantly increasing the penalties associated with violations of the legislation (the maximum fine increased from CAN\$5,000 to CAN\$5,000,000, while failure to recall unsafe drugs could result in a two-year jail sentence).

Curiously, though, and in marked contrast to Bill C-51 of 2008, Vanessa's Law contained no provisions to improve the level of transparency in pharmaceutical research and regulation when it was first introduced into Parliament (Herder et al., 2014). Clinicians, legal scholars, and other advocates pointed out this critical omission in Vanessa's Law, and following debate in the House of Commons and expert testimony before the Standing Committee on Health, Bill C-17 was amended to include a number of transparency-related measures. Many of the details would need to be worked out through yet-to-be drafted regulations. Given Health Canada's track record as a secretive institution, significant concerns remained about whether and how these transparency measures would be implemented (Herder, 2014, 2016; Fierlbeck, 2016). However, Vanessa's Law, including the newly added transparency provisions, was enacted by Parliament without any further changes on 5 November 2014.

The transparency provisions of Vanessa's Law can be described as fitting into three categories. First, the minister of health gained new discretionary powers to share so-called "confidential business information" (CBI) under particular circumstances without notice or consent from the party that claimed ownership over that information. For example, if the minister believed there was a serious risk to human health, CBI could be shared in an effort to avoid or mitigate that risk. As well, even when no such risk appeared to exist, the minister had the discretion to share CBI to a person who "protects or promotes human health" or public safety, provided the person utilizes the CBI for that purpose (as opposed to, say, a commercial purpose). These discretionary provisions gave the minister the immediate ability to share unpublished safety and efficacy data related to therapeutic products – data which Health Canada had long refused to share on the grounds that it was CBI (Herder, 2016). By incorporating the regulator's understanding of what constituted CBI into the Food and Drugs Act, Vanessa's Law also opened up the possibility of altering Health Canada's long-standing practices by giving the federal cabinet the power to pass new regulations specifying when certain information ceases to be CBI. This definitional power was the second transparency measure included in the legislation. Similarly, the third transparency provision in Vanessa's Law stipulated that companies must make publicly available certain information about the clinical trials and other studies they sponsor in the course of developing a drug.

The force of these new statutory provisions, however, was limited by obstacles in their manner of implementation. Although access to clinical trial data was granted for "a person who carries out functions relating to the protection or promotion of human health or the safety of the public" (Protecting Canadians from Unsafe Drugs Act [Vanessa's Law], section 21.1 [3]), the underlying information was still not allowed to be publicly shared. In 2015, Dr. Navindra Persaud was granted access by Health Canada to unpublished data, including several clinical trials for Diclectin, a treatment used for nausea during pregnancy (see chapter six). This information was, however, only granted on condition that he sign a confidentiality agreement recognizing that the data should be considered confidential business information and requiring that he not share it with any patients or other medical experts (Herder & Lemmens, 2016). As noted in chapter two, the specific parameters of transparency are critical; that Vanessa's Law did not specify the *terms* on which clinical data could be accessed introduced a level of uncertainty about what access would look like in practice – uncertainty which Health Canada had the discretion to resolve. And Health Canada chose to use that discretion in a way that would discourage researchers from accessing clinical data and limit what they could do with data once obtained.

In March 2016, Health Canada published a draft guidance aimed at amending eligibility for access to drug information. It required researchers to sign a strictly worded confidentiality agreement stipulating that they had made efforts to obtain this information from "all other possible sources" before making their request (Herder, Lemmens, Lexchin, Mintzes, & Jefferson, 2016). These clauses, however, seemed incompatible with the spirit, wording, and purpose of Vanessa's Law.

As Health Canada continued to impose restrictions on researchers wanting to access clinical trial data, an assistant professor at the University of Maryland School of Pharmacy, Peter Doshi, challenged Health Canada on the interpretation of the terms for the release of clinical trial data in 2016. Doshi had asked Health Canada to release clinical trial information on the human papilloma virus (HPV) vaccines and the antiviral medication Tamiflu. When Health Canada would not release this information to Doshi without his signed non-disclosure confidentiality agreement, Doshi took Health Canada to court, arguing that signing a confidentiality agreement was against the spirit of Vanessa's Law (Weeks, 2018). On 9 July 2018, Federal Court Justice Sébastien Grammond ruled that Health Canada's decision was "unreasonable" and that it "entirely disregards one of the main purposes of Vanessa's Law, namely to improve clinical-trial transparency" (*Doshi v. Attorney General of Canada*, 2018). Health Canada has not appealed the decision.

While the Federal Court's decision acknowledged that there may be circumstances where confidentiality could be required, it stands in principle as an important ruling in favour of pharmaceutical data transparency. Beyond emphasizing the importance of transparency to Vanessa's Law, the court ruled that denying researchers' access to data violated their freedom of expression, as protected under Canada's Charter of Rights and Freedoms.

Meanwhile, Health Canada was in the midst of putting into place an online portal for the public release of "clinical information" on the strength of the legislative power to redefine what is (and what is not) CBI. In 2017, Health Canada published proposed draft regulations to support the public release of clinical information in drug submissions and medical device applications. Feedback received during the public comment period was quite critical, and in response, Health Canada published a revised draft guidance document in April 2018 covering the public release of clinical trial information. This document did not have the force of law, but it demonstrated the direction Health Canada was taking at the time concerning clinical trial data transparency. Health Canada acknowledged that disclosure of clinical trial data has many benefits, including the ability to "enable independent re-analyses of data, foster new research questions, and benefit Canadians by helping them make informed decisions about their health" (Health Canada, 2019). As before, the guidance document was criticized for the exemptions that could limit public disclosure of clinical trial data. Under the new regulations, once a decision to approve or reject a drug or device has been made, Health Canada would post clinical data provided by pharmaceutical companies as part of their regulatory submission. Two categories of information would continue to be regarded as CBI after a regulatory decision to approve or reject the product in question, namely: "(a) information that the manufacturer did not use in the drug submission to support the proposed conditions of use or purpose for the drug; or (b) information that describes tests, methods or assays that are used exclusively by the manufacturer" (Health Canada, 2019). But apart from those exceptions, all summary-level data generated in the course of clinical studies would be publicly disclosed via the new portal.

By March 2019, Health Canada finalized the regulations, and the portal went live (Adhopia, 2019; Lexchin, Herder, & Doshi, 2019). While CBI exemptions as described earlier are still not disclosed, the implementation of the portal allowing free access to clinical trial data submitted for drug approval, now considered by default not to be CBI once a regulatory decision has been made, arguably makes Health Canada a world leader in clinical trial data transparency. Having set a new standard for clinical trial data transparency, this model now imposes a certain expectation for other drug regulatory agencies to do the same (Mantel, 2019). The portal, now online at https://clinical-information.canada.ca /search/ci-rc, will normally include all clinical trial data for new products submitted to Health Canada once an authorization decision has been reached. Clinical trial data information for older drugs will be made available on a case-by-case basis following the judgement of *Doshi v. Attorney General of Canada* (2018). At the time of writing, disclosures of clinical data connected to over 100 drug approvals had been posted on the portal. The question that remains is whether independent researchers, health-care providers, journalists, and others – both in Canada and abroad – will rise to the challenge of scrutinizing this wealth of information now that it has finally become available.

Conclusion

In this chapter, we have provided an overview of the history of access to clinical trial data in Canada. For decades, Canada has been somewhat of a laggard in its regulation of pharmaceutical policy. Although there were some minor policy developments throughout the twentieth century, it was not until Vanessa's Law was proclaimed that significant policy change occurred. Vanessa's Law introduced a number of new measures in order to enhance the regulation of pharmaceuticals, including several provisions designed to improve the level of transparency of clinical trial data. Running up against decades of institutional practice in favour of confidentiality, the new law's transparency provisions had little impact initially, but signs of institutional change are finally beginning to appear.

It is difficult to encapsulate the main factors that transformed Health Canada when it comes to transparency of clinical trial data. During the first reading of Vanessa's Law, the law did not even include amendments to improve clinical trial data transparency. The advocacy work of legal and academic experts (for example, Herder et al., 2014), along with the work of MP Terence Young in sponsoring the bill, allowed last minute amendments to the law aimed at improving clinical trial data disclosure. Historically, Health Canada has been hesitant to implement any reform that could create tension within its networked governance, where corporate influence has been implicitly dominant. That Health Canada was dragging its feet in terms of implementing clinical trial data disclosure as required by Vanessa's Law was no surprise, but it brought significant backlash, not only from legal and academic experts but also from the Federal Court. Health Canada's institutional resistance against such reform brought a Federal Court judgement (*Doshi v. Attorney General of Canada*, 2018), underscoring the need for Health Canada to become proactive in terms of clinical trial data disclosure. Not only does Health Canada now allow greater clinical trial data transparency when the information can help protect and promote patients' health, but Health Canada has also embraced the more progressive vision of considering the bulk of submitted clinical trial data as public rather than commercial information and agreed to disclose the lion's share of this information through a public portal (after anonymization for reasons of patient privacy).

One question that arises is whether other regulatory agencies will follow Health Canada's lead, apart from the European Medicines Agency, which has implemented a similar approach. Creating a data sharing mechanism can bring many benefits to the public, as it has the ability to better assess the risks and benefits of different drugs, increase the likelihood and speed of finding cures and remedies, and avoid unnecessary clinical trials that can cause human harm and research waste. The issue here is political rather than technical: under what circumstances can greater transparency be successfully introduced into new regulatory legislation? The policy lesson arising from Canada's experience provocatively suggests the utility of *not* focusing on transparency as a key objective. Articulating a policy reform strategy that identifies transparency at the outset provides a clear target for oppositional interests to set in their crosshairs. The pre-eminent focus of the Food and Drugs Act reform was largely one of safety, a measure that pharmaceutical firms also had a stake in maintaining; as such, the industry did not vigorously dispute the reforms. Yet, the process of revising regulatory frameworks also requires a close working relationship between regulators and stakeholders beyond industry (including lawyers, academics, and advocates). As the process of policy revision is a public process, it provides an opportunity for other voices to influence the secretive relationship between industry and Health Canada. In this way, once the process of policy review was established, the epistemic community supporting transparency were better able to place this issue on the table for public discussion, notwithstanding Health Canada's reluctance to accommodate them. Thus, regulatory reform per se provides a window of opportunity to achieve greater transparency, but the way in which it is introduced and implemented will unquestionably be critical for its success.

REFERENCES

Adhopia, V. (2019, 13 March). Health Canada starts releasing drug and medical device data: Drug and device clinical trial data to be posted on new clinical information portal. *CBC News*. Retrieved from https://www.cbc.ca/news /health/health-canada-drug-device-database-1.5054838

Brown, N., & Beynon-Jones, S.M. (2012). "Reflex regulation": An anatomy of promissory science governance. *Health, Risk & Society, 14*(3), 223–40. https://doi.org/10.1080/13698575.2012.662633

Davis, C., & Abraham, J. (2013). *Unhealthy pharmaceutical regulation: Innovation, politics and promissory science.* Basingstoke, UK: Palgrave Macmillan.

Doern, G.B., & Prince, M.J. (2012). *Three bio-realms: Biotechnology and the governance of food, health, and life in Canada.* Toronto, ON: University of Toronto Press.

Doshi v. Attorney General of Canada, 2018 FC 710.

Fierlbeck, K. (2016). Reforming the regulation of therapeutic products in Canada: The Protecting of Canadians from Unsafe Drugs Act (Vanessa's Law). *Health Reform Observer / Observatoire Des Réformes De Santé, 4*(2), 5. https://doi.org/10.13162/hro-ors.v4i2.2681

Government of Canada. (2008, 8 April). Bill C-51: An Act to amend the Food and Drugs Act and to make consequential amendments to other Acts, first reading, 56–7. 39th Parliament, 2nd Session. Retrieved from https://parl.ca/DocumentViewer/en/39-2/bill/C-51/first-reading

Graham, J.E. (2005). Smart regulation: Will the government's strategy work? *CMAJ, 173*(12), 1469–70. https://doi.org/10.1503/cmaj.050424

Graham, J.E., & Jones, M. (2010). Rendre évident: Une approche symétrique de la réglementation des produits thérapeutiques. [Determining evidence: A symmetrical approach to the regulation of therapeutic products.] *Sociologie et sociétés, 42*(2), 153–80. https://doi.org/10.7202/045360ar

Graham, J.E., & Nuttall, R.K. (2013). Faster access to new drugs: Fault lines between Health Canada's regulatory intent and industry innovation practices. *Ethics in Biology, Engineering & Medicine: An International Journal, 4*(3), 231–9. https://doi.org/10.1615/EthicsBiologyEngMed.2014010771

Greyson. (2011, 4 April). The mystery of the missing CIHR trials policy. *Social Justice Librarian.* Retrieved from https://sjlibrarian.wordpress.com/2011/04/04/the-mystery-of-the-missing-cihr-trials-policy/

Habibi, R., & Lexchin, J. (2014). Quality and quantity of information in Summary Basis of Decision documents issued by Health Canada. *PLoS ONE, 9*(3), e92038. https://doi.org/10.1371/journal.pone.0092038

Health Canada. (2019). Public release of clinical information: Guidance document. Retrieved from https://www.canada.ca/en/health-canada/services/drug-health-product-review-approval/profile-public-release-clinical-information-guidance/document.html

Hébert, P.C. (2007). Progressive licensing needs progressive open debate. *CMAJ, 176*(13), 1801. https://doi.org/10.1503/cmaj.070703

Herder, M. (2014, 23 June). The opacity of Bill C-17's transparency amendments. *Impact Ethics.* Retrieved from https://impactethics.ca/2014/06/23/the-opacity-of-bill-c-17s-transparency-amendments/

Herder, M. (2015). Denaturalizing transparency in drug regulation. *McGill Journal of Law & Health, 8*(2), S57–S143. Retrieved from https://mjlhmcgill .files.wordpress.com/2017/07/mjlh_8_2_herder.pdf

Herder, M. (2016). Reinstitutionalizing transparency at Health Canada. *CMAJ, 188*(3), 218–19. https://doi.org/10.1503/cmaj.150765

Herder, M., Gibson, E., Graham, J., Lexchin, J., & Mintzes, B. (2014). Regulating prescription drugs for patient safety: Does Bill C-17 go far enough? *CMAJ, 186*(8), E287–92. https://doi.org/10.1503/cmaj.131850

Herder, M., & Lemmens, T. (2016). Memorandum re: Health Canada's "draft guidance" on section 21.1(3)(c) of the Food and Drugs Act. Dalhousie University Schulich School of Law Working Paper No. 25. Retrieved from https://digitalcommons.schulichlaw.dal.ca/cgi/viewcontent.cgi?article =1024&context=working_papers

Herder, M., Lemmens, T., Lexchin, J., Mintzes, B., & Jefferson, T. (2016, 6 June). Pharmaceutical transparency in Canada: Tired of talk. *BMJopinion.* Retrieved from https://blogs.bmj.com/bmj/2016/06/06/pharmaceutical-transparency -in-canada-tired-of-talk/

Jepson, G. (2009). Drug, food and device regulation in Canada 2008: The year in review. *Regulatory Focus: Journal of the Regulatory Affairs Professionals Society,* January, 16–21.

Jones, M., & Graham, J.E. (2009). Multiple institutional rationalities in the regulation of health technologies: An ethnographic examination. *Science and Public Policy, 36*(6), 445–55. https://doi.org/10.3152/030234209X460980

Kermode-Scott, B. (2004). Canadian health ministry faces criticism for its secrecy. *BMJ, 328*(7450), 1222. https://doi.org/10.1136/bmj.328.7450.1222-f

Krleža-Jerić, K. (2005). Clinical trial registration: The differing views of industry, the WHO, and the Ottawa Group. *PLoS Medicine, 2*(11), e378. https://doi.org /10.1371/journal.pmed.0020378

Krleža-Jerić, K., Lemmens, T., Reveiz, L., Cuervo, L.G., & Bero, L.A. (2011). Prospective registration and results disclosure of clinical trials in the Americas: A roadmap toward transparency. *Revista Panamericana De Salud Publica / Pan American Journal of Public Health, 30*(1), 87–96.

Leeson, H. (2002). *Constitutional jurisdiction over health and health care services in Canada.* Discussion paper No. 12. Commission on the Future of Health Care in Canada. Retrieved from https://qspace.library.queensu.ca/bitstream /handle/1974/6884/discussion_paper_12_e.pdf

Lemmens, T., & Gibson, S. (2014). Decreasing the data deficit: Improving post-market surveillance in pharmaceutical regulation. *McGill Law Journal / Revue de droit de McGill, 59*(4), 943–88. https://doi.org/10.7202/1026134ar

Lexchin, J. (1984). *The real pushers: A critical analysis of the Canadian pharmaceutical industry.* Toronto, ON: New Star Books.

Lexchin, J. (2013). Health Canada and the pharmaceutical industry: A preliminary analysis of the historical relationship. *Healthcare Policy / Politiques De Sante, 9*(2), 22–3. https://doi.org/10.12927/hcpol.2013.23621

Lexchin, J. (2016). *Private profits versus public policy: The pharmaceutical industry and the Canadian state.* Toronto, ON: University of Toronto Press.

Lexchin, J., Herder, M., & Doshi, P. (2019). Canada finally opens up data on new drugs and devices: Other regulators should take note of Health Canada's substantive reforms. *BMJ, 365*(11), i1825. https://doi.org/10.1136/bmj.l1825

Malleck, D. (2015). *When good drugs go bad: Opium, medicine, and the origins of Canadian drug laws.* Vancouver, BC: UBC Press.

Mantel, B. (2019, 11 October). Canada's decision to make public more clinical trial data puts pressure on FDA. *NPR.* Retrieved from https://www.npr.org/sections/health-shots/2019/10/11/769348119/canadas-decision-to-make-public-more-clinical-trial-data-puts-pressure-on-fda

McIver, S., & Wyndham, R. (2013). *After the error: Speaking out about patient safety to save lives.* Toronto, ON: ECW Press.

Ogilvie, M. (2009, 12 April). MP on mission to root out truth of daughter's death. *Toronto Star.* Retrieved from https://www.thestar.com/news/insight/2009/04/12/mp_on_mission_to_root_out_truth_of_daughters_death.html

Spelsberg, A., Prugger, C., Doshi, P., Ostrowski, K., Witte, T., Hüsgen, D., & Keil, U. (2017). Contribution of industry funded post-marketing studies to drug safety: Survey of notifications submitted to regulatory agencies *BMJ, 356,* j337. https://doi.org/10.1136/bmj.j337

Tuffs, A. (2007). Thalidomide: The true story? *BMJ, 334*(7600), 933. https://doi.org/10.1136/bmj.39199.637986.59

Weeks, C. (2018, 13 July). Judge rules Health Canada cannot withhold clinical trial data. *The Globe and Mail.* Retrieved from https://www.theglobeandmail.com/canada/article-judge-rules-health-canada-cannot-withhold-clinical-trial-data/

Wiktorowicz, M.E., Lexchin, J., Moscou, K., Silversides, A., & Eggertson, L. (2010). Keeping an eye on prescription drugs, keeping Canadians safe: Active monitoring systems for drug safety and effectiveness in Canada and internationally. Toronto, ON: Health Council of Canada. Retrieved from http://publications.gc.ca/collections/collection_2011/ccs-hcc/H174-21-2010-eng.pdf

Young, T.H. (2009). *Death by prescription.* Toronto: Key Porter Books.

6 The Limits of Transparency and the Role of Essential Medicines

NAV PERSAUD

If the main purpose of clinical research is to improve health, greater transparency of clinical research should also serve to ameliorate health. Transparency can serve a variety of ends, such as promoting confidence in clinical research and maintaining the integrity of researchers; ultimately, transparency should improve health if it is integral to clinical research. In this chapter, I provide four examples illustrating that improved transparency for clinical study information has not always resulted in health improvements. I then discuss reasons transparency has not yet helped promote health in substantial ways, and suggest a potential means to ensure that the considerable resources needed to promote transparency actually can improve health by focusing on essential medicines. I also discuss important *indirect* benefits of transparency in addition to direct improvements in health.

I argue in this chapter that transparency is insufficient to achieve health improvements. The substantial and important advances in clinical research transparency made recently in Canada must be followed by changes in public policy and clinical practice; otherwise, questions will be raised about the purpose of transparency. Transparency can be used to hold powerful institutions to account, but power and influence can frustrate attempts to act on uncovered information and thus indirectly undermine efforts to promote transparency.

"Same Data, Opposite Conclusions"

Four examples demonstrate that improved transparency for clinical study information may fail to translate into health improvements. These cases are the use of antidepressants for adolescents with depression, oseltamivir for the prevention of serious complications of influenza, doxylamine-pyridoxine for nausea and vomiting during pregnancy, and long-acting opioids for the treatment of chronic non-palliative pain.

Study 329 was reported in 2001 as showing that paroxetine was effective and safe when used to treat adolescents with depression (Keller et al., 2001). After Herculean efforts to obtain information about this clinical trial, an independent group of researchers published a 2015 report of the same study that indicated the medicine is not effective and that it *increases* the risk of suicidality (Le Noury et al., 2015). The differences in the two reports relate to differences in the application of pre-specified outcomes and the tallying of adverse events recorded in study documents. No change in the prescribing of antidepressants to adolescents after the 2015 report has been measured. It appears that the opposing conclusion of the report did not alter the care of adolescents with depression. A table summarizing the differences between the two Study 329 reports is maintained on a website created by the authors of the 2015 report. Titled "Same Data, Opposite Conclusions," the table contrasts the implications of the two reports (Le Noury et al., n.d.). According to this table, the first report "misled doctors into prescribing a drug that is ineffective [and] unsafe for adolescents," while the later report "corrects the record [and] reveals that the data did not support the conclusion of the original study." The first report had a direct impact on *health* by altering prescribing, while the second, based on efforts to promote transparency, merely corrected the *literature*.

Oseltamivir was stockpiled by various governments in case of an influenza pandemic based on results of seventeen published trials that indicated it prevented serious complications of influenza in the context of a pandemic. A systematic review that included twenty unpublished studies concluded that oseltamivir does not prevent serious complications of influenza (Jefferson et al., 2014). Oseltamivir is still being stockpiled for a pandemic, and it is still being prescribed. It is not clear that the use of this medicine has been changed by the newly available information (see chapter three in this volume for a more detailed discussion of this case).

Doxylamine-pyridoxine is the first-line treatment for nausea and vomiting during pregnancy in Canada (Campbell, Rowe, Azzam, & Lane, 2016). The medicine was approved decades ago in Canada, and a new trial was completed in 2009 as part of the manufacturer's application for approval in the United States (Koren et al., 2010). A re-analysis of that trial indicated that the medicine is not effective (Persaud, Meaney, El-Emam, Moineddin, & Thorpe, 2018), and the Motherisk Program at Toronto's Hospital for Sick Children that conducted the original study and also provided patients and clinicians advice about its use was closed down amid controversy (Glauser, 2019). Doxylamine-pyridoxine continues to enjoy place of pride as the first-line treatment for nausea and vomiting during pregnancy in Canada and the United States (Campbell et al., 2016). It is commonly prescribed in Canada, and its prescribing rate is increasing in the United States (while alternative treatments are used in other countries).

The opioid crisis that killed more than 4,000 Canadians and more than 60,000 Americans in 2017 started after long-acting opioids were approved and publicly funded in the late 1990s and the early 2000s (Public Health Agency of Canada, 2018; US Centers for Disease Control and Prevention [CDC], 2018). These long-acting opioids were illegally marketed as having a lower abuse potential, according to a 2007 court case in the United States (District Court for the Western District of Virginia, 2007; Meier, 2007). Despite the guilty finding, which clearly showed that clinical studies never provided any justification for the claim that long-acting opioids had a lower abuse potential compared with other opioid products, prescribing rates of long-acting opioids continued to increase and remain more the double the rate prescribed in the 1990s (CDC, 2018; Ontario Drug Policy Research Network, 2016). After approximately two decades of heavy opioid prescribing, rates only started to gradually decrease around 2016, which may be reason for cautious optimism, even though rates remain high.

Potential Reasons Transparency Does Not Always Help

Delays in the availability of information about clinical studies can decrease the utility of the information for several reasons. Once a medication becomes entrenched in clinical practice, both clinicians and patients may be reluctant to make changes regardless of what new information indicates. This factor may be operative in all four examples. The newly available information may be viewed with scepticism, since it may be in conflict with a previous report; clinicians and patients may therefore be less likely to act on apparently controversial information compared with information that had been available from the beginning. Information about old clinical studies may be rejected as "old news," even if critical information was not previously available.

Clinicians worry about the volume of information from clinical studies that they need to review in order to remain current. Multiple reports of the same study increases the amount of information to digest. We should thus not expect clinicians to welcome additional reports of a trial that has already been reported. Producers of clinical practice guidelines also may not have the time or resources to handle multiple reports of the same study. Similarly, patients are confused by medical controversies and may choose to ignore them in favour of a clear recommendation from a trusted source, even if that source is not correct.

While increased transparency can call into question claims about treatments that are widely spread by the pharmaceutical industry using considerable resources, the countervailing effects of industry marketing and lobbying may overpower any effect of improved transparency. Moreover, regulators have disincentives to make changes based on information gleaned by activities aimed at promoting transparency. Reversing regulatory decisions may increase scrutiny on regulators and could undermine public confidence in them. Products are rarely withdrawn by regulators, and withdrawals are almost never carried out in response to questions about efficacy or effectiveness. Thus transparency, despite calling into question the effectiveness of a medicine, is unlikely to result in a regulatory change.

Just a Matter of Time?

Increased transparency may translate into health improvements in the future. Time may be needed to adapt to the unprecedented improvements in access to information made over the last decade, especially to changes made by the European Medicines Agency. New tools and processes may be needed to ensure that transparency leads to improved health. Similarly, medical journals, producers of clinical practice guidelines, and other actors may need time and support to accommodate these changes. Examples of increased transparency resulting in health improvements may already exist.

On the other hand, regulators are currently charged with reviewing all available information. Regulatory processes and guidelines exist for reviewing information that becomes available after a product is approved. However, regulators have reviewed information gleaned through efforts to promote transparency and decided not to make changes. Guidelines are in place outlining when articles should be retracted (Committee on Publication Ethics, 2019), yet there has been no retraction even after study conclusions are proven unjustified based on newly available information (Le Noury et al., n.d.). Clinical practice guidelines are intended to be updated based on current information. But efforts to make information about clinical studies more easily available does not seem to change clinical practice guidelines. It appears that more than just the passage of time is needed.

Other Forms of Transparency and Non-health Benefits of Transparency

Failures of clinical trial transparency to translate into health improvements might indicate that the value of other laudable efforts to improve transparency should be carefully examined. Efforts are underway to increase transparency concerning payments to physicians by the pharmaceutical and medical device industries. The Affordable Care Act in the United States required disclosures starting in 2014. These payments are not known to benefit patients, and they are intended to alter the care that clinicians provide based on the interests of the pharmaceutical companies (Spurling et al., 2010); even small gifts can alter physician behaviour (Institute of Medicine, 2009). Increased transparency could mitigate the negative effects of industry payments to doctors, either by deterring clinicians from accepting them or by causing patients and others to scrutinize decisions made by clinicians who have received payments.

It is not clear, however, that increased transparency about physician-industry relationships actually results in better care or improved health. While payments to clinicians are correlated with clinical decisions such as prescribing habits, the disclosure of these payments is not known to affect clinical decisions. There may be other important benefits of transparency, such as maintaining trust in the medical profession, but it is thus unclear that increased transparency will result in health improvements. Similarly, payments to patient organizations from industry are concerning, as they affect the activities of these groups (including lobbying for approval and public funding of pharmaceuticals). Industry payment disclosure may or may not help promote health. Improving access to information about how regulators like Health Canada operate may facilitate more informed decisions by health-care providers and by patients. On the other hand, improved transparency may have little or no effect if the information is available on government websites that few people access or is poorly communicated by the regulator (as Lexchin describes in chapter seven of this volume).

There may, of course, be benefits to increased transparency other than health improvements. Transparency may be worth pursuing even if it has no effect on health. Patients may take comfort in knowing whether their clinician has received payment from industry, even if the disclosure of those payments has no effect on the care received. There seems to be an intrinsic value in knowing, for example, that a patient organization is being funded by industry, even if that disclosure does not change any decision. Similarly, there seems to be inherent value in a regulator being clear about its regulatory actions, even if that openness does not have any direct effect on health. This type of transparency can increase public confidence in the government.

Transparency could help reduce the amount spent on medicines. Total drug spending in Canada in 2017 was estimated at CAN$33 billion (or CAN$934 per person annually), which is much more than similar high-income countries (Canadian Institute for Health Information [CIHI], 2017). Transparency for procurement processes and actual prices (as described in chapter two) might help reduce pharmaceutical spending, even if it does not impact health directly. Reduced drug spending could indirectly improve health, either by making medicines more easily available or by freeing up resources to support other interventions that promote health.

"Research waste" refers to research resources being used up without worthwhile achievement. One important cause of research waste is a failure to prioritize important topics for research. For example, pharmaceutical companies may be interested in finding small differences between similar medicines, but these studies have little or no value to others. Increasing transparency requires considerable resources, including time. As efforts to increase transparency intensify in response to encouraging changes, it may be timely now to select priorities for this work.

A Potential Solution: Essential Medicines Lists

Ultimately, increased transparency is presumed to lead to better health-related decisions by clinicians and patients, such as decisions about whether or not to take a specific medicine. Clinical studies are supposed to help determine which medications are best under what circumstances, but the unavailability of information about clinical studies can lead to poorly informed decisions.

The World Health Organization (WHO) established a model list of essential medicines in 1977, which is revised every two years (World Health Organization [WHO], 2015, 2018). Countries can adapt the WHO's template to their own circumstances, and to date 137 countries representing 5.8 billion people have done so (Persaud et al., 2019). In some countries, essential medicines lists are used to determine which medicines are available in health-care institutions, such as hospitals, and which ones are publicly funded. The content of essential medicines lists is thus an important determinant of health globally.

Efforts to increase transparency could be focused on essential medicines lists and the related processes. Transparency could help improve essential medicines list processes at several different levels. Transparency for clinical study information could be required before any medicine is added to the WHO's model list of essential medicines. Medicines currently listed could be removed if complete information about clinical studies is not made available by study sponsors. Complete information about essential medicines, including flags for missing information, could be maintained in a publicly available database such as the one maintained in partnership with the WHO (https://essentialmeds.org). This information would help countries decide which medicines to include in their national lists.

The essential medicines lists of different countries can be compared and explanations for differences sought. While the WHO recommends that each country adapt its essential medicines list to its own circumstances based on the priority health needs of its population, differences in priority health needs do not appear to explain differences in essential medicines lists (Persaud et al., 2019). A large number of differences exist between essential medicines lists of similar countries, and most medicines are listed by a small number of countries (Persaud et al., 2019). Country characteristics account for a small fraction of the variation in essential medicines lists. Publicly reporting these differences, especially where no good explanation exists, could help to improve essential medicines lists (Persaud et al., 2019).

Transparency can also be applied within countries. Information could be made available about whether or not individual clinicians prescribe from the list and whether prescribing differences are explained by industry interactions or payments. One example of an efficient platform for sharing prescribing data within a country is OpenPrescribing.net in the United Kingdom (Walker et al., 2018). While guidance from the WHO already affirms the importance of transparency in the process of medicine selection (for example, through publicly posting criteria for selecting medicines and through disclosing potential conflicts of interest for committee members), advances in transparency can help to inform further bolstering of essential medicines list processes (WHO, 2015, 2018). For example, publicly posting the information considered when deciding whether to add a particular medicine to an essential medicines list could increase confidence in the process by opening up the details of the process to scrutiny.

A number of important limitations to focusing transparency efforts on essential medicines lists can be seen. More than fifty countries do not have an essential medicines list, so the residents of those countries may not realize any direct benefit from improved essential medicines list processes. The essential medicines list concept has existed for more than forty years, and yet some countries have never decided to develop one. Increased transparency related to essential medicines may actually decrease the likelihood that some countries will develop an essential medicines list. Improvements in the WHO's list may or may not translate into improvements in country-level lists, since each country can decide whether to adopt the changes made by the WHO. Individual countries may or may not decide to change their essential medicines processes based on increased transparency, and efforts to improve processes in more than a hundred countries would be resource intensive.

Despite these important limitations, focusing transparency efforts on essential medicines lists seems more prudent than many alternatives.

Regulators in Europe and North America have demonstrated a limited appetite for changing regulatory decisions made about specific products based on information revealed through efforts to improve transparency. Even if these regulators reform their approach, a relatively small fraction of the global population would be directly affected.

Conclusion

Ideally, increased transparency would directly lead clinicians and patients to make better decisions. The four examples noted at the beginning of this chapter suggest that this outcome is not what actually happens. Producers of clinical practice guidelines seem largely unmoved by new information. The best hope, therefore, may be to change an international norm, and the norm that seems to be the most relevant to advances in transparency is the WHO's model list of essential medicines and guidance from the WHO about essential medicines list processes.

Increasing transparency has the potential to improve health. Important advances in transparency are a reason for optimism, although health improvements have not always been realized. Prioritizing and coordinating transparency efforts could help to ensure that increases in transparency translate into improvements in health. Essential medicines lists are already an important determinant of health globally, and essential medicines lists can be improved through increased transparency.

REFERENCES

Campbell, K., Rowe, H., Azzam, H., & Lane, C.A. (2016). The management of nausea and vomiting of pregnancy. SOGC Clinical Practice Guideline. *Journal of Obstetrics and Gynaecology Canada, 38*(12), 1127–37. https://doi.org/10.1016/j.jogc.2016.08.009

Canadian Institute for Health Information (CIHI). (2017). *Prescribed drug spending in Canada, 2017: A focus on public drug programs.* Ottawa, ON: CIHI. Retrieved from https://www.cihi.ca/sites/default/files/document/pdex2017-report-en.pdf

Committee on Publication Ethics. (2019). Retraction guidelines. Retrieved from https://publicationethics.org/retraction-guidelines

District Court for the Western District of Virginia, Abingdon Division. (2007, 8 May). *United States v. The Purdue Frederick Company, Inc. (Purdue).* Agreed statement of facts. Retrieved from http://i.bnet.com/blogs/purdue-agreed-facts.pdf

Glauser, W. (2019, 14 May). New service proposed for expectant mothers after Motherisk closure. *CMAJnews.* Retrieved from https://cmajnews.com

/2019/05/14/new-service-proposed-for-expectant-mothers-after-motherisk
-closure-cmaj-109-5755/

Institute of Medicine (IOM), Committee on Conflict of Interest in Medical
Research, Education, and Practice. (2009). *Conflict of interest in medical research,
education, and practice.* Washington, DC: National Academies Press. Retrieved
from https://www.ncbi.nlm.nih.gov/books/NBK22942

Jefferson, T., Jones, M., Doshi, P., Spencer, E.A., Onakpoya, I., & Heneghan, C.J.
(2014). Oseltamivir for influenza in adults and children: Systematic review of
clinical study reports and summary of regulatory comments. *BMJ, 348,* g2545.
https://doi.org/10.1136/bmj.g2545

Keller, M.B., Ryan, N.D., Strober, M., Klein, R.G., Kutcher, S.P., Birmaher, B., …
McCafferty, J.P. (2001). Efficacy of paroxetine in the treatment of adolescent
major depression: A randomized, controlled trial. *Journal of the American
Academy of Child & Adolescent Psychiatry, 40*(7), 762–72. https://doi.org/10.1097
/00004583-200107000-00010

Koren, G., Clark, S., Hankins, G.D.V., Caritis, S.N., Miodovnik, M., Umans,
J.G., & Mattison, D.R. (2010). Effectiveness of delayed-release doxylamine
and pyridoxine for nausea and vomiting of pregnancy: A randomized placebo
controlled trial. *American Journal of Obstetrics & Gynecology, 203*(6), 571.e1–7.
https://doi.org/10.1016/j.ajog.2010.07.030

Le Noury, J., Nardo, J.M., Healy, D., Jureidini, J., Raven, M., Tufanaru, C., &
Abi-Jaoude, E. (2015). Restoring Study 329: Efficacy and harms of paroxetine
and imipramine in treatment of major depression in adolescence. *BMJ, 351,*
h4320. https://doi.org/10.1136/bmj.h4320

Le Noury, J., Nardo, J.M., Healy, D., Jureidini, J., Raven, M., Tufanaru, C., &
Abi-Jaoude, E. (n.d.). Restoring Study 329: Scientific integrity through data
based medicine. Retrieved from https://study329.org/

Meier, B. (2007, 10 May). In guilty plea, OxyContin maker to pay $600 million.
New York Times. Retrieved from https://www.nytimes.com/2007/05/10/business
/11drug-web.html

Ontario Drug Policy Research Network (ODPRN). (2016). *Opioid use and related
events in Ontario.* Toronto, ON: ODPRN. Retrieved from http://odprn.ca/wp
-content/uploads/2016/11/ODPRN-Opioid-Use-and-Related-Adverse-Events
-Nov-2016.pdf

Persaud, N., Jiang, M., Shaikh, R., Bali, A., Oronsaye, E., Woods, H., …
Heneghan, C. (2019, 1 June). Comparison of essential medicines lists in 137
countries. *Bulletin of the World Health Organization, 97*(6), 394–404C. https://
doi.org/10.2471/BLT.18.222448

Persaud, N., Meaney, C., El-Emam, K., Moineddin, R., & Thorpe, K. (2018).
Doxylamine-pyridoxine for nausea and vomiting of pregnancy randomized
placebo controlled trial: Prespecified analyses and reanalysis. *PLoS One,
13*(1), e0189978. https://doi.org/10.1371/journal.pone.0189978

Public Health Agency of Canada, Special Advisory Committee on the Epidemic
of Opioid Overdoses. (2018). National report: Apparent opioid-related
deaths in Canada, January 2016 to September 2017. Ottawa, ON: Public
Health Agency of Canada. Retrieved from https://www.canada.ca/en/public
-health/services/publications/healthy-living/national-report-apparent-opioid
-related-deaths-released-march-2018.html

Spurling, G.K., Mansfield, P.R., Montgomery, B.D., Lexchin, J., Doust, J.,
Othman, N., & Vitry, A.I. (2010). Information from pharmaceutical companies
and the quality, quantity, and cost of physicians' prescribing: A systematic
review. *PLoS Medicine, 7*(10), e1000352. https://doi.org/10.1371/journal.pmed
.1000352

US Centers for Disease Control and Prevention (CDC). (2018, March 29). U.S.
drug overdose deaths continue to rise; increase fueled by synthetic opioids.
Press release. Retrieved from https://www.cdc.gov/media/releases/2018
/p0329-drug-overdose-deaths.html

Walker, A.J., Croker, R., Bacon, S., Ernst, E., Curtis, H.J., & Goldacre, B. (2018).
Is use of homeopathy associated with poor prescribing in English primary
care? A cross-sectional study. *Journal of the Royal Society of Medicine, 111*(5),
167–74. https://doi.org/10.1177/0141076818765779

World Health Organization (WHO). (2015). Essential medicines. List prepared
April 2015. Retrieved from http://www.who.int/medicines/services
/essmedicines_def/en/

World Health Organization (WHO). (2018). Essential medicines selection:
National medicines list/formulary/standard treatment guidelines. Retrieved
from http://www.who.int/selection_medicines/country_lists/en/#B

7 Speak No Secrets: (Non)transparency in Health Canada's Communications about Pharmaceutical Regulation

JOEL LEXCHIN

Introduction

There are three levels of transparency in government regulation: First, the rules that form the basis for regulation must be publicly available. Second, the data and information that are the results of regulations must be publicly released. Finally, the way that the government applies the regulations in reaching a final decision needs to be communicated effectively and publicly, and the effectiveness of those communications in achieving their objectives needs to be evaluated to be sure that people understand what is being said and that the messages, if necessary, are having the desired effect. Without transparency at all three levels, it is not possible for the public to be assured of why and how decisions that affect their lives are being made. It is this final aspect of transparency that this chapter will consider when it comes to pharmaceutical regulation. Transparency is key to people having confidence in what Health Canada has to say about how it deals with pharmaceutical policy issues. Without that confidence, many people will be apprehensive each time they put a pill in their mouths or get an injection in their arms. As this chapter will show, Health Canada's communication practices have been problematic for a long time. Although the situation has been slowly improving over the past decade, there are still many areas where significant improvements wait to be made. Specifically, in this chapter I will consider *how much information* Health Canada communicates, the *manner* in which it communicates, and the *type of information* it communicates in the following four areas: regulation of the conduct of clinical trials, drug approvals, drug safety, and drug promotion. Finally, I will explore reasons for the style of communication that Health Canada has adopted.

Conduct of Clinical Trials

Clinical Trial Inspections

Regulations allowing Health Canada to inspect clinical trials came into effect in early 2002 (Health Products and Food Branch Inspectorate [HPFBI], 2002). Although Health Canada aims to inspect 2 per cent of ongoing clinical trials annually, in 2006–07 it only managed to achieve half that figure, or forty inspections versus a targeted eighty (Shuchman, 2008), probably because it did not allocate sufficient resources to the task (Auditor General of Canada, 2006). An auditor general's report in 2011 documented a continuing shortfall in the number of inspections undertaken – fifty-two in 2009 and fifty in 2010 – largely because of a lack of resources and a reallocation of resources to other programs (Auditor General of Canada, 2011). Previously, program managers at Health Canada had told the auditor general that they considered there was an insufficient level of activity at Health Canada when it came to investigating clinical trials (Auditor General of Canada, 2006).

Health Canada says that it uses "risk-based criteria" to select the trials to be inspected, but these criteria are vague and merely state that they include the number of subjects enrolled and the number of trials conducted at a specific location (Health Products and Food Branch [HPFB], 2004). Therefore, it is unknown whether Health Canada is actually monitoring the trials where the subjects are at the greatest risk. Moreover,

> Health Canada does not regularly collect all of the information necessary to assess these factors and to make comparative risk-based decisions. Because clinical trial sponsors are not required to submit up-to-date information on clinical trial sites, inspectors must call each site directly to find out the current status of the clinical trial site and the number of participants enrolled ... Thus, inspectors have up-to-date information only for sites that they call and are unable to compare the risks posed by all sites. (Auditor General of Canada, 2011, p. 9)

New interim risk-based criteria for trial inspections were developed and piloted by Health Canada for use during 2012–13 in conjunction with the development of a new site selection process (HPFB, 2014), but as of late 2020, only vague generic information about these new criteria or how they are being applied was available.

Health Canada was once much less transparent in the information it publicized about its inspections compared to the United States. When the US Food and Drug Administration (FDA) found serious problems, the results of its inspection and its warning letter to the company were posted on its website, albeit with some delay and certain information redacted (Shuchman, 2008). By contrast, Health Canada only provided summary statistics about its inspections but no information about individual sites, corrective actions required, the drugs involved, the names of the doctors running the trials, or the names of the companies (HPFBI, 2012a; McLean & Bruser, 2014a, 2014b).

In 2014, Health Canada told the *Toronto Star* that "confidential and/or proprietary information is removed" from the summary reports (McLean & Bruser, 2014a). According to the *Star*, "over the past 12 years, Health Canada found at least 33 clinical trials had critical problems and were 'non-compliant.'" The *Star* asked for details of these and other inspections in July 2014, but two months later Health Canada refused, stating that providing records "would require an exhaustive manual paper file review." As McLean & Bruser (2014a) note, "the regulator also said the release of these clinical trial inspection reports could only come after consultation with third parties, typically the doctors running the trials and drug companies. The Canadian regulator refused to say how many clinical trials it has shut down or stopped, if any."

Health Canada started publishing reports about its inspections, with the first one covering 2002 (HPFBI, 2003) and a second one covering the period 2003–04 (HPFBI, 2004). After that, there was a prolonged silence. In March 2008, I began an effort to find out when the next report would be released, a project that dragged on for over three years. The report finally appeared on 28 March 2012 and covered 2004–11 (HPFBI, 2012a). Since then, Health Canada has become more proactive and now has a website that posts the results of clinical trial inspections and contains information about multiple components of the inspection, including whether the sponsor was compliant or non-compliant. However, if the sponsor were to be non-compliant, there continues to be minimal information about what measures Health Canada would require. For example, in the case of AO Spine North America, the following is all that appears: "Proposed corrective actions were requested and are pending" (Health Canada, 2016a).

Monitoring of Phase IV Studies

The degree to which Phase IV studies (those done after a drug has been approved and is being marketed) are monitored is also a significant cause for concern. According to the Senate Standing Committee on Social Affairs, Science and Technology (2012), about 70 per cent of all studies are run in a community setting and have therefore been approved by a for-profit research ethics board (REB). It is likely that an even greater percentage of Phase IV studies are done in this setting. Moreover, Phase IV studies are often used by industry not to generate new scientific data but as a way to generate interest about the drug among doctors involved in the trials and get them familiar with prescribing the product (Kessler, Rose, Temple, Schapiro, & Griffin, 1994). Previously, Health Canada said its inspection process can be applied to these studies "as needed" (HPFB, 2004), but what that means is not spelled out, and none of the inspection reports provided information if any studies of this type were inspected.

Drug Approvals

Summary Basis of Decision

"Transparency" is a term that is often thrown around when it comes to drug regulation. When Health Canada uses the term, the meaning it gives is reassuring:

> Canadians also want to better understand the decision-making process undertaken by the regulator. Health Canada must provide greater and more meaningful transparency by enabling easier access to information, as well as providing information in a format that is easy to understand and provides value to the end user. (Health Canada, 2012)

Understanding decision-making means two things: providing the information that was used to make the decision and – the focus of this chapter – disclosing in detail *the reasoning process* behind the decision. In practice, it means that Health Canada should make public the reports from its reviewers about the quality of the information.

The closest Health Canada has currently come to releasing its reviewers' reports are the Summary Basis of Decision (SBD) documents, a project that began in 2005. The SBD is issued after a new drug is approved, and explains the scientific and benefit/risk information that was considered prior to approving the product. Particularly valuable for health-care professionals is the third section, which contains a description of the pre-market clinical trials examined by Health Canada and a summary of the final benefit/risk assessment for the product. Health Canada's position is that, as a result of this initiative, "Canadian healthcare professionals and patients will have more information at their disposal to support informed treatment choices" (Health Canada, 2004).

An analysis of all 161 SBDs (containing the results of 456 clinical trials) released from the beginning of the project until the end of April

2012 showed that clinical trial information was presented in a haphazard manner, with no apparent method to its presentation. In the vast majority of SBDs (126 of 161), at least one-third of the potential information about patient trial characteristics (for example, age, sex, whether they were inpatients or outpatients) and the benefits and risks of tested treatments is missing. While basic details of clinical trials were more frequently described, any omissions or ambiguities in this component were especially troubling given the straightforward nature of the information that needed to be conveyed, for example, the number of patients per trial arm, whether the trial took place at a single site or multiple sites, and if a unique trial identifier was included (Habibi & Lexchin, 2014). Without this type of basic information, it is impossible to understand how Health Canada reached its decision about allowing new products onto the market.

Priority Reviews

The lack of communication is especially troubling when it comes to drugs approved through Health Canada's priority review process. In an effort to ensure that promising therapies for serious illnesses can reach Canadians in a timely manner, Health Canada has created a priority review pathway. This pathway is intended for drug submissions "for a serious, life-threatening or severely debilitating disease or condition for which there is substantial evidence of clinical effectiveness that the drug provides ... effective treatment, prevention or diagnosis of a disease or condition for which no drug is presently marketed in Canada; or ... a significant increase in efficacy and/or significant decrease in risk such that the overall benefit/risk profile is improved over existing therapies, preventatives or diagnostic agents for a disease or condition that is not adequately managed by a drug marketed in Canada" (HPFB, 2009, p. 2). The company seeking approval still has to submit a complete new drug submission, but the review period is reduced to 180 days from a standard 300 days.

Since 1995, Health Canada has used this process for about 25 per cent of the submissions that it receives (Lexchin, 2018). The use of a priority review carries both resource and safety implications. Although the priority and standard approval pathways are equivalent in terms of the amount of data reviewed, the former is done in 180 days compared to 300 days for the latter, meaning that the priority pathway is more resource intensive, possibly drawing resources from other Health Canada activities. More importantly, drugs reviewed through the priority process are more likely to receive safety warnings once they are on the market compared to drugs with a standard approval (Lexchin, 2012). Despite these concerns, priority reviews would still be justified if they actually meant that therapeutically important new drugs reached patients more rapidly – but that does not appear to be the case for most of the products given a priority review. From 1995 to 2016, inclusive, Health Canada approved 623 new drugs, of which 509 (81.7 per cent) were evaluated for their therapeutic innovation by independent bodies. Health Canada used an accelerated review pathway for 159 of the 509 drugs, whereas only 55 were judged to be therapeutically innovative by one or both of the independent reviews (Lexchin, 2018). Health Canada's rationale behind its seemingly liberal use of priority reviews is not known, since its reviewer reports are not made public.

Notice of Compliance with Conditions

A second mechanism for getting drugs on the market more rapidly is the Notice of Compliance with conditions (NOC/c). The goal of this policy is to "provide effective treatment, prevention or diagnosis of a disease or condition for which no drug is presently marketed in Canada; or a significant increase in efficacy and/or significant decrease in risk such that the overall benefit/risk profile is improved over existing therapies" (Health Canada, 2016b). In many cases, "promising evidence of clinical effectiveness" is based solely on a surrogate marker, that is, an outcome that is thought to be linked to increased life expectancy or a better quality of life. For example, lowered blood pressure is a surrogate marker that is linked to a lower risk of a stroke or heart attack. In return for NOC/c status, companies sign a Letter of Undertaking to complete confirmatory clinical studies (studies that definitively establish efficacy) and submit their results to Health Canada. A failure to complete these studies, or negative results from the studies, could lead to the marketing authorization being cancelled. However, as of November 2019, there were six drugs that have been sold for more than ten years without completing the required studies (Lexchin, 2019). Full details about the trials necessary to fulfil the conditions are not made publicly available, and there is no published information even about whether trials have been undertaken or about their current progress status.

Bill C-17

Bill C-17 (commonly referred to as Vanessa's Law), which was signed into law in November 2014, offered a further opportunity to improve transparency. However, the legislation does not explicitly require Health

Canada to publish the rationale for decisions concerning all drugs approved for sale or drugs refused for reasons of safety and/or efficacy, or the names of drugs that are suspended or recalled (Herder, Gibson, Graham, Lexchin, & Mintzes, 2014). A press release issued by the government on the passage of Bill C-17 said that the regulatory decisions about drugs refused market authorization will be published (Government of Canada, 2014). As of January 2021, Bill C-17 has not led to the release of reviewers' reports.

Health Canada held a consultation between March and June 2015 on the proposed interpretation and implementation of its new powers to release clinical study reports that were conferred under Bill C-17. This consultation offers an example of the extent of Health Canada's commitment to communication. Twenty-five stakeholders responded to the request to provide input, including those from industry, health-care professional associations, and academia. According to Health Canada, "all comments were considered and the final Guide incorporates changes to improve the clarity and precision of language to better reflect the legislative provisions" (Health Canada, 2015). But exactly how many of the comments were used is unclear. Health Canada's remarks about comments on how to define confidential business information and what information Health Canada made public all ended with phrases such as "Health Canada is considering comments received as the Department moves forward on further policy and process developments and will provide more information to stakeholders in the coming months" (Health Canada, 2015).

From the fall of 2017 to the spring of 2018, Health Canada engaged with a reference group of stakeholders, of which I was one, to develop regulations regarding the extent of information about safety and efficacy from pre-market clinical trials that it started to publicly release at the end of February 2019. Information on drugs approved prior to the finalization of the regulations is now also being released based on a prioritization of requests. However, even in this new mood of openness, there are still issues with the way that Health Canada communicates. Health Canada has a web page that gives summaries of its stakeholder meetings and engagement activities, including with the reference group (Health Canada, 2018a), which is a positive development. But its "What we heard" web page (Health Canada, 2018b) that summarizes responses to its white paper "Public Release of Clinical Information in Drug Submissions and Medical Device Applications" is problematic. Health Canada has a pie chart that breaks down the number of submissions by stakeholder groups, for example, academics, industry, and so on. What the pie chart initially didn't convey was that some single submissions were signed by multiple individuals. For example, one submission that I was involved with was endorsed by over 120 academics, something that was completely hidden from anyone visiting the website. When this problem was pointed out to Health Canada, its response was to add an asterisk to the pie chart that reads: "Note: the numbers below reflect unique submissions from each stakeholder group; some submissions were submitted on behalf of multiple individuals or organizations."

As Lexchin, Herder, and Doshi (2019) note, the Canadian regulations and the resulting portal that provides access to information mirror policies adopted by the European Medicines Agency (EMA) in 2010 and 2014, which grant access to clinical study reports on request and authorize the publication of study reports submitted by drug companies. In several important ways, Health Canada has gone beyond the European regulator. Its reforms are grounded not just in policy but also in legislation, strengthening its position should its approach be challenged in court, as the EMA's has been. Health Canada also allows anyone to download the data without registration, something EMA's policy now limits to residents of the European Union.

Drug Safety

Safety Warnings

Health Canada documents about what triggers a safety action are quite vague and provide little transparency or specifics regarding how decisions are made. For example, Health Canada (2007) states: "The determination of the seriousness of risk (probability of health hazard and probability of occurrence) and urgency of risk communication is based on sound scientific judgement." Further, Health Canada's Marketed Health Products Directorate (MHPD; 2004) earlier explained that "regulatory actions ... are taken according to the regulatory framework in place. This implies an evaluation of the signal and the appropriate benefit-risk review of the information available."

Chris Turner, the former head of the MHPD, the part of Health Canada charged with monitoring the safety of drugs already marketed, wrote a letter to the *Toronto Star* defending Health Canada's drug safety program, saying: "Health Canada has highly trained specialists who use Canadian adverse reaction data as well as other sources of information to systematically monitor, analyse and act on safety issues" (Turner, 2012). But another unnamed Health Canada official is quoted as telling the *Toronto Star*: "It is primarily the [drug company's] responsibility to monitor the safe use of their products" (Bruser & Bailey, 2012).

Communicating Safety Issues

The 2011 auditor general's (AG) report investigated how well Health Canada ensures the safety of the drugs that it approves (Auditor General of Canada, 2011). In eleven out of twenty-four cases where it was necessary to issue risk communications to the public, Health Canada took more than two years to assess the potential safety issue, update the drug's label (where necessary), and issue the risk communication. Even more worrisome, Health Canada had no standards for monitoring the effectiveness of its communication strategies with either the public or health-care professionals, although it told the AG that it was taking steps to do so (Auditor General of Canada, 2011). A 2006 survey of the general public showed that citizens are generally unaware of, and do not consider, Health Canada Public Advisories and Warnings and its website as important sources of new drug safety information. Only 1 per cent made use of the former, and 3 per cent of the latter, and just 8 per cent of consumers reported having used the Health Canada website for this purpose over a six month period (Decima Research Inc., 2003). With such low use, their effectiveness is clearly in question, although the public may receive information in other ways. Use by health-care professionals is somewhat better, but they too seldom used these sources.

Inspections of Drug Manufacturing Facilities

Health Canada has long had a system for the inspection of drug manufacturing facilities – Good Manufacturing Practices (GMP) – co-developed with the cooperation of the pharmaceutical industry. Up until 2016, the only report about the results of Health Canada's inspection program covered the period 2006 to 2011 (HPFBI, 2012b). The document broke down the findings into gross categories, such as the number of inspections performed, the percentage of inspections where various problems were found, and the most common problems. There was no information about any specific inspection; no comment about what actions, if any, were taken to correct the problems; and nothing about the individual products involved. In order to find information about problems in specific Canadian manufacturing facilities, it was necessary to file a Freedom of Information Act request with the FDA in the United States. The FDA inspects not only domestic plants but also foreign plants that ship drugs into the United States. According to the *Toronto Star*, FDA inspections previously found serious manufacturing violations in forty Canadian plants since 2008 (Bruser & McLean, 2014). This information was available because the FDA makes inspection dates and results available to the public on its website, whereas Health Canada did not give any details of the problems, if any, that it found during individual inspections and wouldn't make public "the names of the 20-plus companies that have been cited since 2012 for severe manufacturing violations" (Bruser & McLean, 2014). Health Canada told the *Toronto Star* that it would need to consult with the companies in question before releasing that type of information.

Several months after the *Toronto Star* story appeared, Health Canada released inspection reports showing that "nearly one-third of all Canadian drug plants inspected since 2013 have terms and conditions on their licences" (McLean & Bruser, 2014b). However, there were still ongoing gaps in what Health Canada was willing to make public.

> While the disclosures show the date and location of the inspection, and whether the inspection led to regulatory action, Health Canada has not yet released details of the problems it found in all but one case. [The story in the *Toronto Star* did not say what that case was.]
>
> And while the new data shows that 13 facilities received a non-compliant rating and no longer have a licence, Health Canada refused to say whether in these cases it revoked the licence or the company voluntarily shut down post-inspection. (McLean & Bruser, 2014b)

As with its clinical trial inspection system, Health Canada is now posting individual manufacturing inspection reports on its website with reasonably detailed descriptions of problems that the inspections uncovered. But once again, if a non-compliant rating was issued, there is nothing to indicate what measures the company needed to undertake to become compliant.

Drug Promotion

Lack of Regulatory Oversight by Health Canada

The Food and Drugs Act and Regulations give the government the authority over the promotion of prescription drugs and ban direct-to-consumer advertising (DTCA). But despite having the nominal control over promotion, over the past century Health Canada has never shown much interest in exercising that power. Health Canada's position has been that "it's not our policy to treat advertising as the definitive source of information with respect to drugs" (Cocking, 1977). No penalties were imposed by Health Canada on any pharmaceutical company for illegal advertising between 1978 and 1984 (Lexchin, 1984), and there is no public record of any since then. Several companies prosecuted for illegally marketing unapproved uses in the United States sell the same products in Canada, but a Health Canada spokesperson told the *Toronto Star* that it "has not been made aware of any specific similar issue in Canada and has not received complaints concerning these companies promoting off-label uses of their products in Canada." Despite repeated requests by the *Star*, "Health Canada provided no evidence it has ever investigated, prosecuted or fined a single drug company for off-label promotions" (Bruser, McLean, & Bailey, 2014).

The Regulatory Advertising Section within the MHPD, the part of Health Canada charged with regulating drugs already on the market, oversees regulated advertising activities, but the exact nature of its activities is opaque. Despite an extensive search on Health Canada's website, I found no information about the number of personnel in the section or its level of resources.

Starting in 2015, Health Canada has been posting complaints about advertising on a website (Health Canada, 2020a), but details about the nature of the alleged violation are virtually non-existent (for example, one entry notes a "complaint regarding the advertising of unauthorized products including claims for serious disease"). There is no information given about how a decision is made to uphold or dismiss a complaint, and if the complaint is upheld, information about any penalties or other actions is minimal (for example, "Compliance letter sent to request stop sale and advertising of unlicensed product; Ongoing follow-up to confirm the stop sale and non-compliant materials are modified/removed/discontinued").

Pharmaceutical Advertising Advisory Board

In practice, Health Canada has turned over the day-to-day regulation of promotion to a combination of an independent external group with strong industry representation and the pharmaceutical industry itself. The former is the Pharmaceutical Advertising Advisory Board (PAAB), which has the responsibility for advertising/promotion systems, that is, the media presentation of promotion in all forms – print, audio, visual, audio/visual, and later electronic and computer means of communication. Advertisements in any of these forms have to be submitted to the PAAB for preclearance to ensure compliance with the provisions of its code before they can be used (Pharmaceutical Advertising Advisory Board [PAAB], 2018).

Despite the nominal independence of the PAAB from industry, its board includes a representative of the Canadian Association of

Medical Publishers; Canadian Generic Pharmaceutical Association; Food, Health & Consumer Products of Canada; Innovative Medicines Canada; and BIOTECanada, meaning that five of the ten members come from organizations that, in one way or another, benefit from advertising. Importantly, the PAAB's code is not legally binding; its decisions are not legally enforceable; and, as a voluntary, independent body, the PAAB is not accountable for its actions to government or any other organization. The PAAB rules on an average of five complaints per year, and will occasionally refer complaints about advertisements to Health Canada for final resolution. The PAAB publishes its decisions about complaints on its website in the *PAAB Newsletter,* but their location is not immediately evident from the organization's website homepage, and clicking on the button labelled "PAAB Code" does not lead to complaints as might be expected. Aside from the minutes of annual meetings between Health Canada and the PAAB (and other agencies concerned with drug promotion; PAAB, n.d.), there are no communications from Health Canada about how it views the effectiveness of the PAAB. However, it would appear that the PAAB's operation is acceptable to Health Canada, as it continues to be an ex-officio member of the board.

Innovative Medicines Canada

All other forms of promotion, including interactions between sales representatives and doctors, gift giving, and the sponsorship of meetings are de facto under the control of Innovative Medicines Canada (IMC), the umbrella organization representing the multinational companies operating in Canada (Innovative Medicines Canada, 2020). From 2008 to 2016, there were fifteen complaints about possible violations of the IMC code, of which six were upheld. Like the PAAB, IMC publishes its rulings on complaints on its website, but unlike the PAAB, the page is relatively easy to locate. Since 2015, detailed reasons about the rulings are available, but before that they were sporadically published. The validity of complaints is decided by the Industry Practices Review Committee (IPRC). Health Canada has no role on the IPRC. There is no information on the Health Canada website about its interactions with IMC regarding the regulation of promotion.

Direct-to-Consumer Advertising

The one area of prescription drug promotion where Health Canada does retain authority is for direct-to-consumer advertising (DTCA). DTCA is generally regarded as the mention of the name of a drug and its indications in the same piece of promotional material. While this practice is not allowed in Canada, Health Canada does permit "help-seeking" advertisements, where a condition is mentioned and the readers or viewers are advised to see their doctor, as well as "reminder" advertisements that give the name of the product but not its use. By the mid-2000s, companies were spending in excess of CAN$20 million annually on these two forms of promotion, primarily in the form of TV advertising (Mintzes, Morgan, & Wright, 2009).

From 2000 to 2006, Health Canada received eighty complaints about DTCA and judged that only six (8 per cent) were not in violation of the law (*CanWest MediaWorks Inc. v. Attorney General of Canada*, 2006), but the internal discussion behind these decisions is hidden from public view and continues to be hidden as a review of ten complaints about DTCA shows. Health Canada often took prolonged times, in some cases years, to respond to complaints, and then either did not make decisions public or issued perfunctory responses claiming that an advertisement was a help-seeking message and not DTCA (Lexchin & Mintzes, 2014). The lack of public disclosure about regulatory decisions does little to encourage complainants to come forward. Lack of public access to information on regulatory decisions also means that media companies may unknowingly participate in advertising activities very similar to those that were previously judged to be illegal, or members of the public may be unaware about exposure to advertising later judged to be unacceptable.

Explanations for Health Canada's Communication Style

Health Canada's poor communication style is multifactorial in origin. First and foremost, Health Canada's relationship with the pharmaceutical industry is a reflection of how the Canadian government treats industry in general. In my book, *Private Profits vs Public Policy: The Pharmaceutical Industry and the Canadian State* (Lexchin, 2016), I use the insights from Davis and Abraham (2013) to show how the Canadian state, as represented by the federal government, has sought cooperation with the pharmaceutical industry. Often, it has gone beyond cooperation and actively promoted industry's interests through legislation and policies, even when industry's interests conflicted with those of the public. In some areas, it has voluntarily turned over de facto regulatory power to industry.

The alliance of interests between the state and industry has not been static, and has markedly increased over the past two decades. As the neoliberal agenda gained momentum in the mid-1980s, the deregulation trend in Canada accelerated, further deepening the relationship between

Health Canada and the pharmaceutical industry. Neoliberalism heralded a prioritization of intellectual property rights over public values, affecting drug-pricing policies, incentives offered for research and development (R&D), and Canadian foreign policy on access to drugs for countries in the Global South. It is crucial to emphasize the point that neoliberalism is not merely another incarnation of laissez-faire capitalism whereby the state stands back and gives the market free rein. Neoliberalism involves the active participation in *facilitating* markets, that is, the state adopts a bias in favour of corporations. It would be a mistake to see the Canadian government as a passive victim of external pressure; rather, it actively cooperated in declining to adopt stricter regulatory measures and in relinquishing national authority over intellectual property rights.

Neoliberalism is focused on the regulatory power of the marketplace and supports the diminishing role of the state in protecting its citizens by letting industry set its own regulatory standards and policing them. This acceleration in deference to the industry is best understood in the context of corporate bias. The state did not completely surrender its regulatory role, but attempts to exert more authority were undertaken in a half-hearted manner that avoided confrontation with industry and actually strengthened industry's position.

Other factors affecting the transparency of Health Canada's communications follow on from its relationship with industry. To start, Health Canada has consistently treated information that originates with pharmaceutical companies or that might conceivably affect the economic health of these companies as confidential business information. Subsection 20(6) of the Access to Information Act could actually allow Health Canada to release much of the data it currently keeps secret on the grounds that "disclosure would be in the public interest as it relates to public health ... and, if the public interest in disclosure clearly outweighs in importance any financial loss or gain to a third party ... any prejudice to its competitive position or any interference with its contractual or other negotiations" (Access to Information Act, 1985). However, for reasons that are not clear, Health Canada never chose to try and use this section of the act.

Even Health Canada's decision to release clinical trial information, described earlier, has its limitations. Health Canada has created two exemptions to its policy, one for information that the manufacturer did not use in the drug submission to support the proposed conditions of use or purpose for the drug and a second for information that describes tests, methods, or assays that are used exclusively by the manufacturer (Health Canada, 2019). However, Health Canada ignores important consequences of withholding information about analyses of possible future indications for a product from the public. If trial results are negative, companies are unlikely to pursue the indication and will not submit the results of the trial. If those trials remain unpublished, then information about the drug being ineffective or unsafe for that indication will not be available to clinicians or patients. The use of selective serotonin reuptake inhibitors (SSRIs) for the treatment of depression in children and adolescents is one example of harms that can arise when negative findings are not published. SSRIs were (and still are) used off-label for this problem. The published literature suggested a favourable risk/benefit ratio for some of the drugs in this class, but when the unpublished data was considered, the conclusion was that, for most of the drugs, the risks could outweigh the benefits.

Turning to the second exemption, restricting the release of this type of information means that there cannot be any independent examination of the tests, methods, or assays. In effect, people outside Health Canada are being asked to trust both the information provided by the manufacturers to the agency and how Health Canada has evaluated that information without access to details on the content, approach, reliability, or validity of the test, method, or assay.

Specifically related to Health Canada's communication style about safety issues is the significant imbalance in personnel and resources between the two directorates that approve drugs and biologics (Therapeutic Products Directorate; and Biologics and Genetic Therapies Directorate) and the Marketed Health Products Directorate that monitors the safety of products already on the market. As of the end of March 2020, the former two directorates had over three times more money and personnel allocated to them compared to the MHPD (Health Canada, 2020b).

Finally, Health Canada's style of communication may reflect the organization's lack of comfort with transparency in general, as can be seen in its responses to Access to Information requests. It took Health Canada over nineteen months (request filed 15 December 2014, final response 5 August 2016) to release information to me that had previously been publicly available on its website. In September 2011, Toronto doctor Nav Persaud filed a request with Health Canada for clinical trial information about a drug used in the treatment of pregnancy-related morning sickness (see chapter six); he waited over a year to get a 359-page document, of which 212 pages were completely redacted (Bruser, McLean, & Mendleson, 2015).

Conclusion

Health Canada has improved the amount of information about various aspects of drug regulation that it releases in some areas, but the *manner* in which it communicates continues to be decidedly non-transparent for multiple possible reasons. Its communications are not timely; it does not explain its decision-making; and when it does, the explanations are vague and contain almost no details. In some areas, such as the regulation of DTCA, Health Canada is almost completely silent and does not evaluate the effectiveness of its communications. This poor record of communication reinforces the industry's ghost-management strategies that Gagnon (in chapter eight) documents, because there is a paucity of other information to challenge what industry is producing.

The Canadian Association of Journalists deemed Health Canada the most secretive of all government departments and, in 2004, awarded Health Canada its fourth annual "Code of Silence" award for showing "remarkable zeal in suppressing information" and "concealing vital data about dangerous drugs" (Kermode-Scott, 2004). Although Health Canada is showing leadership in releasing clinical study reports, in many other aspects of its communication practices that Code of Silence award is still largely deserved.

REFERENCES

Access to Information Act (R.S. 1985, c. A-1). Retrieved from https://laws-lois
   .justice.gc.ca/eng/acts/a-1/
Auditor General of Canada. (2006). *2006 November report of the Auditor General
   of Canada to the House of Commons.* Chapter 8: Allocating funds to regulatory
   programs – Health Canada. Ottawa, ON: Office of the Auditor General of
   Canada. Retrieved from https://www.oag-bvg.gc.ca/internet/English/parl
   _oag_200611_08_e_14976.html
Auditor General of Canada. (2011). *2011 Fall report of the Auditor General of
   Canada to the House of Commons.* Chapter 4: Regulating pharmaceutical
   drugs – Health Canada. Ottawa, ON: Office of the Auditor General of
   Canada. Retrieved from https://www1.oag-bvg.gc.ca/internet/English/parl
   _oag_201111_04_e_35936.html
Bruser, D., & Bailey, A. (2012, 26 September). ADHD drugs suspected of
   hurting Canadian kids. *Toronto Star.* Retrieved from https://www.thestar.com
   /news/canada/2012/09/26/adhd_drugs_suspected_of_hurting_canadian
   _kids.html
Bruser, D., & McLean, J. (2014, 11 September). Canadians kept in dark about
   defective drugs. *Toronto Star.* Retrieved from https://www.thestar.com/news
   /canada/2014/09/11/canadians_kept_in_dark_about_defective_drugs.html
Bruser, D., McLean, J., & Bailey, A. (2014, 26 June). Dangers of off-label drug
   use kept secret. *Toronto Star.* Retrieved from https://www.thestar.com/news
   /canada/2014/06/26/dangers_of_offlabel_drug_use_kept_secret.html

Bruser, D., McLean, J., & Mendleson, R. (2015, April 24). Toronto doctor asks Health Canada about pregnancy drug, gets 212 pages of censored information. *Toronto Star*. Retrieved from https://www.thestar.com/news /canada/2015/04/24/toronto-doctor-asks-health-canada-about-pregnancy -drug-gets-212-pages-of-censored-information.html

CanWest MediaWorks Inc. v. Attorney General of Canada. (2006). Affidavit of Ann Sztuke-Fournier. 05-CV-303001PD2. Ontario Superior Court of Justice. Retrieved from https://whp-apsf.ca/pdf/health_can/HCaffidavitsSztuke -Fournier.pdf

Cocking, C. (1977, June 18). The abuse of prescription drugs. *Weekend Magazine*, 16–19.

Davis, C., & Abraham, J. (2013). *Unhealthy pharmaceutical regulation: Innovation, politics and promissory science*. Basingstoke, UK: Palgrave Macmillan.

Decima Research Inc. (2003). Public opinion survey on key issues pertaining to post-market surveillance of marketed health products in Canada. POR# 298-02. Ottawa, ON: Health Canada.

Government of Canada. (2014). Harper government announces passage of Vanessa's Law – Modernized laws for drugs and medical devices mark a new era in Canadian patient safety. Retrieved from https://www.canada.ca/en/news /archive/2014/11/harper-government-announces-passage-vanessa-law -modernized-laws-drugs-medical-devices-mark-new-era-canadian-patient-safety.html

Habibi, R., & Lexchin, J. (2014). Quality and quantity of information in Summary Basis of Decision documents issued by Health Canada. *PLoS One, 9*(3), e92038. https://doi.org/10.1371/journal.pone.0092038

Health Canada. (2004). Issue analysis summary: Summary Basis of Decision – draft 7. Ottawa, ON: Health Canada.

Health Canada. (2007). Draft guidance document – Triggers for issuance of risk communication documents for marketed health products for human use. Retrieved from http://publications.gc.ca/collections/collection_2007 /hc-sc/H164-48-2007E.pdf

Health Canada. (2012). *Regulatory roadmap for health products and food*. Ottawa, ON: Health Canada. Retrieved from https://www.canada.ca/content/dam /hc-sc/migration/hc-sc/ahc-asc/alt_formats/pdf/activit/mod/roadmap -feuillederoute-eng.pdf

Health Canada. (2015). Consultation on the amendments to the Food and Drugs Act: Guide to new authorities – What we heard. Retrieved from https://www.canada.ca/en/health-canada/services/drugs-health-products /legislation-guidelines/consultation-amendments-food-drugs-act-guide-new -authorities-what-we-heard.html

Health Canada. (2016a). Clinical trial inspection report card summary. Retrieved from https://www.drug-inspections.canada.ca/gcp/fullReportCard -en.html?lang=en&gcpid=4462d630-3d96-4cd1-9365-60e242af6208

Health Canada. (2016b). Guidance document: Notice of compliance with conditions (NOC/c). Ottawa, ON: Health Canada. Retrieved from https://www.canada.ca/content/dam/hc-sc/migration/hc-sc/dhp-mps/alt_formats/pdf/prodpharma/applic-demande/guide-ld/compli-conform/noccg_accd-eng.pdf

Health Canada. (2018a). Public release of clinical information – Stakeholder meetings and engagement activities. Retrieved from https://www.canada.ca/en/health-canada/programs/consultation-public-release-clinical-information-drug-submissions-medical-device-applications/meeting-table.html

Health Canada. (2018b).What we heard: Reponses to the public consultation on the white paper "Public release of information in drug submissions and medical device applications." Retrieved from https://www.canada.ca/en/health-canada/programs/consultation-public-release-clinical-information-drug-submissions-medical-device-applications/what-we-heard.html

Health Canada. (2019). Guidance document on public release of clinical information: Profile page. Retrieved from https://www.canada.ca/en/health|-canada/services/drug-health-product-review-approval/profile-public-release-clinical-information-guidance.html

Health Canada. (2020a). Health product advertising incidents. Retrieved from https://www.canada.ca/en/health-canada/services/drugs-health-products/regulatory-requirements-advertising/health-product-advertising-complaints.html

Health Canada. (2020b). Resource distribution: Drug approvals vs drug safety 2004–2020. Retrieved from https://shpm.info.yorku.ca/files/2020/09/Health-Canada-funding-distribution-2004-2020.pdf

Health Products and Food Branch (HPFB). (2004). Summary report of the inspections of clinical trials conducted in 2003/2004. Ottawa, ON: Health Canada.

Health Products and Food Branch (HPFB). (2009). Guidance for industry: Priority review of drug submissions. Ottawa, ON: Health Canada. Retrieved from https://www.canada.ca/en/health-canada/services/drugs-health-products/drug-products/applications-submissions/guidance-documents/priority-review/drug-submissions.html

Health Products and Food Branch (HPFB). (2014). Final update and response to OAG recommendations for the regulation of pharmaceutical drugs. Retrieved from http://www.hc-sc.gc.ca/ahc-asc/pubs/hpfb-dgpsa/oag-bvg-eng.php

Health Products and Food Branch Inspectorate (HPFBI). (2002). Inspection strategy for clinical trials. Ottawa, ON: Health Canada.

Health Products and Food Branch Inspectorate (HPFBI). (2003). Summary report of the inspections of clinical trials conducted under voluntary phase. Ottawa, ON: Health Canada.

Health Products and Food Branch Inspectorate (HPFBI). (2004). Summary report of the inspections of clinical trials conducted in 2003/2004. Ottawa, ON: Health Canada.

Health Products and Food Branch Inspectorate (HPFBI). (2012a). Summary report of inspections of clinical trials conducted from April 2004 to March 2011. Ottawa, ON: Health Canada. Retrieved from https://www.canada.ca /en/health-canada/services/drugs-health-products/compliance-enforcement /good-clinical-practices/reports/summary-report-inspections-clinical-trials -conducted-april-2004-march-2011.html

Health Products and Food Branch Inspectorate (HPFBI). (2012b). Summary report of the drug good manufacturing practices (GMP) inspection program April 1, 2006 to March 31, 2011. Ottawa, ON: Health Canada.

Herder, M., Gibson, E., Graham, J., Lexchin, J., & Mintzes, B. (2014). Regulating prescription drugs for patient safety: Does Bill C-17 go far enough? *CMAJ, 186*(8), E287–92. https://doi.org/10.1503/cmaj.131850

Innovative Medicines Canada. (2020). Code of ethical practices. Retrieved from http://innovativemedicines.ca/ethics/code-of-ethics/

Kermode-Scott, B. (2004). Canadian health ministry faces criticism for its secrecy. *BMJ, 328,* 1222. https://doi.org/10.1136/bmj.328.7450.1222-f

Kessler, D.A., Rose, J.L., Temple, R.J., Schapiro, R., & Griffin, J.P. (1994). Therapeutic-class wars – Drug promotion in a competitive marketplace. *New England Journal of Medicine, 331,* 1350–3. https://doi.org/10.1056 /NEJM199411173312007

Lexchin, J. (1984). *The real pushers: A critical analysis of the Canadian drug industry.* Vancouver, BC: New Star Books.

Lexchin, J. (2012). New drugs and safety: What happened to new active substances approved in Canada between 1995 and 2010? *Archives of Internal Medicine, 172*(21), 1680–1. https://doi.org/10.1001/archinternmed.2012.4444

Lexchin, J. (2016). *Private profits vs public policy: The pharmaceutical industry and the Canadian state.* Toronto, ON: University of Toronto Press.

Lexchin, J. (2018). Health Canada's use of expedited review pathways and therapeutic innovation, 1995–2016: Cross-sectional analysis. *BMJ Open, 8,* e023605. https://doi.org/10.1136/bmjopen-2018-023605

Lexchin, J. (2019). Health Canada's use of its Notice of Compliance with conditions drug approval policy: A retrospective cohort analysis. *International Journal of Health Services, 49*(2), 294–305. https://doi.org/10.1177 /0020731418821007

Lexchin, J., Herder, M., & Doshi, P. (2019). Canada finally opens up data on new drugs and devices: Other regulators should take note of Health Canada's substantive reforms. *BMJ, 365*(11), i1825. https://doi.org/10.1136/bmj. l1825

Lexchin, J., & Mintzes, B. (2014). A compromise too far: A review of Canadian cases of direct-to-consumer advertising regulation. *International Journal of Risk and Safety in Medicine, 26*(4), 213–25. https://doi.org/10.3233/JRS-140635

Marketed Health Products Directorate (MHPD). (2004). How adverse reaction information on health products is used. Ottawa, ON: Health Canada.

McLean, J., & Bruser, D. (2014a, 16 September). Drug-testing rules broken by Canadian researchers. *Toronto Star*. Retrieved from https://www.thestar.com /news/canada/2014/09/16/drugtesting_rules_broken_by_canadian _researchers.html

McLean, J., & Bruser, D. (2014b, 5 November). Canadian drug companies violating the law. *Toronto Star*. Retrieved from https://www.thestar.com/news /canada/2014/11/04/canadian_drug_companies_violating_the_law.html

Mintzes, B., Morgan, S., & Wright, J.M. (2009). Twelve years' experience with direct-to-consumer advertising of prescription drugs in Canada: A cautionary tale. *PLoS One*, *4*(5), e5699. https://doi.org/10.1371/journal.pone.0005699

Pharmaceutical Advertising Advisory Board (PAAB). (2018). Code of advertising acceptance. Retrieved from http://www.paab.ca/paab-code.htm

Pharmaceutical Advertising Advisory Board (PAAB). (n.d.). Resources: meetings. Retrieved from http://www.paab.ca/resources/category/meetings

Shuchman, M. (2008). Clinical trials regulation – how Canada compares. *CMAJ*, *179*(7), 635–8. https://doi.org/10.1503/cmaj.081271

Standing Senate Committee on Social Affairs, Science and Technology. (2012). *Canada's clinical trial infrastructure: A prescription for improved access to new medicines*. Ottawa, ON. Retrieved from https://sencanada.ca/Content/SEN /Committee/411/soci/rep/rep14nov12-e.pdf

Turner, C. (2012, 28 September). Re: ADHD drugs suspected of hurting Canadian kids, Sept. 26. Letter to the Editor. *Toronto Star*, A22.

8 The Political Economy of Influence: Ghost-Management in the Pharmaceutical Sector

MARC-ANDRÉ GAGNON

Ghost-Managing the Social Determinants of Value

In 2014, TransCanada Corporation (now TC Energy Corporation) pushed for the construction of different pipeline projects, including Keystone XL in the United States and Energy East in Eastern Canada. In November 2014, five strategy documents detailing the communication campaign organized by the public relations firm Edelman to help TransCanada gain social support (and political approval) for Energy East were leaked (Edelman, 2014). The documents called for a budget to recruit 35,000 "activists" supporting the project through "grassroots" advocacy by using social media, especially by paying numerous bloggers and key opinion leaders to defend the interests of TransCanada Corporation. The documents explained how to transform public opinion and the economic preferences of the population by creating the illusion that a mass movement in favour of the pipeline existed. One of the five leaked documents even elucidated that it is necessary to take some lessons from the Keystone XL, where the industry mobilized a million activists and generated more than 500,000 pro-Keystone comments during the public comment period. The leaked documents pointed out:

> It's not just associations or advocacy groups building these programs in support of the industry. Companies like ExxonMobil, Chevron, Shell and Halliburton (and many more) have all made key investments in building permanent advocacy assets and programs to support their lobbying, outreach and policy efforts. (Goldenberg, 2014)

The documents also indicated the need to pressure opponents of Energy East: "Add layers of difficulty for our opponents, distracting them from their mission and causing them to redirect their resources"

(Goldenberg, 2014). The idea was to create spurious issues forcing opponents to divert their resources to irrelevant matters. Documents also indicated the need to build partnerships with universities in order to produce scientific claims about the low environmental risks of the projects.

The leaked documents are of great interest because they show how important it is for companies to invest not only in their public image but also in their capacity to shape the social debates surrounding their industry by expending vast amounts of resources to influence public opinion, media, and science in favour of specific corporate interests. The production of influence over social structures seems to be a central component for projects' commercial success. Note that it does not matter if the project is a good one or not: if the project is "good" for the community as a whole, the company still needs to invest massive resources to convince a sceptical population of its value. If the project is "bad" because risks are being externalized to the community, a good communication campaign can potentially make the project socially acceptable in spite of the externalized risks.

The capacity of a company to build profit depends not only on the production of value (the production of social wealth for the community) but also on its ability to influence and shape habits of thought in the community in line with its interests. A dominant firm needs to produce not only value but also what we could call the *social determinants* of that value. In many industrial sectors, a firm without the capacity to shape social structures and habits of thought in favour of its interests is unlikely to enter or remain among the dominant companies of corporate capitalism, such as getting into or staying in the Fortune 500 (the list of the 500 largest global companies).

What would happen if dominant corporations like TransCanada were not able to invisibly "ghost-shape" the social determinants of value? Their market value might simply collapse. Following the works of Thorstein Veblen, one should consider the possibility that what dominant corporations capitalize is partly their power to directly or indirectly shape the societal structures and habits of thought. The capacity to shape social determinants of value and habits of thought seems pivotal in industrial sectors where risk assessment is central to determining the corporate earning capacity: from oil and gas, tobacco, food and beverages, chemicals, or pharmaceuticals, ghost-shaping of the social determinants has become a central issue on which little attention has been devoted. In the case of pharmaceuticals, the behind-the-scenes strategies deployed by corporations to maximize earnings seem to have become the central activity of most dominant drug companies.

Building on a concept developed by Sismondo (2007, 2018), this chapter explores what we could call the "ghost-management" of the economy. The chapter focuses on the pharmaceutical sector. One can argue that, beyond the political economy of production and distribution, we find a *political economy of influence* in which dominant interests invest significant resources to influence and reshape social structures according to their interests. In more theoretical terms, the questions of importance are twofold: What is being capitalized by pharmaceutical companies? And how can we understand the nature of capital accumulation when investments are aimed more at transforming habits of thought and social structures than at producing therapeutically significant products? By analysing how ghost-management has become central to drug companies' earning capacity, it becomes possible to better understand how transparency could play a role in defusing opportunities for dominant pharmaceutical companies to maximize their gains in ways that can harm communities and patients.

The hidden nature of this political economy of influence also brings to the forefront the issue of transparency as a potential tool to better understand the ways and means of ghost-management in a corporate sector. What needs to be made transparent? What should be the objectives for transparency? By identifying the main strategies used by pharmaceutical companies for ghost-managing their earning capacity, it becomes easier to understand when, how, and why these strategies might not align with what is desirable for communities and patients. By better understanding ghost-management, we can also better understand how and why policies to improve transparency can help to restrain corporate strategies that might increase corporate earnings by creating harms and risks for communities and patients.

Building on the works of Thorstein Veblen and Sergio Sismondo, this chapter analyses the different types of corporate strategies for ghost-managing the social determinants of value in the pharmaceutical sector. After discussing how we need to rethink the nature of profit and capital accumulation, the chapter provides a quick overview of different ways corporations influence and shape habits of thought through various forms of capture, from scientific to regulatory. With each type of capture, the chapter analyses the role transparency could take to allow a better understanding of the ongoing dynamics at play. While the chapter emphasizes that a tangible understanding of corporate capitalism must systematically include an analysis of corporations' ghost-management of the social determinants of value, it shows that such an understanding becomes impossible without specific tools and policies that improve transparency over existing corporate practices in the pharmaceutical sector.

Rethinking Capital Accumulation

Interestingly, the analysis of how corporations capitalize their social power over the community is absent from dominant economic analysis. According to contemporary mainstream microeconomics textbooks, the capital of companies is assumed to be the means of production, which produces social wealth, and the profit of capital is assumed to be the result of the social wealth produced by these companies. From there, we find another economic assumption: maximizing profits necessarily maximizes the social wealth of a community. The dominant economic theory acknowledges that monopolistic capacities can exist, but it is considered an exception to the rule, and the revenues obtained this way are called "rents" instead of "profits."

Thorstein Veblen was the first scholar to analyse the co-production of value and its social determinants by distinguishing the earning capacity of the businessman[1] and the social productivity of the industry (Veblen, 1996, 1908a, 1908b). For Veblen, capital is a pecuniary concept that relates to the predatory world of the businessman. The latter maximizes his earning capacity not by increasing his productivity but by maximizing his control over the community, mostly through strategies of sabotage and by reshaping habits of thought and social structures (Gagnon, 2007).

Analysing the early twentieth century American economy, Veblen contended that knowledge and technology have always been the main productive economic assets of a community (Veblen, 1908a). Veblen also analysed the ways and means of industrial control by business interests during the era he called the "New Order."[2] He considers that control over industrial knowledge, and over the material means to put this knowledge to use, constitutes the core of capital's earning capacity as a form of control over the community. From a Veblenian point of view, capitalism's contemporary transformations should not be viewed in terms of new forms of productivity but, instead, in terms of the new ways and means for business interests to extend their control over the knowledge and technology of a community.

Businessmen do not participate in production, but rather develop control over the collective capacity of production (including technological knowledge) and thereby gain an upper hand on political power and on the population's habits of thought. Businessmen's motives are not to maximize production, but to maximize pecuniary gains through pecuniary transactions of buying and selling. In fact, their pecuniary interests are better served by restraining production and artificially creating scarcity. For Veblen, business practices are thus predatory practices of industrial sabotage, and the business trade must be considered not as a positive or zero-sum game but as a negative-sum game (Veblen, 2002, pp. 54–5): "[This state of affairs] has some analogy with the phenomena of blackmail, ransom and any similar enterprise that aims to get something for nothing." The businessman interferes in strategic interstices of the industrial system, and depending upon its sabotage capacity, he can reclaim a more or less important ransom, which could be understood in contemporary economic theory as a monopolistic rent.

This logic applies particularly well to the pharmaceutical sector. The blackmail capacity of a drug company owning a patent monopoly over a life-saving drug is obviously of huge magnitude. For example, with only one product for a very rare disease, Alexion Pharmaceuticals managed to rank 314th among the world's largest corporations in terms of market value in 2015; its chief executive officer (CEO), Leonard Bell, was the highest paid CEO of the pharmaceutical industry in 2014, with a total compensation of US$196 million. The earning capacity of the company is completely disproportional to its therapeutic contribution to the community. Any such earning capacity with no equivalent counterpart in terms of wealth creation to the community is what Veblen calls the "intangible assets" of the corporation.

For Veblen, "intangible assets" comprise not only the direct and indirect predatory means to restrain production but also any institutional settings or social structures that provide earning capacities to business concerns. They can be "habits of life settled by usage, convention, arrogation, legislative action or what not" (1908b, p. 116); or "preferential use of certain facts of human nature – habits, propensities, beliefs, aspirations and necessities" (Veblen 1908b, p. 123). Veblen goes further (1901, p. 223): "Whatever ownership touches, and whatever affords ground for pecuniary discretion, may be turned to account for pecuniary gain and may therefore be comprised in the aggregate of pecuniary capital." Capital is not only an instrument for sabotage; it is any dimension of human life that can translate into higher earnings for businesses.

For Veblen, the capitalized value of a corporation rests upon the control over the community that the owned asset secures, be it in the sphere of production or distribution. If this intangible control is direct (for example, through advertising to manipulate the desires and habits of the common man), the control is first and foremost structural, and rests on established social structures and habits of thought. The example of Pfizer illustrates this point: Pfizer's market value of US$257 billion (as of January 2019) depends not on its productivity but primarily on its capacity to restrain others' production through patent monopolies. This capacity is not based on direct power to compel the population to act a certain way; instead, it is based on the fact that the community accepts the legitimacy of the current regime of intellectual property rights, without which Pfizer's market value would collapse.

With Veblen, one should consider that the organization of the economy has to be understood as *the design of dominant interests shaping the social structures according to their own interests.* Thus, any institutional reality can be capitalized, be it social, legal, political, cultural, psychological, religious, technical, or anything else that can grant an earning capacity, any capacity for vested interests to gain something for nothing. In other words, a successful communication campaign that would increase the profits on pharmaceutical products to the detriment of the community is capitalized by the company as much as its control over strategic means of production. Veblen (1997, p. 191) puts it this way: "It is always sound business to take any obtainable net gain, at any cost and at any risk to the rest of the community."

Capital infiltrates the social structures in every interstice to obtain differential earning capacities. By defining capital as capitalized putative earning capacity without reference to productivity, Veblen integrates power – any institutional form of power – in the economy. From this perspective, political economy would provide greater insight on the real dynamics of capitalism if it focused on the dynamics of corporate power and control over the social structures and the community in general, and on the means corporations use to (ghost)manage the development of their influence over the community.

Ghost-Managing the Social Determinants of Value

While the works by Thorstein Veblen are full of rich insights to understand the nature and evolution of corporate capitalism, his works remains a bit dated and challenging to use as a coherent analytical framework. A hundred years later, it is necessary to refine the analysis of how corporations build intangible assets and maximize market value by transforming social structures according to their interests. This section suggests that the corporate strategies used to influence social structures in order to maximize market value can be broken down into different categories.

Miller and Harkins (2010) identified four main corporate strategies to create intangible assets in the food and alcohol industry: science capture, media capture, civil society capture, and policy capture. My own empirical work has focused on the pharmaceutical sector, and I have expanded the categories developed by Miller and Harkins into seven categories in order to have a more comprehensive framework to analyse the political economy of influence in the pharmaceutical sector (Gagnon, 2016): these seven forms of capture are scientific, professional, technological, regulatory, market, media, and civil society. Note that Carpenter and Moss (2014) consider that capture prevails by degrees (strong or weak capture) rather than by its presence or absence. The word "capture" is used to describe attempts to capture elements of these categories by different corporate strategies of influence. The categories' suggested aim is to better understand the imperceptible political economy of influence that is constitutive of the contemporary dynamics of capital accumulation in the pharmaceutical sector.

Scientific Capture

Attempts to capture science by corporate interests are increasingly documented (Krimsky, 2004; Mooney, 2006; McGarity & Wagner, 2008; Matheson, 2008; Michaels, 2008; Wiist, 2010; Mirowski, 2011; Gøtzsche, 2013; Sismondo, 2018). The social authority of scientific discourse makes science an excellent target to shape the social determinants of value. The pharmaceutical sector effectively demonstrates the need to capture science in different ways. A new drug can gain financial success only if it is possible to convince prescribers about the product's benefits and the low risks associated with the product. Ghostwriting has become a usual strategy for scientific capture in the medical literature (US Senate Committee on Finance, 2010a; Lacasse & Leo, 2010). The extent of ghostwriting at play goes beyond the basic issue of plagiarism. The notion of "ghost-management" was developed to show the extent of the use of ghostwriting and refers to a whole system of management behind closed doors used to influence scientific results in favour of corporate interests (Sismondo, 2007; Sismondo & Doucet, 2010; Gagnon, 2012). I explain elsewhere that corporate influence over medical science is normally based on three different strategies: (1) inflating the number of favourable scientific publications; (2) suppressing the scientific results that could harm sales; and (3) neutralizing independent academics and whistle-blowers (Gagnon, 2012).

Many studies found in medical journals are written by ghostwriters or medical writing agencies paid for by drug companies. These publications form part of carefully thought-out publication plans that are essential to the success of promotional campaigns and the market launch of a new drug (Sismondo, 2009). For example, internal documents from Pfizer revealed that, between 1998 and 2000, the company directly initiated the writing of at least 85 scientific articles on the antidepressant drug sertraline (Zoloft). During this period, the entire scientific literature on this active substance consisted of only 211 articles (Sismondo, 2007). In this way, Pfizer produced a raft of articles showing the drug in a positive light, lessening the impact of the critical studies. In the same way, Wyeth (now owned by Pfizer) generated about 50 articles in favour of hormone replacement therapy (Fugh-Berman, 2010). Merck developed a ghost-writing campaign to promote its now-infamous drug rofecoxib (Vioxx): 96 articles were published, some of which omitted to mention patient deaths in the drug's clinical trials (Ross, Hill, Egilman, & Krumholz, 2008). GlaxoSmithKline ran a secret campaign to skew the literature in favour of its antidepressant drug paroxetine (Paxil). The campaign was called "Case Study Publication for Peer-Review," or CASPPER for short, in reference to the well-known "friendly ghost" (Edwards, 2009).

The second strategy is to restrain the disclosure of unfavourable results. Pharmaceutical companies consider that private-sector clinical research produces private, confidential results as part of their intellectual property. They assume the right not to publish certain results in the name of trade secrecy. Because they are not compelled by political and health authorities to make public the data obtained in clinical trials, drug companies can select what data they want to see published (Goldacre, 2013). Pharmaceutical companies not only selectively produce data about their products but they also selectively produce ignorance about the same products.

For example, major pharmaceutical companies have systematically failed to publish unfavourable studies on the "new generation" of antidepressants, known as selective serotonin reuptake inhibitors (SSRIs). Of the seventy-four clinical trials that were conducted on these antidepressants, thirty-eight produced positive results, while the other thirty-six showed the drugs to have questionable or no efficacy. However, while 94 per cent of the positive studies were published, only 8 per cent of the unfavourable studies were published as negative results, and 15 per cent of the negative studies were published in terms that suggested the results were positive (Turner, Matthews, Linardatos, Tell, & Rosenthal, 2008). Doctors reading the scientific literature got a biased view of the "benefits" of SSRIs, which explains why they so readily and systematically prescribed these antidepressants to their patients. The scientific data show that for 70 per cent of the patients taking SSRI antidepressants, the drug is no more effective than a placebo (Fournier et al., 2010), but unlike a placebo, SSRIs are associated with serious adverse effects (for example, an increased risk of suicide). It is fair to argue that the selective production of ignorance has become constitutive of how pharmaceutical companies do science today.

A third strategy is to intimidate and neutralize independent researchers who produce studies that show the product in an unfavourable light. For example, Merck's internal emails, which came out during lawsuits over the harm caused by its drug rofecoxib (Vioxx), revealed that the company had drawn up a hit list of "rogue" researchers who had criticized Vioxx. One email recommended that the researchers on the hit list had to be "discredited" and "neutralized." "Seek them out and destroy them where they live" read one of the emails. This intimidation was the result of the work of an entire team that systematically monitored everything said about the product (Rout, 2009). Similarly, in the case of the anti-diabetic drug rosiglitazone (Avandia), which was withdrawn from the market in 2010 for safety reasons, a report by the US Senate explained that the main strategy of GlaxoSmithKline executives when confronted with the publication of negative clinical results was to downplay the importance of these results and to intimidate independent researchers (US Senate Committee of Finance, 2010b). In Canada, the long *Report of the Committee of Inquiry on the Case Involving Dr. Nancy Olivieri* (Thompson, Baird, & Downie, 2001) depicts in detail how Dr. Olivieri's reputation was systematically attacked and discredited after blowing the whistle on the undisclosed adverse effects of deferiprone, on which Dr. Olivieri was running clinical trials for the company Apotex.

It is important to understand that, in a sector like pharmaceuticals, these strategies are no exception: a company that would refrain from these strategies in the name of ethics would simply lose their market share (Gagnon, 2013). If profits are affected by the scientific literature about the risks of the product (be it for pharmaceuticals, tobacco, genetically modified organisms [GMOs], sugar, pipelines, and so on), it is more than likely that dominant corporations in the sector will deploy strategies to capture science in order to build their intangible assets.

Professional Capture

Beyond scientific capture, it is important to understand that many companies deploy additional strategies to capture the technical experts of a specific sector, like engineers or health-care professionals. It is important to differentiate this strategy from scientific capture, since it has sometimes very little to do with science and more to do with promotional campaigns. In the United States, while the pharmaceutical industry spent US$24 billion in research and development in 2004, it spent US$58 billion in promotional campaigns (Gagnon & Lexchin, 2008), of which US$54 billion was spent targeting health-care professionals, including US$43 billion spent specifically targeting physicians. This figure represents an average promotional spending of US$61,000 per physician annually to influence their prescribing habits. In addition to standard promotion, the data collected through the Physician Payments Sunshine

Act in the United States about the disclosure of financial relationships between drug and medical device companies and physicians showed that drug manufacturers directly paid US$9.35 billion to 627,000 physicians in 2018, which represents a yearly average of US$15,000 per physician (Chen, Cortez, & Wayne, 2014).

The investment in professional capture in the pharmaceutical sector is financially greater than anything being invested in research and development. In other words, the main activity of drug companies is not to produce drugs; it is to produce and control narratives shaping medical knowledge in a way that favours their interests. The production of the social determinants of value (medical knowledge and social demand for drugs) is much more important here than producing value (the drugs). "Key opinion leaders" and promotional campaigns geared towards professionals have the capacity to shape expert opinion and influence professionals on controversial issues. Professional capture thus seems central to developing intangible assets in specific industrial sectors.

Technological Capture

The notion of technological capture is important when considering that the dominant corporations in many sectors are the driving engines of technological change in the context of important technological path dependency. Core companies often compete to establish the technological standards in their sector or to develop patent portfolios to increase their bargaining capacity against competitors. In two books, *Inventing the Electronic Century* (Chandler, 2001) and *Shaping the Industrial Century* (Chandler, 2005), Alfred D. Chandler provides a conceptual approach that allows us to interpret the dynamics for the technological capture of a sector. Chandler's basic idea is that the competitive strength of industrial firms in market economies rests on *learned organizational capabilities*:

> In modern industrial economies, the large enterprise performs its critical role in the evolution of industries not merely as a unit carrying out transactions on the basis of flows of information, but, more important, as a creator and repository of product-related embedded organizational knowledge. (Chandler, 2005, p. 6)

In a new industrial sector, for example, the *first movers* are the first enterprises to develop an integrated set of capabilities essential to commercialize the new products in volume for national or world markets. They benefit from their integrated capabilities, which become their learning bases to develop their control of the networks of production and distribution, to improve existing products and processes or to adapt to new conditions, such as those of war or depression. This way, the first movers, and those who in some way manage to catch up for their late arrival in the industry, become "core companies," or dominant firms, that set the technological direction in which the whole industry evolves:

> The concentrated power of technical, often proprietary, and functional knowledge embedded in the first movers' integrated learning bases is such that a relatively small number of enterprises define the evolving paths of learning in which the products of new technical knowledge are commercialized for widespread public consumption. The barriers to entry thus prevent startups from creating effective integrated learning bases essential to compete in the industry. (Chandler, 2005, p. 9)

These dynamics are evident in the pharmaceutical sector, in which most startup companies cannot even consider competing with core companies and live only in the hope of being acquired by a core company (Economist, 2014).

Furthermore, because patents make technical knowledge proprietary, developing technical capacity often takes the form of "kicking away the ladder" for smaller companies who would like to enter a market. In fact, the race for patents has become a race for strategic patenting, consisting of patenting as many elements as possible in their broadest scope, in order to provide patent holders greater potential rights over future innovations. Such patent portfolios allow the construction of "patent thickets," or "patent gridlocks" (Heller, 2008a), which are barriers to entry based on the threat of patent litigations against any new competitors. As such, patents are used in business sectors as a barrier to entry and restraint on competition rather than an incentive to innovate.

In the pharmaceutical sector, technological capture can often take the form of evergreening strategies to extend patents and protection over existing drugs. For example, 78 per cent of the drugs associated with new patents in the United States were not new drugs, but existing ones (Feldman, 2018). For example, AbbVie secured more than 100 patents for its drug adalimumab (Humira) alone (Edney, 2019). Patents not only create barriers to entry to competitors once the product is on the market; they can also hinder innovation. For example, while patents can increase revenues for specific drug companies, they can also stifle innovation as a whole. Peter Ringrose, former chief science officer at Bristol Myers Squibb, claimed that his company would not investigate some fifty potential cancer-causing proteins because patent holders would either decline to cooperate or demand large royalties (quoted in Heller, 2008b). Two

Nobel laureates, Joseph Stiglitz and John Sulston, have concluded that, because of the intellectual property regime, medical research is "hindered by out-of-date laws" and that obstructive patents on genes and medical techniques can in fact "impede innovation, lead to monopolization, and unduly restrict access to the benefits of knowledge" (quoted in Jenkins & Henderson, 2008). In fact, in order to foster therapeutic innovation in the medical sciences, some academic research centres now embrace open science and refuse to patent their discoveries (Gold, 2016).

When doing research in a sector ruled by patents, an important share of the cost of innovation involves the assembly of dispersed bits of intellectual property and the acquisition of necessary licenses. Nicholas Naclerio, former head of the BioChip Division at Motorola, has suggested that the surge in biotech patenting did not bring about therapeutic innovation but "a bewildering web of lawsuits – and it may only get worse." He continued: "If we want to make a medical diagnostic with 40 genes on it, and 20 companies hold patents on those genes, we may have a big problem. It isn't at all clear how this is going to work out" (quoted in Gibbs, 2001). Heller and Eisenberg (1998, p. 698) define such underuse of a resource, when multiple owners each have a right to exclude others from that scarce resource, the "Tragedy of the Anticommons." For Heller (2008a), such examples show that, if everyone invests in the litigation process, innovation is tossed aside, gridlock sets in, and many lose out – except the dominant patent holders restraining innovation.

In the United States, in May 2019, Senators John Cornyn (Rep) and Richard Blumenthal (Dem) proposed legislation that would give the Federal Trade Commission greater power against patent thickets in the pharmaceutical industry. In his colourful language, Senator Blumenthal synthesized what technological capture through patent thickets could mean in the pharmaceutical sector: "Using practices that would make the robber barons of the Gilded Age blush, Big Pharma has crushed competition and stifled access to cheaper generic drugs to squeeze billions out of families, businesses and the government" (quoted in Edney, 2019). For dominant pharmaceutical companies selling brand-name drugs, intellectual property rights like patents or data exclusivity are central to their earning capacity, and they will do everything they can to preserve market exclusivity. Using the appropriation of technical knowledge through patent portfolios, technological capture is a central intangible asset in the pharmaceutical sector.

Regulatory Capture

Following Carpenter and Moss (2014, p. 13), regulatory capture can be defined as "the result or process by which regulation, in law or application, is consistently or repeatedly directed away from the public interest and towards the interests of the regulated industry, by the intent or action of the industry itself." In the political economy of influence, influencing laws and regulations are key objectives for many companies. An obvious way in which corporations invest in influencing policy-makers is through lobbying on their own account or via heavyweight trade associations. According to the Center for Responsive Politics, based on data from the Senate Office of Public Records, the number of lobbyists at the federal level in the United States (Congress and federal agencies) was 11,652 in 2018, and total declared spending on lobbying was US$3.45 billion. The pharmaceutical sector ranked as the top lobbying industry in 2018, with declared spending of US$282 million, followed by the insurance sector (US$158 million), and electronics (US$147 million) (Center for Responsive Politics, 2020).

Since the Citizens United decision by the US Supreme Court in 2010, corporations are allowed to spend as much as they want to convince people to vote for or against a political candidate. According to the 5 to 4 Supreme Court decision, if the funds are not being spent in coordination with a political campaign, they "do not give rise to corruption or the appearance of corruption." Following the decision, independent expenditure-only committees (also called super political action committees [PACs]) were created to raise unlimited sums of money to overtly advocate for or against political candidates (see chapter two in this volume). In 2012, super PACs amassed US$828 million. For many, such political funding can be compared to open forms of corruption (Lessig, 2011).

In addition to direct lobbying, revolving doors (White, 2005) and ubiquitous conflicts of interests in government and academia should also be considered as important means of regulatory capture. For example, a growing literature describes how private interests manage to shape public law, especially in the case of international trade agreements (Drahos & Braithwaite, 2002; Sell, 2003; Brunelle, 2007; Lexchin & Gagnon, 2013). The pharmaceutical sector counted 1,021 revolving door lobbyists (industry lobbyists who previously worked with government). It is the industry with the most revolving door lobbyists, followed by electronics (828), and general manufacturing and distribution (677) (Center for Responsive Politics, 2020). While this chapter cannot review all strategies and dimensions of regulatory capture, it seems evident that such strategies are a central feature in the accumulation of intangible assets for dominant corporations.

Market Capture

The category of market capture, already analysed by Thorstein Veblen, refers to any capacity for corporations to develop market power or restrain market competition. The building of monopolistic capacity through cartel agreements, mergers and acquisitions, cooperation agreements, or through specific forms of corporate structures (trusts, holdings, conglomerates) are the main elements that could be included under this category.

Cartels abounded in the 1930s, but declined after the Second World War. From 1955 to 1985, the US Department of Justice discovered only a few cases of international price-fixing agreements, including a case of price fixing in antibiotics, and between 1985 and 1994, no cases were discovered. Since 1994, a cartel revival has been observable as twenty international cartels were found. Two of those cartels were in pharmaceutical products: one in lysine (an essential amino acid), which managed to increase world prices by 70 per cent on that substance, and another in vitamins (Connor, 2008). In fact, it was the discovery of the cartel in lysine that brought antitrust authorities to open investigations in other sectors. The investigations of the lysine cartel revealed how easy it was to organize a price-fixing agreement, and it created a public uproar by exposing the sharp disdain such firms had for their customers. For example, in an FBI tape of one session of the cartel, ADM's president and lysine cartel leader, James Randall, explains: "We have a saying in our company: our competitors are our friends, our customers are the enemy" (Gagnon, 2009).

Such "traditional" price-fixing agreements remain illegal according to competition policies in most industrialized countries: they are normally prosecuted by law, and should not be considered central within the structure of corporate capitalism. However, other strategies, like mergers and acquisitions, or cooperation agreements, are central to market capture. With more than US$2.5 trillion in deals announced worldwide, 2018 became a record year for corporate mergers and acquisitions (Grocer, 2018). Mergers and acquisitions are a typical case of goodwill creation that does not increase production capacity. For example, in the case of pharmaceuticals, mergers and acquisitions are often used to slash spending in research and development. As the *Economist* (2014) explained, "some in Wall Street see pharma research as value-destroying and an obvious target for cuts." In a nutshell, the destruction of innovation capacity in the pharmaceutical sector is considered to be an excellent way to build the intangible assets for the shareholders.

Collaboration agreements between companies are becoming very important, especially in knowledge-based sectors. In the pharmaceutical sector, it was found that, among the sixteen largest pharmaceutical companies worldwide, at least eighty-two collaboration agreements existed in 2008, which means that each dominant firm had on average more than ten cooperation agreements with other dominant firms (Gagnon, 2009).

In 2017, by using the Cortellis database,[3] it was possible to identify 296 collaboration agreements between the thirteen largest companies. The result is that the sector is organized less like a competitive market and more like a network of cooperation. Market competition in the pharmaceutical sector becomes an elusive concept when compared to the reality of organized systematic cooperation. While there is no official cartel agreement, we find ourselves confronted with the multiplication of quasi-cartel agreements, which results in the same consequence – increased monopolistic capacities as a form of intangible assets.

Media Capture

Media can play an important role in creating intangible assets, as is detailed in the leaked communication plan for TransCanada Corporation (TC Energy). It can play a direct role in lobbying and policy-making, as it provides a capacity to connect with public opinion and elite opinion, and it can help to target and destroy industry critics (Miller & Harkins, 2010). Literature on media institutions and processes accounts for the different mechanisms by which media are influenced and captured by corporate interests. Such mechanisms include advertising, public relations, influence of media ownership, and attacks on critics (McChesney, 2008).

In the United States, annual spending in pharmaceutical direct-to-consumer advertising went from US$1.3 billion in 1997 to US$6 billion in 2016, and the number of television commercials increased almost tenfold in the same period (Schwartz & Woloshin, 2019). Experts in corporate public relations (PR) are becoming more and more active in shaping the news concerning corporate interests. It is estimated that, for every working journalist in the United States, there are now 4.6 PR people, up from 3.2 a decade ago (Edgecliffe-Johnson, 2014). A report from the United Kingdom estimated that 41 per cent of press articles and 52 per cent of broadcast news items contain PR materials that play an agenda-setting role or make up the bulk of the story (Lewis, Williams, Franklin, Thomas, & Mosdell, 2008).

Miller and Dinan (2009) emphasized a neglected dimension of media capture by analysing the use and role of media in securing regulatory capture through the sophisticated use of seemingly independent organizations as echo chambers for corporate messages or through direct attempts to take over the means of communication. Many think tanks presenting themselves as independent non-profit organizations act as lobbying organizations for their corporate funders. Miller and Harkins (2010) describe the example of the Social Issues Research Centre (SIRC), an "independent non-profit organization" producing "balanced" research on lifestyle issues such as drinking, diet, and phar-maceuticals. The "social scientists" staffing the SIRC also work for the market research company MCM Research, whose website used to ask: "Do your PR initiatives sometimes look too much like PR initiatives? MCM conducts social/psychological research on the positive aspects of your business. The results do not read like PR literature, or like market research data. Our reports are credible, interesting and entertaining in their own right. This is why they capture the imagination of the media and your customers" (quoted in Ferriman, 1999).

The line between journalism and lobbying is becoming quite blurred, especially in the era of the internet and social media. Confessore (2003) calls the massive lobbying disguised as journalism "journo-lobbying":

> Lobbying firms that once specialized in gaining person-to-person access to key decision-makers have branched out. The new game is to dominate the entire intellectual environment in which officials make policy decisions, which means funding everything from think tanks to issue ads to phony grassroots pressure groups. But the institution that most affects the intellec-tual atmosphere in Washington, the media, has also proven the hardest for K Street to influence – until now. (Confessore, 2003, p. 32)

Civil Society Capture

Civil society refers here to charities, non-governmental organizations, trade unions, social movements, and other groups. The technique of creating front groups (sometimes called astroturf organizations) has a long history in the era of corporate capitalism (Miller & Dinan, 2008). Some companies, like Pfizer, are known to be very proactive in develop-ing means to capture civil society (Drahos & Braithwaite, 2002). Pfizer has prioritized the funding and creation of think tanks all over the world. Former Reagan administration official, Catherine Windels, was in charge of "Worldwide Policy Mobilization at Pfizer" and is sometimes described as the "godmother of think tanks" (Powerbase, 2010). During her twenty-two-year career at Pfizer, she helped create new think tanks and networks of think tanks in Europe, Canada, Africa, and Asia, and worked closely with many leading institutes in the United States. Among other positions, she is the former secretary treasurer of the very influen-tial Fraser Institute in Canada.

However, the creation of front groups for lobbying purposes is only one technique to capture civil society. Many grassroots organizations in civil society can be captured or influenced by corporate groups, espe-cially when they rely on corporate grants to fund their activities. In the pharmaceutical sector, patient groups can play a key role to get a drug approved and reimbursed by insurers at very high prices. Most patient groups are not created by drug companies, but they often rely on corporate donations to fund their activity. Not surprisingly, they often end up defending the interests of drug companies in spite of claims that their funding does not influence their discourse (Batt, 2017). Note that it is likely these groups did not change their discourse because of their funding. However, one must consider that drug companies will only fund groups who have already embraced the "right" discourse in order to make sure that this "patient voice" has more impact than others in the regulatory debates.

Some companies like GlaxoSmithKline (GSK), Novartis, Roche, and Genentech (now a subsidiary of Roche) detail their financial grants to different charities and patient groups in the United States. According to its website, GlaxoSmithKline (2017a) distributed US$29.4 million to US-based non-profit organizations in 2017. Novartis (2020) spent US$20.4 million on patient organizations in the United States in 2017. Hoffmann-La Roche (2020) disclosed that it gave US$25.5 million to patient organizations in the United States in 2018, and Genentech (2020) paid US$58 million in grants and donations to patient groups and independent medical education initiatives. If the funding pattern of GSK, Novartis, Roche, and Genentech is representative of other companies, and considering that these companies jointly represented 14.3 per cent of the total US$952.5 billion global prescription drug markets in 2018 (Pharmaceutical Technology, 2019), we can estimate that drug companies spent almost a billion USD ($932 million) in grants to patient groups and education in the United States in 2017.

In Canada, in the context of discussions about implementing a national pharmacare, GSK funded patient groups specifically "in project funding to increase the role of the patient voice in the discussion on National Pharmacare" (GSK, 2016) or for advocacy boot camps to train patient advocates in order "to get access to the right treatment at the right time for the right individual" (GSK, 2017b). In many ways, patient organizations have become a central part of the communication strategies used by Big Pharma (McCoy, 2018).

Let the Sun Shine In: Transparency against Ghost-Management

The use of seven categories of capture to analyse intangible assets in the pharmaceutical sector allows us to understand how pervasive corporate power is becoming in the shaping of the social structures in which we live. The ghost-management of the economy is not a secondary matter that can be analysed at the margin. Remember that, in the case of the pharmaceutical sector, drug companies spent around US$66.2 billion in research and development (R&D) in 2017 according to statistics compiled by the Organisation for Economic Co-operation and Development (OECD).[4] The analysis of science capture showed that an important part of this sum is in fact invested in strategies to manage R&D as promotional campaigns. Furthermore, according to our analysis, the US pharmaceutical industry spends around US$54 billion every year in promotional campaigns towards health-care professionals for their products, US$8.4 billion in direct payment to physicians, US$6 billion in direct-to-consumer advertising, US$228 million in lobbying policy-makers, and US$932 million in funding charities and patient groups. Our analysis thus shows that pharmaceutical companies are in fact spending more resources in ghost-management strategies than they spend on research and development. Additional resources are also being spent in different ways to capture the media, technology, or markets. The production of Veblenian intangible assets through the ghost-management of the social determinants of value can thus be understood as the main driving engine for capital accumulation in this sector. Control of ideas, knowledge, habits of thought, and narratives have become central to how dominant corporations thrive in corporate capitalism, in pharmaceuticals or in other industrial sectors. Mapping this political economy of influence by identifying the mechanisms of how dominant interests are ghost-managing the economy is a necessary first step to better understand the dynamics of corporate power in our society. This task is where transparency can be a useful tool to better map these dynamics at work. Transparency is certainly not a miracle remedy to counteract the forces of corporate capitalism, but it can help improve some aspects of research in health and social science to better identify the methods used by corporations to increase their earning capacity through dubious means. In the case of pharmaceuticals, transparency could play a significant role across different types of capture. In particular, transparency could be helpful to better map scientific capture, professional capture, regulatory capture, and civil society capture.

In the case of scientific capture, many corporate strategies focus on selectively producing ignorance through non-disclosure of clinical trial data. Allowing complete transparency of clinical trial data (for example, by making registration in a data repository like clinicaltrials.gov mandatory) would allow researchers to access clinical trial data and monitor what is being said about the products. Researchers could in this way better identify risks about these products and flag misleading claims made about some products. In the case of professional capture, a "physician payments sunshine act" can go a long way to identify material means used by drug companies to influence prescribing habits. The correlation between payments received by physicians and prescribing habits is still unclear, but many studies using open payments databases seem to show that there is a clear positive relationship between the two (see, for example, Carlat, 2014; Yeh, Franklin, Avorn, Landon, & Kesselheim, 2016; Hadland, Rivera-Aguirre, Marshall, & Cerdá, 2019). Is correlation between payments and prescribing habits always positive for all products and all types of specialties? Are the prescribing habits improving or not in terms of risks, benefits, and costs? Without transparency, research cannot be conducted on these questions.

In the case of regulatory capture, transparency can also play a role by identifying lobbying expenditures and listing all encounters between lobbyists and policy-makers. Again, transparency would not be a cure for regulatory capture, but it would open a window to better understand the dynamics at play. Finally, in the case of civil society capture, transparency over grants and gifts could allow a better understanding of the relationship between drug companies and different charities, specifically by identifying patient groups financed by the industry. A systematic application of transparency over these types of relationships could allow more productive consultations with patient groups over public policy issues by better weighting expertise over financial interests (Biossé-Duplan, 2015).

Again, transparency is no panacea in eliminating these different types of capture. However, transparency would allow health policy analysts and social scientists to better understand the political economy of influence at work in order to develop efficient proposals to help reduce the negative effects of these types of capture. Unveiling corporate strategies of social control is a necessary step, but it is not enough. Citizens must also develop their own strategies to efficiently oppose this ubiquitous corporate power in our society. In order to develop such strategies, transparency is certainly one of the main tools that we can put in our toolbox.

NOTES

1 This chapter uses the terms "businessman" or "common man" instead of gender neutral terms only because it is the terminology used by Thorstein Veblen.
2 By the term "New Order," Veblen (1997) refers to the new business order that emerged in the era of robber barons, when industries organized into corporations, cartels, and trusts. This *New Order* is characterized by the collectivization of capital in business enterprises and absentee ownership of corporations.

3 Access to the Cortellis database is available on demand at https://clarivate
   .com/cortellis/.
4 The result is taken from OECD.Stat (https://stats.oecd.org/). We use the result
   obtained for total business expenditure in research and development (BERD)
   in the United States (in current national currency) for the sector "Manufacture
   of basic pharmaceutical products and pharmaceutical preparations."

REFERENCES

Batt, S. (2017). *Health Advocacy Inc.: How pharmaceutical funding changed the breast
   cancer movement.* Vancouver, BC: UBC Press.
Biossé-Duplan, A. (2015, février). Participation des associations de patients à
   l'expertise sanitaire: expérience de la Haute Autorité de Santé. *Les cahiers de
   la fonction publique, 352,* 75–8.
Brunelle, D. (2007). *From world order to global disorder: States, markets and dissent.*
   R. Howard (Trans.). Vancouver, BC: UBC Press.
Carlat, D. (2014). Exploring the link between industry payments to doctors and
   prescribing habits. *BMJ, 349,* g6651. https://doi.org/10.1136/bmj.g6651
Carpenter, D., & Moss, D.A. (Eds.). (2014). *Preventing regulatory capture: Special
   interest influence and how to limit it.* New York, NY: Cambridge University Press.
Center for Responsive Politics. (2020). Databases. *OpenSecrets.Org.* Retrieved
   from https://www.opensecrets.org/
Chandler, A.D. (2001). *Inventing the electronic century: The epic story of the consumer
   electronics and computer science industries.* New York, NY: Free Press.
Chandler, A.D. (2005). *Shaping the industrial century: The remarkable story of the
   evolution of the modern chemical and pharmaceutical industries.* Cambridge, MA:
   Harvard University Press.
Chen, C., Cortez, M.F., & Wayne, A. (2014, 1 October). Drug, device companies
   paid $3.5 billion to U.S. doctors. *Bloomberg.* Retrieved from https://www
   .bloomberg.com/news/articles/2014-09-30/drug-device-companies
   -paid-3-5-billion-to-u-s-doctors
Confessore, N. (2003, December). Meet the press: How James Glassman
   reinvented journalism – as lobbying. *Washington Monthly.* Retrieved from
   https://washingtonmonthly.com/magazine/december-2003/meet-the-press/
Connor, J.M. (2008). *Global price fixing: Our customers are the enemy.* Berlin, DE:
   Springer-Verlag.
Drahos, P., & Braithwaite, J. (2002). *Information feudalism: Who owns the knowledge
   economy?* New York, NY: The New Press.
Economist. (2014, 15 November). Pharmaceutical M&A: Invent it, swap it or
   buy it. *The Economist.* Retrieved from https://www.economist.com/business
   /2014/11/15/invent-it-swap-it-or-buy-it

Edelman. (2014). *Digital grassroots advocacy implementation plan.* Calgary, AB: Edelman. Retrieved from https://www.documentcloud.org/documents /1363082-tc-energy-east-grassroots-advocacy.html#document/p3/a187491

Edgecliffe-Johnson, A. (2014, 19 September). The invasion of corporate news. *Financial Times.* Retrieved from https://www.ft.com/content/937b06c2-3ebd -11e4-adef-00144feabdc0

Edney, A. (2019, 9 May). Senate targets hoarding of drug patents to deter competition. *Bloomberg.* Retrieved from https://www.bloomberg.com/news /articles/2019-05-09/hoarding-drug-patents-to-deter-competition-is-targeted -by-senate

Edwards, J. (2009, 29 November). "'CASSPER' was GSK's friendly ghostwriting program on Paxil. *CBS.* Retrieved from https://www.cbsnews.com/news/cassper -was-gsks-friendly-ghostwriting-program-on-paxil/

Feldman, R. (2018). May your drug price be evergreen. *Journal of Law and the Biosciences, 5*(3), 590–647. https://doi.org/10.1093/jlb/lsy022

Ferriman, A. (1999). An end to health scares? *British Medical Journal, 319,* 716. https://doi.org/10.1136/bmj.319.7211.716

Fournier, J.C., DeRubeis, R.J., Hollon, S.D., Dimidjian, S., Amsterdam, J.D., Shelton, R.C., & Fawcett, J. (2010). Antidepressant drug effects and depression severity: A patient-level meta-analysis. *JAMA, 303*(1), 47–53. https://doi.org /10.1001/jama.2009.1943

Fugh-Berman, A. (2010). The haunting of medical journals: How ghostwriting sold "HRT." *PLoS Medicine, 7*(9), e1000335. https://doi.org/10.1371/journal .pmed.1000335

Gagnon, M.-A. (2007). Capital, power & knowledge according to Thorstein Veblen: Reinterpreting the knowledge-based economy. *Journal of Economic Issues, 41*(2), 593–600. https://doi.org/10.1080/00213624.2007.11507049

Gagnon, M.-A. (2009). *The nature of capital in the knowledge-based economy: The case of the global pharmaceutical industry.* Unpublished doctoral dissertation, York University, Toronto, ON.

Gagnon, M.-A. (2012). Corporate influence over clinical research: Considering the alternatives. *Prescrire International, 21*(129), 191–4. Retrieved from https:// english.prescrire.org/en/81/168/47928/0/NewsDetails.aspx

Gagnon, M.-A. (2013). Corruption of pharmaceutical markets: Addressing the misalignment of financial incentives and public health. *Journal of Law, Medicine & Ethics, 41*(3), 571–80. https://doi.org/10.1111/jlme.12066

Gagnon, M.-A. (2016). Shaping the social determinants of value through economic ghostmanagement: An institutionalist approach to capital accumulation. In T.-H. Jo & F.S. Lee (Eds.). *Marx, Veblen, and the foundations of heterodox economics: Essays in honor of John F. Henry* (pp. 228–51). London, UK: Routledge.

Gagnon, M.-A., & Lexchin, J. (2008). The cost of pushing pills: A new estimate of pharmaceutical promotion expenditures in the United States. *PLoS Medicine, 5*(1), e1. https://doi.org/10.1371/journal.pmed.0050001

Genentech. (2020). Grants and contributions report. Retrieved from https://www.gene.com/good/giving/corporate-giving/grants-contributions

Gibbs, W.W. (2001). Patently inefficient: A new industry is thrashed by waves of litigations. *Scientific American, 284*(3), 34. Retrieved from https://www.scientificamerican.com/article/patently-inefficient/

GlaxoSmithKline (GSK). (2016). Best Medicines Coalition. Retrieved from https://ca.gsk.com/en-ca/responsibility/responsibility-reports-and-additional-data/patient-group-funding/2016-best-medicines-coalition/

GlaxoSmithKline (GSK). (2017a). Advocacy boot camp. Retrieved from https://ca.gsk.com/en-ca/responsibility/responsibility-reports-and-additional-data/patient-group-funding/2017-advocacy-boot-camp/

GlaxoSmithKline (GSK). (2017b). Grants & charitable contributions to US based healthcare organizations, January 1 through December 31, 2017. Retrieved from http://fortherecord.payments.us.gsk.com/hcppayments/archive.html

Gold, E.R. (2016). Accelerating translational research through open science: The neuro experiment. *PLoS Biology, 14*(12), e2001259. https://doi.org/10.1371/journal.pbio.2001259

Goldacre, B. (2013). *Bad Pharma: How drug companies mislead doctors and harm patients*. London, UK: Faber and Faber.

Goldenberg, S. (2014, 18 November). Revealed: Keystone company's PR blitz to safeguard its backup plan. *The Guardian*. Retrieved from https://www.theguardian.com/environment/2014/nov/18/revealed-keystone-companys-pr-blitz-to-safeguard-its-backup-plan

Gøtzsche, P. (2013). *Deadly medicines and organised crime: How big pharma has corrupted healthcare*. London, UK: Radcliffe Publishing.

Grocer, S. (2018, 30 June). A record $2.5 trillion in mergers were announced in the first half of 2018. *New York Times*. Retrieved from https://www.nytimes.com/2018/07/03/business/dealbook/mergers-record-levels.html

Hadland S.E., Rivera-Aguirre, A., Marshall, B.D.L., & Cerdá, M. (2019). Association of pharmaceutical industry marketing of opioid products with mortality from opioid-related overdoses. *JAMA Network Open, 2*(1), e186007. https://doi.org/10.1001/jamanetworkopen.2018.6007

Heller, M. (2008a). *The gridlock economy*. New York, NY: Basic Books.

Heller, M. (2008b, 24 July). Where are the cures? *Forbes*. Retrieved from https://www.forbes.com/forbes/2008/0811/030.html

Heller, M.A., & Eisenberg, R.S. (1998). Can patents deter innovation: The anticommons in biomedical research. *Science, 280*(5364), 698–701. https://doi.org/10.1126/science.280.5364.698

Hoffmann-La Roche. (2020). Working with patient organisations. Retrieved from https://www.roche.com/sustainability/patientorganisations/patient -groups-list.htm

Jenkins, R., & Henderson, M. (2008, 5 July). Medical research is "hindered by out-of-date laws." *The Times.* Retrieved from https://www.thetimes.co.uk /article/medical-research-is-hindered-by-out-of-date-laws-575xsksb5m7

Krimsky, S. (2004). *Science in the private interest: Has the lure of profits corrupted biomedical research.* Oxford, UK: Rowman and Littlefield.

Lacasse, J.R., & Leo, J. (2010). Ghostwriting at elite academic medical centers in the United States. *PLoS Medicine, 7*(2), e1000230. https://doi.org/10.1371 /journal.pmed.1000230

Lessig, L. (2011). *Republic, lost: How money corrupts Congress – and a plan to stop it.* New York, NY: Twelve.

Lewis, J., Williams, A., Franklin, B., Thomas, J., & Mosdell, N. (2008). *The quality and independence of British journalism: Tracking the changes over 20 years.* Mediawise report. Retrieved from http://www.mediawise.org.uk/wp-content /uploads/2011/03/Quality-Independence-of-British-Journalism.pdf

Lexchin, J., & Gagnon, M.-A. (2013). CETA and pharmaceuticals: Impact of the trade agreement between Europe and Canada on the costs of patented drugs. CCPA Briefing Paper. Retrieved from https://www.policyalternatives .ca/publications/reports/ceta-and-pharmaceuticals

Matheson, A. (2008). Corporate science and the husbandry of scientific and medical knowledge by the pharmaceutical industry. *BioSocieties, 3,* 355–82. https://doi.org/10.1017/S1745855208006297

McChesney, R.W. (2008). *The political economy of media: Enduring issues, emerging dilemmas.* New York, NY: Monthly Review Press.

McCoy, M.S. (2018). Industry support of patient advocacy organizations: The case for an extension of the Sunshine Act provisions of the Affordable Care Act. *American Journal of Public Health, 108*(8), 1026–30. https://doi.org /10.2105/AJPH.2018.304467

McGarity, T.O., & Wagner, W.E. (2008). *Bending science: How special interests corrupt public health research.* Cambridge, MA: Harvard University Press.

Michaels, D. (2008). *Doubt is their product: How industry's assault on science threatens your health.* Oxford, UK: Oxford University Press.

Miller, D., & Dinan, W. (2008). *A century of spin: How public relations became the cutting edge of corporate power.* London, UK: Pluto.

Miller, D., & Dinan, W. (2009). Journalism, public relations and spin. In K. Wahl-Jorgensen & T. Hanitzsch (Eds.), *Handbook of journalism studies* (pp. 250–64). New York, NY: Routledge.

Miller, D., & Harkins, C. (2010). Corporate strategy, corporate capture: Food and alcohol industry lobbying and public health. *Critical Social Policy, 30*(4), 564–89. https://doi.org/10.1177/0261018310376805

Mirowski, P. (2011). *Science-mart: Privatizing American science.* Cambridge, MA: Harvard University Press.

Mooney, C. (2006). *The Republican war on science.* New York, NY: Basic Books.

Novartis. (2020). Patient organization funding. Retrieved from https://www .novartis.com/our-company/corporate-responsibility/doing-business -responsibly/transparency-disclosure/patient-group-funding

Pharmaceutical Technology. (2019). The top ten pharmaceutical companies by market share in 2018. *Pharmaceutical Technology.* Retrieved from https://www .pharmaceutical-technology.com/features/top-pharmaceutical-companies/

Powerbase. (2010). Catherine Windels. Retrieved from https://powerbase.info /index.php?title=Catherine_Windels

Ross, J.S., Hill, K.P., Egilman, D.S., & Krumholz, H.M. (2008). Guest authorship and ghostwriting in publications related to rofecoxib: A case study of industry documents from rofecoxib litigation. *JAMA, 299*(15), 1800–12. https://doi .org/10.1001/jama.299.15.1800

Rout, M. (2009, 6 April). Vioxx maker Merck and Co drew up doctor hit list. *The Australian.* Retrieved from https://www.news.com.au/news/drug-company -drew-up-doctor-hit-list/news-story/eb55ca36e081d497730629e6c8559abf

Schwartz, L.M., & Woloshin, S. (2019). Medical marketing in the United States, 1997–2016. *JAMA, 321*(1), 80–96. https://doi.org/10.1001/jama.2018.19320

Sell, S.K. (2003). *Private power, public law: The globalization of intellectual property rights.* Cambridge, UK: Cambridge University Press.

Sismondo, S. (2007). Ghost management: How much of the medical literature is shaped behind the scenes by the pharmaceutical industry? *PLoS Medicine, 4*(9), 1429–33. https://doi.org/10.1371/journal.pmed.0040286

Sismondo, S. (2009). Ghosts in the machine: Publication planning in the medical sciences. *Social Studies of Science, 39*(2), 171–98. https://doi.org/10.1177 /0306312708101047

Sismondo, S. (2018). *Ghost-managed medicine: Big pharma's invisible hands.* Manchester, UK: Mattering Press.

Sismondo, S., & Doucet, M. (2010). Publication ethics and the ghost management of medical research. *Bioethics, 24*(6), 273–83. https://doi.org/10.1111/j.1467 -8519.2008.01702.x

Thompson, J., Baird, P., & Downie, J. (2001). *Report of the Committee of Inquiry on the case involving Dr. Nancy Olivieri, the Hospital for Sick Children, the University of Toronto, and Apotex Inc.* Toronto, ON: Lorimer.

Turner, E.H., Matthews, A.M., Linardatos, E., Tell, R.A., & Rosenthal, R. (2008). Selective publication of antidepressant trials and its influence on apparent efficacy. *New England Journal of Medicine, 358*(3), 252–60. https://doi.org /10.1056/NEJMsa065779

US Senate Committee on Finance. (2010a). *Ghostwriting in medical literature.* Minority Staff report, 111th Congress. Retrieved from https://www.grassley .senate.gov/sites/default/files/about/upload/Senator-Grassley-Report.pdf

US Senate Committee on Finance. (2010b, 20 February). Grassley, Baucus release committee report on Avandia. Press release. Retrieved from https://www.finance.senate.gov/release/grassley-baucus-release-committee-report-on-avandia

Veblen, T. (1901). Industrial and pecuniary employments. *Publications of the American Economic Association, 2*(1, February), 190–235.

Veblen, T. (1908a). On the nature of capital I. *Quarterly Journal of Economics, 22*(4), 517–42. https://doi.org/10.2307/1884915

Veblen, T. (1908b). On the nature of capital II: Investments, intangible assets and the pecuniary magnate. *Quarterly Journal of Economics, 23*(1), 104–36. https://doi.org/10.2307/1883967

Veblen, T. (1996). *The theory of business enterprise.* New Brunswick, NJ: Transaction Publishers. (Original work published 1904)

Veblen, T. (1997). *Absentee ownership: Business enterprise in recent times: The case of America.* New Brunswick, NJ: Transaction Publishers. (Original work published 1923)

Veblen, T. (2002). *The vested interests and the common man.* New Brunswick, NJ: Transaction Publishers. (Original work published 1919)

White, B. (2005). *Congressional revolving doors: The journey from Congress to K street.* Washington, DC: Public Citizen. Retrieved from https://www.citizen.org/wp-content/uploads/Congressional-Revolving-Doors-2005.pdf

Wiist, W. (Ed.) (2010). *The bottom line or public health: Tactics corporations use to influence health and health policy, and what we can do to counter them.* New York, NY: Oxford University Press.

Yeh, J.S., Franklin, J.M., Avorn, J., Landon, J., & Kesselheim, A.S. (2016). Association of industry payments to physicians with the prescribing of brand-name statins in Massachusetts. *JAMA Internal Medicine, 176*(6), 763–8. https://doi.org/10.1001/jamainternmed.2016.1709

9 Data Transparency and Rare Disease: Privacy versus Public Interest?

KANKSHA MAHADEVIA GHIMIRE
AND TRUDO LEMMENS

While there is a growing consensus that increased transparency of clinical trial data is needed to strengthen the reliability of pharmaceutical research and safeguard public health, concerns have been raised about the privacy of human research participants whose information is contained in clinical reports.[1] This argument is made particularly in the context of clinical trials involving rare diseases, where the number of research subjects participating in clinical trials is often small, and as a result, risks of re-identification are arguably higher.

Regulators across jurisdictions, such as in Canada and Europe, are increasingly implementing policies to promote transparency of clinical trial data, while trying to ensure that the privacy interests of those participating in clinical trials are protected. But the manner in which regulators have sought to achieve the balance between increased transparency and adequate protection of privacy varies. For example, recognizing the key role that transparency plays in protecting and fostering public health, the European Medicines Agency (EMA) has made great strides in recent years in increasing the transparency of information on medicinal products held by the agency. It has done so while trying to address privacy-linked concerns.[2] In Canada, access to data held by drug regulators has dramatically improved, particularly as a result of recent case law and amendments in legislation and regulations. But further legislative and regulatory efforts are still needed, in part to prevent measures protecting the privacy of research participants from adding unnecessary limits on the transparency of clinical trial data. As we discuss later, some exceptions to data sharing have also been criticized.

This chapter explores the question of whether concerns about privacy justify limits on data transparency, thereby limiting the benefits derived from transparency of clinical trial data, particularly in the rare disease context. The chapter discusses the range of benefits provided by increased transparency in the rare disease context and examines scholarly discussions on the practical possibilities of data breach. The chapter suggests that the fear of privacy breach is often overstated, and instead must be viewed through the lens of proportionality. Instances of data breach can be mitigated through use of appropriate technical and legal mechanisms. It concludes by recommending legal mechanisms that may be implemented to mitigate privacy-breach concerns, while continuing to facilitate increased transparency of clinical trial data.

The Contemporary Context

The topic of clinical trials and pharmaceutical data transparency has received significant attention in various jurisdictions, including Canada, the United States, and Europe. International organizations, regulators across jurisdictions, scientific organizations, medical journal editors, pharmaceutical companies, and public-private research partnerships focusing on drug development are recognizing the importance of data sharing. Public funding agencies and drug regulators are increasingly introducing transparency obligations, while pharmaceutical companies and public-private partnerships are also developing their own data sharing initiatives. Increasing transparency in clinical trial data is deemed to be important in order to conduct a reliable analysis of drug safety and efficacy, and for improving public health.

But the privacy of human research participants (patients and healthy volunteers), who allow their body to be used as a source of information in this context, continues to be invoked as a risk factor in debates about data transparency. Even those who recognize and emphasize the importance of data transparency suggest at times that sharing details of clinical trial reports may create risks to the privacy of research subjects, and sometimes privacy laws of a country are invoked to impede sharing of clinical trial data.[3] There are often stark differences in opinion about the required and desirable level of transparency – especially between industry and the scientific community. In particular, how much information should be provided, what criteria should be used to evaluate access requests, and what kind of restrictions can be imposed on the use of that data remain the subject of heated debate. In this debate, arguments about risks to research participant confidentiality, and the privacy rights of both research participants and pharmaceutical companies, are invoked to support significant limits on data transparency. Because of the fundamental rights nature of these claims, they carry significant weight and deserve to be carefully scrutinized.

The concerns about privacy are particularly prominent in the context of research involving rare diseases. A disease typically falls under the category of a "rare disease" when it afflicts, as the term suggests, only a small minority of the population. The concept of "rare disease" is defined differently in various jurisdictions. For example, for the European Union (EU), a rare disease is "a life-threatening, debilitating and/or seriously chronic illness affecting fewer than 5 in 10,000 people" (So, Joly, & Knoppers, 2013; Gibson & Lemmens, 2014, pp. 205–6) or fewer than 1 in 2,000 (1:2000; Marešová, Mohelská, & Kuča, 2015, p. 1303; Genetic and Rare Diseases Information Center, 2017). To be categorized as a rare disease in the United States, the disease must affect fewer than 200,000 people in the country, or 1:1333 (So et al., 2013; Gibson & Lemmens, 2014). For Australia's Therapeutic Goods Authority, a rare disease is one that has a prevalence of 1 in 10,000 people or fewer (1:9090). Japan considers a disease rare when it affects fewer than 50,000 patients, a prevalence of 1:2500 (Canadian Organization of Rare Disorders, 2005; Song, Gao, Inagaki, & Tang, 2012). Canada does not yet have a nationwide legislative definition of "rare disease" (Menon, Clark, & Stafinski, 2015; Loorand-Stiver, Cowling, & Perras, 2016). In 2012, Health Canada proposed in a draft *Orphan Drug Framework for Canada* to adopt a definition of rare disease similar to that in the European Union (Health Canada, 2012). Yet, in October 2017, the "federal government deleted ... all references to the ... 2012 Orphan Drug Regulatory Framework" (Rawson & Adams, 2018; see also Forrest, 2017). In the 2019 federal budget, the Canadian government announced funding for rare disease therapies in connection with the creation of a national drug agency; the details are so far lacking (Government of Canada, 2019a). Although "rare diseases" have been defined differently in the European Union, the United States, Australia, and Japan, the one commonality is that only those diseases that afflict a very small population qualify as rare diseases.

Hence, it is not surprising that, typically, in clinical trials involving rare diseases, the number of research subjects participating is small, and as a result, risks of identification are arguably higher (or at least higher than in more traditional drug development). When a drug is developed for a traditional disease, often more than 3,000 people participate in a Phase III trial, and many more people are living with the condition in the general population. For rare diseases, the number of participants will tend to be smaller, and the number of people with the condition in the larger population may at times not be much larger than the number of people participating in the trial. This fact, so it is argued, creates unique risks of identification of those who participated in a trial. Some commentators, research participants, and pharmaceutical companies invoke this situation as an argument to limit data transparency specifically in the rare disease context, citing research participants' privacy-linked concerns.[4]

While the issue of balancing privacy rights and industry interests with the need for increased transparency is widely discussed, the analysis in the context of rare diseases is limited. This chapter explores the question of whether arguments grounded upon the fear of privacy breach favouring limiting data transparency are justified in undermining efforts to increase data transparency, thereby limiting the benefits derived from transparency of clinical trial data. The analysis aims to shed light on the debate between privacy rights *versus* the need for increased transparency. The discussion should help ensure that voluntary data sharing practices and new transparency regulations properly balance the public interest of advancing the safety and accountability of the drug development process through increased transparency with the rights and interests of research participants, particularly the right to privacy in the rare disease context.

In the following section, we will first discuss the range of benefits that increased transparency has the potential to provide, focusing particularly on the rare disease context. The next section maps the scholarly literature discussing the practical possibilities of data breach. The discussion highlights the view that the fear of privacy breach is often overstated and, instead, must be looked at through the lens of *proportionality*. Instances of data breach can be mitigated through the use of appropriate technical and legal mechanisms. The final two sections discuss, and conclude, by recommending (respectively) certain legal mechanisms to mitigate privacy-breach concerns, while continuing to facilitate increased transparency of clinical trial data. Our recommendations aim at balancing research participants' privacy rights and clinical data transparency.

The Rare Disease Context: Necessity for, and Benefits of, Increased Data Transparency

In the context of rare disease research, where privacy concerns are considered more significant, the importance of early data sharing has also been emphasized. Data sharing has been particularly promoted in the area of genomic research, which often focuses on rare diseases and targeted drug development. This section identifies key reasons why increasing transparency of clinical trial data is necessary and beneficial in the rare disease context. These reasons are in addition to the wide range of public benefits that transparency of clinical trials conducted on diseases impacting a large number of people provides, such as enabling evidence-based public health policy-making, providing economic advantages, and improving scientific research.[5] The reasons discussed later are also in addition to the legal, ethical, and social arguments made in favour of increasing the transparency of clinical trial research.[6]

Better Understanding and Treatment of Rare Diseases

Genomics England, a project funded by the UK Department of Health, estimates that "one in seventeen people are born with or develop a rare disease during their lifetime" (Genomics England, n.d.). A majority of rare diseases (nearly 85 per cent) are considered to be life-threatening or serious, and among these, treatments are known for less than 5 per cent (Genomics England, n.d.; Gibson & Lemmens, 2014, p. 211; President's Council of Advisors on Science and Technology, 2012). However, since in many circumstances rare diseases may not be diagnosed, they may be more common than some estimates suggest. In many cases, the methodology used to gather the raw data that gives the prevalence of rare diseases has not been critically examined. More clinical research on rare diseases and their treatments is arguably important to provide further analysis.

When conducting clinical trials involving rare diseases, researchers and research agencies face unique challenges compared to clinical trials conducted on diseases impacting a large number of people. Undertaking rare disease clinical trials is more difficult, as rare diseases affect very few individuals in a population, and some potential participants may also have short lifespans. Both factors limit the availability of individuals who can participate in rare disease–focused clinical trials (Coté, Xu, & Pariser, 2010; Melnikova, 2012; So et al., 2013, pp. 322–3; Gibson & Lemmens, 2014, p. 209; Boon & Moors, 2008). The challenges may be accentuated as individuals' conditions may be heterogeneous and poorly understood (Coté et al., 2010; Melnikova, 2012; So et al., 2013, pp. 322–3).

In light of the challenge of accumulating sufficient data, data sharing becomes uniquely important. It helps overcome or at least attenuate many of the challenges just identified. It thus benefits the people who are afflicted or who may be afflicted in the future by a rare disease (Yakowitz, 2011; So et al., 2013, p. 323). Mining existing clinical, pharmacological, and chemical data can help researchers discover unrecognized connections between existing drugs and potential targets for rare disease treatments (Sardana et al., 2011; Coté et al., 2010; Melnikova, 2012; So et al., 2013, pp. 322–3). The sharing of clinical trial data could therefore enable repurposing of existing medicines for the treatment of rare diseases at reduced costs (So et al., 2013, pp. 322–3). On account of the nature of certain types of rare diseases, for example, Huntington disease, only a few researchers may be directly researching the disease, and hence any incremental step contributing to the understanding or treatment of the disease is a big step forward (Harding, 2018).

Benefit to the Individual

Sharing clinical trial data is also beneficial at the individual level to the research participants for a range of reasons. For example, findings from secondary research using their clinical trial data may benefit them, as secondary research may provide scientific advancements such as improving the understanding of the disease or possibly even developing a treatment or cure. Further, secondary research findings may protect research participants from undergoing unnecessary risks (Bierer, Li, Barnes, & Sim, 2016; Institute of Medicine, 2015b). In the future, for instance, clinical trial patients would not be exposed to known harms that might occur if trials were repeated due to the results of the original trials not being known. The last benefit is a general benefit of data sharing, but, again, it becomes particularly important in the context of scarcity of data.

Scrutiny of Orphan Drugs

Concerns are often raised that pharmaceutical companies may have less incentive to invest in research to develop treatments focusing on rare diseases as there would typically be a limited number of potential buyers, possibly making profit recovery difficult (So et al., 2013, pp. 322–3; Woodcock, 2007; Kesselheim & Treasure, 2017; Tambuyzer, 2010). To address this issue, many jurisdictions, such as the United States and the European Union, have adopted legislative measures incentivizing pharmaceutical companies to develop orphan drugs, that is medicines to treat rare diseases (Gibson & Lemmens, 2014, pp. 205–6; So et al., 2013, pp. 322–3; Gibson & Von Tigerstrom, 2015) such as tax benefits, funding for clinical trials, and/or fast-track approvals (Gibson & Lemmens, 2014, pp. 205–6; Kesselheim & Treasure, 2017; Lexchin, 2015). In the United States, the classification of a drug as falling under the *breakthrough therapy* category has also been used to promote drug development focused on rare diseases (Kesselheim et al., 2016). These measures have arguably been successful, as many orphan drugs have been developed (Gibson & Lemmens, 2014, pp. 205–6; Melnikova, 2012; So et al., 2013, pp. 322–3; Coté et al., 2010; Kesselheim & Treasure, 2017). For example, the US Food and Drug Administration (FDA) reports that nearly 200 orphan drugs enter development each year, and approximately one third of new drugs approved by the FDA are for the treatment of rare diseases (Rockoff, 2013). The pharmaceutical industry's interest in developing orphan drugs has also increased on account of several other factors such as advancements in pharmacogenetics, which has enabled "more common disease to be stratified into rarer disease genotypes"

(Gibson & Lemmens, 2014, pp. 201–3; Collier, 2011; Dolgin, 2010; see also Kesselheim & Treasure, 2017), and the possibility of charging "significant price premiums" (Gibson & Lemmens, 2014, p. 205; Trusheim, Berndt, & Douglas, 2007)[7] in monopolistic markets created by disease stratification (Gibson & Lemmens, 2014, p. 205; Boon & Moors, 2008).

However, large-scale clinical trial data are typically not available for specialized drugs or orphan drugs used by a small population, and developing evidence profiles for orphan drugs or innovative specialized drugs is an inherent challenge in the rare disease context (Gibson & Lemmens, 2014, p. 209; Owen et al., 2008). Consequently, orphan drugs are being approved by relying on clinical trials that are smaller, and potentially less robust in verifying the safety and efficacy of medicines, than those aimed at treating diseases affecting larger populations (Gibson & Lemmens, 2014, p. 209).

This limitation has implications for the integrity of the system. Terms such as "breakthrough" drugs appear to make consumers and physicians overly optimistic about drug efficacy (Kesselheim et al., 2016; Krishnamurti, Woloshin, Schwartz, & Fischhoff, 2015). One research study found that some orphan drugs presented before the European Union for market authorization relied upon methodologically flawed analysis (Picavet, Cassiman, Hollak, Maertens, & Simoens, 2013). Several experts have warned that, in some cases, "the prioritization of rare diseases [has] not [been] based on scientific evidence" (Picavet et al., 2013, p. 2; see also Dupont & Van Wilder, 2011; McCabe, Tsuchiya, Claxton, & Raftery, 2006). Orphan drugs or specialized drugs are being approved more and more rapidly (Gibson & Lemmens, 2014, pp. 209, 211; Kesselheim, Wang, Franklin, & Darrow, 2015) – for a range of reasons, including meeting the urgent demand for treating serious or life-threatening rare diseases (Gibson & Lemmens, 2014, pp. 209, 211; Darrow, Avorn, & Kesselheim, 2014). The rapid approval is often conditional on further post-market testing, but this practice has increased the challenges in balancing the risks with the benefits of orphan drugs, as the drugs are thus entered onto the market without sufficient safety data (Moore & Furberg, 2014). Drugs that are approved in a fast-track manner are more likely to produce unknown side effects, putting the patients' health at risk (Lexchin, 2012; Darrow et al., 2014). Some commentators further emphasize that "rare drug reactions will almost always only be identified after marketing of the drug and broad use of it in different populations" (Hansson, 2012, p. 316; Barry, Koshman, & Pearson, 2014). These limitations and flaws in orphan drugs and specialized drug clinical trials highlight the necessity for closer scrutiny of existing clinical trial data and findings pertaining to the pre- and post-market phase, continuing throughout the life cycle of the drug, and of evidence-generation through secondary research

(Gibson & Lemmens, 2014, p. 214; Hansson 2012, p. 316; Eichler, Pignatti, Flamion, Leufkens, & Breckenridge, 2008).

Canadian Companies' Transparency Policy in Respect of Drugs Treating Rare Diseases

As part of a project funded by the Privacy Commissioner of Canada,[8] a research team the authors were part of undertook a public search for, and review of, the transparency policies of pharmaceutical companies that complete clinical trials in Canada. The goal was to sketch a picture of how clinical trial data are treated by the companies that collect the data and to explore whether they provide sufficient access to data to fulfil the goals of data transparency, in particular with respect to data for studies that relate to rare diseases.[9] Pharmaceutical companies examined were brand-name companies operating in Canada.[10]

The examination uncovered a range of issues with the transparency policies adopted by several pharmaceutical companies, but most importantly, it revealed that some pharmaceutical companies had no transparency policies at all.[11] However, the finding pertinent to the rare disease context – and particularly troubling – was that none of the companies committed to sharing data for trials conducted to study orphan drugs and/or rare diseases; instead, the corporations would frequently cite the fact that a trial related to an orphan drug or rare disease was a reason for not sharing the data for that particular trial. The corporations argued that issues with anonymization and privacy, which arise in the context of orphan drug and rare disease trials, meant that those trials could not be included in their general policy of disclosing clinical trial data; Bayer, for example, holds that data will not be shared when the company believes there is a reasonable likelihood that a participant could be re-identified, and mentions as examples studies of rare diseases or studies with a small number of subjects (Clinical Study Data Request, 2020b). Some companies do state that they will consider disclosing such trials on a case-by-case basis, rather than excluding them entirely. This examination reinforces the need to take legal steps for balancing the privacy rights of research participants with the need for increasing transparency on account of the range of benefits it provides. Privacy-related concerns cannot be used to entirely thwart prudently done data sharing.

How Real Is the "Breach of Privacy" Concern?

In light of the concerns highlighted and the range of potential benefits identified earlier that data sharing can provide in the rare disease context, why are hurdles created that hamper efforts to increase data transparency? Concerns over sharing clinical trial data have primarily been raised from the perspective of safeguarding the privacy of research participants, the commercial interests of pharmaceutical companies, and the academic/research interests of the original researchers and academics.[12] The most prominent reservations that have been expressed about increasing transparency of clinical trial data relate to concerns that research participants may be re-identified, and upon re-identification, possibly face discrimination.[13] These concerns about breach of participants' confidentiality and discrimination are arguably accentuated in clinical trials involving rare diseases since the number of participants involved is typically small, and consequently participants may be more easily identifiable (Silverman, 2018; So et al., 2013, p. 323; Lapham, Kozma, & Weiss, 1996; Geelen, Horstman, Marcelis, Doevendans, & Van Hoyweghen, 2012; McCormack et al., 2016, pp. 1406–7; Garrison et al., 2016). Moreover, clinical trials for rare disease may take place across multiple jurisdictions due to the limited number of participants in a single jurisdiction, which can further complicate the privacy landscape (Mascalzoni, Paradiso, & Hansson, 2014). But are these privacy-linked fears practically valid and sufficient to limit the sharing of clinical research data, consequently depriving research participants of the range of benefits that may potentially be derived from data sharing? This question is explored in the following section.

Willingness of Research Participants to Share Clinical Trial Data

Several empirical studies have demonstrated that some participants are willing to share their clinical trial data on account of the benefits they believe will be derived from secondary research, subject to certain conditions, such as appropriate governance and management and safeguards against privacy breaches (McCormack et al, 2016, p. 1404; Harding, 2018; El Emam et al., 2007, p. 7), and to usage being limited to "legitimate" purposes, such as research that advances knowledge about the disease or its treatment (El Emam, 2018). Not surprisingly, patients' concerns typically pertain to their identifiable data (rather than their anonymized data), and they tend to be more willing to share their anonymized data (El Emam, 2018). However, participants' willingness to share their data varies, influenced by factors such as the characteristics and seriousness of the disease they have, the length of time they may have before succumbing to the disease, the sometimes potentially embarrassing and intimate details they may have had to share with the original researchers (which they fear may be revealed), and their individual experiences with research (McCormack et al., 2016, p. 1404; El Emam,

2018). Participants may also be hesitant to permit clinical trial data to be used for non-research purposes (El Emam, 2018). Although some participants may be willing to share, they are concerned about the potential misuse of their data.

Privacy-Related Fears Overstated

While many researchers and bioethics and legal experts concur that adequately protecting research participants' privacy is an important obligation of researchers, some contend that the concerns over breach of research participants' privacy are often overstated (Rasi, 2013; Hirschler, 2013) and that it is an issue of perception rather than a real concern (El Emam, 2013; Krleža-Jerić et al., 2016). In most clinical trials, they argue, appropriate safeguards are sufficient to protect privacy, and the prospect of re-identification using clinical trial data is minimal (Yakowitz, 2011; Rubinstein & Hartzog, 2016, p. 705; Cavoukian & El Emam, 2011; Benitez & Malin, 2010; El Emam, 2013; Krleža-Jerić et al., 2016). The Canadian Institutes of Health Research observe that "researchers who study health services or the health of populations rarely have any direct interest in knowing the specific identities of the people they study. Their focus is on aggregate trends" (Canadian Institutes of Health Research [CIHR], 2002, p. 8).

Some researchers and experts acknowledge that, despite technological advancements and efforts taken to secure participant privacy, including the process of anonymization, risk of exposure may remain, but the risk is low if effective governance protocols and adequate technical safeguards are implemented (Council of Canadian Academies Expert Panel, 2015, pp. xix, 98; Rubinstein & Hartzog, 2016, p. 708; Bambauer, 2012; Institute of Medicine, 2015a). Risks may occur on account of "accidental release of identifiable data to the public or unauthorized researchers, when proper security and privacy protocols are not followed (e.g., through loss of computer equipment); illicit access to identifiable data (e.g., through hacking); and inadvertent access to identifiable data by those working inside data organizations" (Council of Canadian Academies Expert Panel, 2015, p. xix). Nelson (2015, p. 4) has identified several instances of data breach in the health-care sector, but observes that, in the majority of cases, breaches occurred because of human error or negligence rather than limitations in technology resulting in hacking.[14] The Council of Canadian Academies Expert Panel (2015) finds that "breaches rarely happen at institutions with databases set up specifically for maintaining large volumes of health and health-related data for research and administrative purposes. They are much more likely to occur when researchers or employees are accessing data directly from health-care centres" (p. xix). The panel further contends that risks of re-identification can be reduced through the implementation of best practices in de-identification (p. xix). Rubinstein and Hartzog (2016) emphasize that "there is no perfect anonymity" and "no such thing as perfect de-identification" (pp. 708, 751; see also Bambauer, 2012).

But, in light of the numerous benefits provided by sharing, both to the public and potentially to the research participant, these authors and others argue, a reasonably low threshold of risk must be tolerated (Rubinstein & Hartzog, 2016, p. 708; Ohm, 2010; Wu, 2013; Yakowitz, 2011). As Bambauer (2012) observes, "good enough is, generally, good enough" (see also Rubinstein & Hartzog, 2016, p. 708; Council of Canadian Academies Expert Panel, 2015, p. xxi; El Emam, 2018).

Emphasis Must Be on Proportionality

In line with suggestions made by various authors and official reports such as the report of the Council of Canadian Academies Expert Panel (2015), we suggest that, at the policy level, the concern about privacy should be explored through the lens of proportionality, thereby balancing the benefits of sharing clinical trial data with the "real" risks to privacy and those created by hiding data and resulting problems with medicines (Council of Canadian Academies Expert Panel, 2015, pp. xix–xx, 133; Hansson, 2012, pp. 313, 318; Katzan et al., 2000; Hill & Buchan, 2001; Tu et al., 2004, p. 1420). As Lexchin and colleagues (2017) contend, the objections against transparency raised on the grounds of confidential information should be analysed in light of the important consequences of withholding this information from the public. The Council of Canadian Academies Expert Panel (2015, p. 133) has equally stressed that "interference with privacy can be justifiable so long as the degree of interference is proportionate to the wider social benefit and is needed to achieve that social benefit."

Clearly, when the number of research participants in a study is low, and the number of people with the condition in the general population is also very low, it becomes more likely that connections to the identity of specific research participants can be made. The principle of proportionality does invite us, however, to look at the incontestable benefits that access to data offer.

We want to suggest further that, as part of the proportionality analysis, the risk of identifying individuals has to be situated in the context of other "data" sharing practices that already take place, particularly those in the rare disease context. Increasingly, patient advocacy and health information websites contain testimonies of people who self-identify as members of specific disease groups. They often share experiences related to their illness, including at times their experience with specific forms of medication. It would seem ironic that, in the name of privacy, we limit data sharing in the context of rigorous clinical trials that aim to provide reliable information about safety and efficacy of medication, while ignoring the voluntary sharing of information by patients in other contexts that may have an impact on health-care practices.

Transparency-Enhancing Projects

While several drug companies have moved aggressively to create regulatory and legal barriers to data sharing, arguing that it may undermine participant privacy (Lemmens, 2013; MacLeod, 2012; Peddicord, Waldo, Boutin, Grande, & Gutierrez, 2010) or their commercial interests,[15] in various public fora, some companies in the pharmaceutical industry have expressed support for transparency measures and committed to dramatically increasing the amount of clinical trial data and results available to researchers, participants, and the public (EFPIA & PhRMA, 2013). Some pharmaceutical companies are advocating and have even initiated steps towards increasing transparency in clinical trial data, albeit often initially as part of a legal settlement. GlaxoSmithKline's initiative in 2013 is sometimes cited as groundbreaking, as it was the first to provide access to de-identified participant-level data from clinical trial studies sponsored through a single system (Strom, Buyse, Hughes, & Knoppers, 2014; Rockhold, Nisen & Freeman, 2016; Nisen & Rockhold, 2013). From January 2014, GlaxoSmithKline's data request platform was relaunched as ClinicalStudyDataRequest.com. Ten pharmaceutical companies started to participate, and the system transformed into a multi-sponsor site (Clinical Study Data Request, 2020a; Strom et al., 2014). As of 2016, thirteen industry sponsors and over 3,000 trials were listed (Rockhold et al., 2016).

Pharmaceutical companies have also begun to collaborate with academic partners to promote transparency. Examples of these initiatives are the Yale University Open Data Access (YODA) Project, a partnership between Yale University and three companies, and the Project Data Sphere, an initiative by more than thirty pharmaceutical companies and other organizations (Krleža-Jerić et al., 2016; Yale University Open Data Access [YODA] Project, n.d.). An interesting initiative in the Canadian context, which is directly tied to novel forms of drug development, is the Structural Genomics Consortium, an international public-private partnership incorporated as a not-for-profit organization that aims at promoting the discovery of new medicines through open-access research. Its mandate is to study potential drug targets.[16] Various pharmaceutical companies participate in the partnership and agree to abide by the transparency rules of the organization. The consortium deals primarily with preclinical data.

The European Federation of Pharmaceutical Industries and Associations (EFPIA) and the Pharmaceutical Research and Manufacturers of America (PhRMA) released in 2013 a joint "Principles for Responsible Clinical Trial Data Sharing: Our Commitment to Patients and Researchers," in which the organizations committed on behalf of their member companies to sharing "patient-level clinical trial data, study-level clinical trial data, full clinical study reports, and protocols from clinical trials in patients ... with qualified scientific and medical researchers upon request and subject to terms necessary to protect patient privacy and confidential commercial information" (EFPIA & PhRMA, 2013).

Recognizing the range of benefits provided by increased clinical trial data sharing, various international and national agencies, scientific journals, and the research community in general promote publication of research results and access to clinical trial data and clinical reports (Mintzes, Lexchin, & Quintano, 2015). For example, the International Committee of Medical Journal Editors (ICMJE) and various individual journals, such as the *BMJ* (formerly the *British Medical Journal*) and *PLOS*, have committed themselves to promoting transparency. However, the disclosure obligations for authors publishing with these journals may differ, with room for improvement. For example, the *BMJ* does not require data sharing, but rather asks that authors agree to make their data available if and when requested to do so. Research organizations such as the Cochrane Collaboration, the Nordic Trial Alliance, and the European Clinical Research Infrastructure Network (ECRIN-ERIC) have done the same. At the level of international organizations, the World Health Organization (WHO) has clearly taken strong steps to promote transparency (Ohmann et al., 2017; Krleža-Jerić et al., 2016; Taichman et al., 2016; Krleža-Jerić et al., 2005; Krleža-Jerić, Lemmens, Reveiz, Cuervo, & Bero, 2011). To foster sharing, these agencies and organizations have issued guidelines and rules to establish best practices, including the Ottawa Statement, the Tri-Council Policy Statement, the Declaration of Helsinki,[17] the European Medicine Agency 2014 policy, and the WHO's "Joint Statement on Public Disclosure of Results from Clinical Trials" (World Health Organization [WHO], 2017), which had twenty-one signatories[18] as of May 2017. While these policies and guidelines are important steps in fostering sharing, they are, some have argued, limited as they pertain to specific geographical areas, specific types of research or data, or specific types of data generators (for example, pharmaceutical companies) (Ohmann et al., 2017).

Multiple agencies, organizations, and their projects have supported the establishment of data sharing initiatives and repositories that host clinical trials, including ClinicalTrials.gov, CORBEL project, European Open Science Cloud, Multi-Regional Clinical Trials Center of Brigham and Women's Hospital and Harvard University, Vivli project, AllTrials, IMPACT Observatory, and repositories such as Dryad Digital Repository and Figshare (Bierer et al., 2016, p. 2412; Ohmann et al., 2017; European Commission, 2016; So et al., 2013, p. 325; Krleža-Jerić et al., 2016).

Among the most significant legal and regulatory initiatives are those undertaken in the United States and Europe. In the United States, the FDA Amendment Act of 2007 introduced strict trial registration and results reporting requirements, accompanied by significant financial penalties for non-compliance.[19]

In Europe, the EMA has tried to push the transparency agenda even further, announcing in November 2012 that it would introduce a prospective data release policy that would result in making clinical trial data from EMA-approved drugs publicly available on a website (European Medicines Agency [EMA], 2021b). The EMA data access policy, ultimately adopted in October 2014, provides for prospective release of clinical trial data (EMA, 2021a) – but with some discretionary power for industry to redact certain data (see chapter three of this volume). Continuing the process, the EMA has been endeavouring to improve de-identification in clinical trial data and increase clinical trial data sharing.

More recently, data transparency has significantly improved in Canada as a result of the 2018 Federal Court decision by Justice Sébastien Grammond in *Peter Doshi v. Canada (AG)*. In this case, Justice Grammond ordered the disclosure, without conditions of confidentiality, all study reports and all data sets, including participant-level data, for three vaccines and two pharmaceutical products to researcher Peter Doshi. Doshi had requested Health Canada for access to such data under Vanessa's Law in order to conduct a secondary analysis. The judge did not rule out the possibility that circumstances could arise in which some level of confidentiality may be imposed on a case-by-case basis "with respect to specific categories of information." Perhaps this clause could be invoked in exceptional circumstances when data disclosure would result in all-too-easy identification of participants in a clinical trial involving a rare disease. At the time of the decision, Health Canada had already been working on draft regulations to implement Vanessa's Law transparency provisions, to which Justice Grammond refers. These regulations were brought into force in 2019 (see chapter five of this volume). However, the regulations have one key drawback. They contain two exceptions to the release of information from clinical trials and other studies submitted in support of a drug, biologic, or medical device submission. The following are the two exceptions:

1 information that the manufacturer did not use in the drug submission to support the proposed conditions of use or purpose for the drug; or
2 information that describes tests, methods or assays that are used exclusively by the manufacturer. (Government of Canada, 2019b)

These exceptions threaten to undermine the fundamental purpose of the regulations, which is to make transparent hidden pharmaceutical evidence about the safety and efficacy of drugs, biologics, and medical devices once a regulatory decision has been made. They appear to run counter to the spirit of Vanessa's Law, which enshrines transparency.[20]

Suggestions and Steps Initiated to Increase Transparency while Protecting Patient Privacy

This section discusses three legal mechanisms aimed at balancing the protection of research participants' privacy rights with increased transparency of clinical trial data:[21] (1) obtaining appropriate informed consent from research participants; (2) research ethics committees/boards (RECs/REBs), with adequate representation of a range of stakeholders at the level of REBs and utilizing REBs to foster data sharing on ethical grounds; and (3) the use of terms of use (ToU) agreements (similar to as prescribed by the EMA). The first two mechanisms are particularly interconnected.

Informed Consent: Merits, Challenges, and Suggestions

A frequently suggested legal mechanism proposes that secondary research of clinical trial data can be made dependent on research participants' informed consent. Various justifications have been provided to insist upon this requirement. Some legal experts argue that explicit informed consent is a non-negotiable prerequisite for disclosure and secondary use of clinical trial data, as disclosure or usage without prior consent is an interference with the participants' privacy rights (Brown, Brown & Korff, 2010, pp. 238, 242, 244–5; Mariner, 2009). Medical research is typically not considered an aspect of participant care because it may not directly benefit the participant whose data are being used, and hence future secondary use of data for purposes other than originally intended must, according to this view, be subject to explicit informed consent (Ploem, 2006, pp. 52–3; Brown et al., 2010, pp. 239, 256). Some have cautioned that, while privacy statutes typically permit, in exceptional circumstances, certain types of disclosures in the public interest without the requirement of prior consent, such as situations where there is "clear and present, or immediate, risk to the public" (Brown et al., 2010, p. 256), such disclosures must not be treated as standard practice (Brown et al., 2010, pp. 239–40). They argue that, even if medical research is clearly beneficial to the public, it is not a sufficient justification to use participants' data without their prior informed consent (Brown et al., 2010, pp. 239–40, 256). Some therefore insist that research participants should not only have a right to consent but also the right to withdraw their consent at any time[22] (Gertz, 2008). By contrast, Hansson (2012, pp. 320–2) argues that, in respect of registries and biobanks, "specific or even a broad consent to each access or use of tissue [should not be] required" and that research participants must be informed so as to maintain participant trust and respect their autonomy. Hansson defends this position primarily on the grounds that "individual informed consent is neither possible nor desirable if one wants to attain an optimal standard of quality care, since allowing people to drop out negates the possibility of universality" (pp. 321–2).

The strategy of informed consent raises a range of questions, including whether and when consent should be obtained (upfront, prior to participating in the trial, or as an ongoing requirement); whether the approval should be general or limited to specific purposes; and whether approval always needs to be obtained in writing or if it can also be oral (CIHR, 2002, pp. 8–9). Some argue that a broad consent obtained at the time the participant enters the trial is sufficient (Hansson, 2012, p. 320; Caulfield & Kaye, 2009; Wendler, 2006; Hansson, 2009; Sheehan, 2011); however, broad consent must "include unspecified or generally specified purposes in the future" (Hansson, 2012, p. 320). Some experts and research participants (McCormack et al., 2016, pp. 1404–5) take an opposing view and insist that the strategy of obtaining a general approval only at the time of entering the trial is not sufficient to protect participants' privacy rights, as it does not sufficiently enable the participant to control use of their data. These objectors also suggest that such a strategy may be used as a method of pressure, that is, if a participant does not acquiesce to secondary research use they may be refused entry into the trial, rendering the consent meaningless (Rubinstein & Hartzog, 2016, p. 730; Solove, 2013). Further, some have raised concerns that, although governments make efforts to obtain upfront consent from research participants, the manner in which consent is sought is often not appropriate because "the patients are not adequately informed about possible secondary uses of their medical data for medical research, are not asked to give clear, specific, free and informed consent, are not even offered unambiguous and effective opt-outs, and are misled about the level of anonymization of their data and the likelihood of re-identification" (Brownet al., 2010, p. 256). Alternatively, some favour informed consent being obtained on an ongoing basis, with the language of the approval specifically identifying a particular research purpose. Concerns regarding consent are further complicated in respect of heritable diseases, such as Huntington disease, because participants' decision to permit the use of their clinical trial data may impact other family members susceptible to the disease (Harding, 2018).

One suggestion is to obtain consent on an ongoing basis through the strategy of "dynamic consent." This term "is ... used to describe personalized, online consent and communication platforms" (Budin-Ljøsne et al., 2017; Fletcher, Gheorghe, Moore, Wilson, & Damery, 2012). Dynamic consent differs from specific consent in that consent can be obtained on an ongoing basis for varying purposes, such as new research objectives not originally foreseen (Kaye et al., 2015; Budin-Ljøsne et al., 2017, p. 3), and participants may also have the option to change their consent if they desire to do so in the future (Budin-Ljøsne et al., 2017, p. 3). Dynamic consent platforms can also be used for other purposes, such as requesting participants to continue to upload data and researchers to update participants on a regular basis (p. 3).

Yet, some caution that certain key hurdles are faced in the efforts to obtain informed consent on an ongoing basis, and more so in the context of "retrospective studies that rely on already-existing, historical or archival data, including sample survey data" (CIHR, 2002, pp. 8–9). Some empirical studies find that obtaining consent in writing after participants have been discharged from hospital or after the clinical trial ends results in particularly low consent response rates (Armstrong, Kline-Rogers, & Jani, 2005). Consent rates may be low for a variety of reasons – participants may have died, or some participants may not have been contacted in writing on account of administrative issues. If no response is received from a participant, it is unclear if it is because the request for consent never reached them, they did not want to participate, or they have refused consent (CIHR, 2002, pp. 8–9; Chen et al., 2005; Armstrong et al., 2005; Tu et al., 2004; Lowrance, 2003). Some empirical studies find that seeking consent on an ongoing basis may result in selection bias (Tu et al., 2004; Armstrong et al., 2005). Concerns have also been raised that ongoing consent requirements may impose substantial costs on the original researcher (Armstrong et al., 2005; Tu et al., 2004).

Others caution that a key disadvantage to seeking informed consent (whether at the time of joining the trial or on ongoing basis) is that "consumers only have a limited ability to make meaningful decisions regarding their own privacy due to the incredible volume, impenetrability, and interconnectedness of data collection and transfers" (Rubinstein & Hartzog, 2016, p. 730; Solove, 2013). Furthermore, in certain cases, strict implementation of a traditional requirement to seek consent may be "impracticable, impossible or self-defeating" (CIHR, 2002, pp. 8–9) on account of "the sheer size of the populations studied; ... the creation of even greater privacy risks by having to link otherwise de-identified data with nominal identifiers in order to communicate with individuals so as to seek their consent; ... [and] the difficulty of contacting individuals directly when there are no ongoing relations with them" (CIHR, 2002, pp. 8–9; Gowans et al., 2011; Ploem, 2006, pp. 52–3). It should be noted that the argument about the sheer size of the research population is less of an issue in the context of rare diseases.

While many experts concur that participant consent is necessary, in light of the challenges in obtaining informed consent – upfront or on an ongoing basis – some suggest that additional methods to protect privacy are needed. Consent cannot, from a practical perspective, be a tool to ensure privacy protection in the context of every individual secondary use of data: the need for informed consent has to be balanced with the practical difficulties faced in obtaining that consent (CIHR, 2002, pp. 8–9), which also have implications for the reliability of the research (selection bias). In the context of biobanks, Austin and Lemmens (2009) recommend that the overemphasis on *consent* must be reduced, and instead of exploring the issue of informed consent through the apparent dichotomy of "strict application of informed consent" *versus* "a more pragmatic application of informed consent to facilitate research," focus should be on good governance. The authors argue:

> The traditional standard of informed consent to participate in a biobank can be met but only where there is a governance structure ensuring consistent information practices and policies across multiple future research projects ... [S]pecific research uses of research samples and associated data in the biobank do not necessarily require informed consent but do require a governance structure that can regulate privacy risks such as the risk of re-identification. Both scenarios – consent at the outset of the collection and no-consent for future use – therefore require a governance structure in order to protect the important interests at stake. (Austin & Lemmens, 2009, p. 111)

We suggest that, particularly in the context of the concern about potential privacy breaches resulting from the transparency of clinical trial data, *the distinction between the consent involved in the general collection and storage of data (consent to a governance structure) and the consent for specific research uses is crucial.* If, as Austin and Lemmens argue, informant consent is not crucial for secondary use of data, the focus should be on providing sufficient information about the type of governance that will surround the collection of data and the overall reasons for this data collection. It thus seems key to ensure that people involved in clinical trials for rare diseases are informed about the likelihood of further data access and the importance of such access.

REBs / Independent Review Panels

Researchers' requests for access to clinical trial data are typically reviewed and approved, often subject to conditions, by specialized independent data review panels or by REBs. This process raises questions regarding who the individuals responsible for approving the request are and which stakeholders should be involved in approving the request. The Institute of Medicine (2015a) explains that, typically, independent review panels comprise experts in "clinical research, clinical trials, biostatistics, and clinical medicine who have no conflicts of interest in deciding whether a data requester receives access. Some panels also have members with expertise in law and ethics." The report further observes that independent review panels established by pharmaceutical companies do not include, *but should include,* the following stakeholders: "representation of clinical trial participants, their communities, disease advocacy groups, or the public" (Institute of Medicine, 2015a). It argues that the public can provide critical diverse perspectives and innovative suggestions that increase data sharing while protecting patient privacy (Institute of Medicine, 2015a). However, concerns have been raised that, when patient advocacy groups are funded by pharmaceutical companies, their actions and demands are sometimes influenced by this relationship, and the practice biases patient advocacy groups in favour of pharmaceutical companies (Moynihan & Bero, 2017; Lin, Lucas, Murimi, Kolodny, & Alexander, 2017; see also Taylor & Denegri, 2017).

Krleža-Jerić (2018) insists that, to mitigate the influence of pharmaceutical companies through patient advocacy groups and limit conflicts of interest arising from such relationships, it is necessary that advocacy groups not sponsored by pharmaceutical companies, such as Pharma-Watch, be involved in the decision-making process.

Since data sharing can be considered an ethical obligation, REBs[23] should also be more extensively involved in fostering data sharing.

REBs could be requested to impose data sharing as a precondition for approval of any research study.[24] For example, the 2017 Transparency International report, *Clinical Trial Transparency*, suggests that "Regulatory Authorities for Ethics Committees, which give approval to conduct a clinical trial, can act as a bottleneck for ensuring trial registration. Mandating registration as part of the ethics approval process would necessitate that trials are registered before the trial can begin" (Bruckner, 2017, p. 11). We recommend that REBs go beyond insistence on clinical trial registration to also insist that data be made publicly available and that consent forms (as discussed earlier) contain specific language to that effect. The consent forms should contain language explaining the importance of data sharing and giving a reasonable assessment of the risk of de-identification that could result from access to data. De-identification, in the context of rare disease research, is a particularly important issue, and a thorough explanation of the risk can prevent future complaints about privacy issues.

Terms of Use Agreements

Health Canada adopted terms of use (ToU) agreements pursuant to the new Regulations Amending the Food and Drug Regulations (Public Release of Clinical Information) and Regulations Amending the Medical Devices Regulations (Public Release of Clinical Information), which came into force in May 2019 (Government of Canada, 2019b, 2019c). The objective of these regulations is to increase public access to clinical trial data submitted to Health Canada by proactively making data available on a website (see chapter five of this volume). In order to access the data, an individual needs to sign the ToU agreement, which primarily "require[s] that end users agree not to use the publicly released data for commercial purposes or attempt to identify clinical trial subjects or individuals" (Government of Canada, 2019b). However, the data available through the ToU agreement is limited due to the exceptions carved out by Health Canada.[25] We argue that Health Canada should remove such limitations on data sharing, which undermine transparency, and focus instead on better protecting the shared data by modelling its data sharing on EMA's two-tiered data sharing regime of registration processes and ToU agreements.

The proactive publication regime created in the European Union by the EMA, via the Publication Policy 0070, structures the disclosure regime to provide for two levels of access to published clinical data based on two-tiered levels of registration processes and ToU agreements that govern the access to and use of clinical reports, depending on the intended use.[26] On the broadest level, the two levels of access provided are on-screen only access for general use and downloadable and printable access to identified users for research purposes.

The on-screen access to clinical reports for general use requires a simple and limited registration process consisting of creating an ID and password, and agreeing to general ToU for general information and non-commercial purposes. Clinical reports under this access model are made available in a "view-on-screen-only" mode. The downloadable access to clinical reports is available to identified users for academic and other non-commercial research purposes, based on a more comprehensive registration process that involves providing identity-related information, including the affiliation and position within the organization of the user. It also requires a ToU agreement for academic and other non-commercial research purposes. This level of access allows clinical reports to be downloaded, saved, and printed.

The EMA's ToU agreements are particularly meritorious as they "provide unfettered access to data for research purposes and use of the data for research, including comparative effectiveness research" (Herder & Lemmens, 2015b). According to Herder and Lemmens, the key advantage of the ToU agreement is that access to data is provided without imposition of confidentiality in respect to the data as long as the data are used for research purposes. To ensure good governance, researchers are required to identify themselves and declare the purpose behind their research (Herder & Lemmens, 2015a). Further, to protect participant privacy and commercially confidential information (CCI), both sets of ToU agreements contain provisions to ensure that users of information do not attempt to re-identify trial subjects or other individuals with the information; or use the clinical reports to support a market authorization (MA) application, or extensions or variations to an MA, or for any other unfair commercial use. In order to emphasize the prohibition of its use for commercial purposes, a watermark is applied to the published information.

Conclusion

Increased transparency in clinical trial data – for ongoing clinical trials as well as in respect of drugs approved/rejected by the regulatory authorities – is as (if not more) important in the context of rare diseases as it is in other areas of medical research. Transparency even provides particular benefits in the rare disease context, as we discussed earlier. It is acknowledged that the question – how access to data can be reconciled with adequate protection of research participant privacy – is particularly pertinent in the context of research involving rare diseases, as the number of research subjects participating in such clinical trials is often very low, and the risk of re-identification arguably high or at least higher than in more traditional drug development. But fears over breach of research participants' privacy are often overstated, and appear more an issue of perception than a real concern. We discussed how, in most clinical trials, existing safeguards are sufficient to protect privacy, and the prospect of re-identification using clinical trial data remains minimal. The policy level concern as to whether the privacy concerns outweigh the benefit of increased transparency of data should be explored through the lens of proportionality, which balances the benefits of sharing clinical trial data with the "real" risks of privacy breaches. However, potential negative implications of access to data for patients should be addressed, and efforts must be undertaken to mitigate privacy-linked concerns while increasing data transparency. For this reason, three legal mechanisms are recommended.

The first, participant consent, is generally necessary for the collection, storage, and use of personal health information, and can be a valuable legal tool in protecting patient privacy rights. But obtaining informed consent upfront, and even more on an ongoing basis (during the clinical trial and after), raises a host of challenges in practical terms, some having the potential to impede efforts to share data. Excessive reliance on informed consent for privacy protection impacts the reliability of research and provides insufficient protection. While informed consent remains important, we emphasize that the informed consent process should focus on the mode of governance of health information access and on providing clear information about the importance of data sharing. Informed consent is only one of the tools to mitigate privacy-linked concerns. Participants' consent for use of their data for secondary research purposes should be obtained upfront before the research participant begins the trial, rather than on an ongoing basis. In the informed consent process, all major privacy-linked concerns should be discussed and connected to the benefits that increased transparency can provide. Additionally, other legal mechanisms – such as implementing a good governance structure – must also be employed.

The second recommendation pertains to independent review panels or, in the absence of specialized committees, REBs. Review panels or REBs should receive, analyse, and approve requests for data access with a reasoned decision provided within a stipulated time period. A minimum level of detail with respect to all requests and decisions must be maintained in a publicly accessible register to improve public accountability. Additionally, the panel or REB's reasons for permitting or rejecting requests must be open to public scrutiny. The independence of a panel and an REB is critical.

The constitution of independent review panels and REBs must be defined to ensure all stakeholders are appropriately represented. Independent review panels and REBs must have representation from a range of interests when analysing requests for access to data, including representation from clinical trial participants, their communities, advocacy organizations, particularly those *not* sponsored by pharmaceutical companies, and the public, as well as researchers who are experts in the field. Decision-making must be safeguarded against conflicts of interest while achieving a diverse yet balanced representation of interests and concerns. Accordingly, individuals representing stakeholders other than the applicable pharmaceutical company or research institution must not be directly or indirectly dependent on that pharmaceutical company or research institution for their personal livelihood, and they must not have financial interests in the research or the drug.

REBs should also play a significant role at the time of the initial collection of data. REBs should insist that consent forms contain specific information about the purpose of data collection and the possible privacy implications of the future transparency of data. REBs should also insist on trial registration as a precondition for approval of the research and on sharing of data. Reference to these obligations should be made in the consent forms.

The third legal mechanism is the use of ToU agreements. The ToU agreement prescribed by the EMA can be seen as a possible model. Under the ToU, access to data should be provided without the imposition of confidentiality in respect to data as long as data are used for research purposes. To ensure good governance, researchers should be required to identify themselves and declare the purpose behind their research (Herder & Lemmens, 2015a). Specifically, to protect participant privacy, ToU agreements must contain provisions stipulating that users of information must not attempt to re-identify trial subjects or other individuals from the information; or use the clinical reports to support an MA application, or extensions or variations to an MA, or for any other unfair commercial use. In order to emphasize the prohibition of its use for commercial purposes, a watermark should be applied to the published information.

These mechanisms endeavour to address privacy-linked concerns while increasing clinical trial data sharing, which is necessary and highly beneficial in the rare disease context. It is recommended that the mechanisms be legally implemented through regulatory measures. In the interim, REBs and pharmaceutical companies should take steps to voluntarily adopt and implement these mechanisms. Research participants should insist upon compliance with these mechanisms as a condition to their participation in clinical trials, particularly those involving rare diseases.

NOTES

1 This chapter is based on Lemmens et al., 2020.
2 For a discussion of the European Medicines Agency's transparency po-
   lices, see Lemmens et al., 2020.
3 For example, see Minssen, Neethu, and Bogers (2019) for a discussion on
   the interplay between European Union transparency policies and privacy
   law, specifically the General Data Protection Regulation (EU) 2016/679.
4 For a discussion on the most commonly cited privacy-linked concerns, see
   Lemmens et al., 2020.
5 For a discussion on the wide range of public benefits, see Lemmens et al.,
   2020.
6 For a discussion on the legal, ethical, and social arguments, see Lemmens
   et al., 2020.
7 For a discussion on pricing of older, unpatented yet essential orphan drugs
   and future orphan drugs, see Roberts, Herder, & Hollis, 2015.
8 For a discussion of this project, see Lemmens et al., 2020.
9 A table summarizing the transparency policies of Canadian pharmaceutical
   companies that are publicly available and were analysed for the purposes
   of the report is attached to Lemmens et al., 2020.
10 A full list of the pharmaceutical companies that were identified, which
   both operate in Canada and develop new pharmaceuticals, is attached
   to Lemmens et al., 2020. For details of the methodology adopted, see
   Lemmens et al., 2020.
11 For a discussion on the range of issues identified, see Lemmens et al., 2020.
12 For a discussion on the range of arguments raised in respect of these
   various aspects, see Lemmens et al., 2020.
13 For a discussion on the concerns raised on re-identification and discrimination, see Lemmens et al., 2020.
14 For a further discussion on security breaches of personal health information,
   see also El Emam et al., 2007, pp. 3–6.
15 For a discussion on arguments raised in respect of commercial interest, see
   Lemmens et al., 2020.
16 For more information, see the Structural Genomics Consortium's website
   at https://www.thesgc.org/about.
17 The Declaration of Helsinki was developed by the World Medical
   Association (WMA) and adopted at the 18th WMA General Assembly held
   in Helsinki, Finland, in 1964. It has since been updated several times, the
   latest at the 64th WMA General Assembly in Fortaleza, Brazil, in October
   2013 (World Medical Association, 2018).
18 European Commission for Horizon 2020 Societal Challenge Health
   Demographic Change and Wellbeing (joined on 27 October 2017); EDCTP

(joined on 5 July 2017); Indian Council of Medical Research; Inserm; Research Council of Norway; UK Department for International Development (DFID; joined on 31 May 2017); UK Medical Research Council; UK National Institute of Health Research (joined on 8 August 2017); ZonMw (joined on 10 July 2017); Aeras (joined on 13 June 2017); CEPI; Drugs for Neglected Diseases Initiative (DNDi); Epicentre; FIND (joined on 26 May 2017); Global Alliance for TB Drug Development (TB Alliance; joined on 13 June 2017); Institut Pasteur; Médecins Sans Frontières; Medicines for Malaria Venture (MMV; joined on 24 May 2017); PATH; Bill & Melinda Gates Foundation; Wellcome Trust.

19 Food and Drug Administration Amendments Act of 2007, Pub L No 110-85, § 801, 121 Stat 823, 904-22.
20 For a discussion of the exceptions, see Lemmens et al., 2020.
21 For a discussion on various other suggestions made to achieve balance, see Lemmens et al., 2020.
22 For a discussion on the challenges involved with providing the right to withdraw, see Kaye, 2012, p. 422.
23 For a description of research ethics boards (REBs), refer to CIHR, 2002, pp. 11–12.
24 For a discussion on research ethics boards (REBs), including shortcomings, see Austin & Lemmens, 2009, p. 244; see also Lemmens & Vacaflor (2018).
25 For a discussion on the exceptions, see Lemmens et al., 2020.
26 For a discussion on critiques of the policy when it was released for public comments, see Gibson & Lemmens, 2014.

REFERENCES

Armstrong, D., Kline-Rogers, E.M., & Jani, S.M. (2005). Potential impact of the HIPAA privacy rule on data collection in a registry of patients with acute coronary syndrome. *ACC Current Journal Review, 14*(8), 6–7. https://doi.org /10.1016/j.accreview.2005.08.012
Austin, L.M., & Lemmens, T. (2009). Privacy, consent, and governance. In K. Dierickx & P. Borry (Eds.), *New challenges for biobanks: Ethics, law and governance* (pp. 111–22). Antwerp, BE: Intersentia.
Bambauer, D.E. (2012). The myth of perfection. *Wake Forest Law Review Online, 2*(22). Retrieved from http://wakeforestlawreview.com/2012/04/the-myth -of-perfection/
Barry, A.R., Koshman, S.L., & Pearson, G.J. (2014). Adverse drug reactions: The importance of maintaining pharmacovigilance. *Canadian Pharmacists Journal, 147*(4), 233–8. https://doi.org/10.1177/1715163514536523
Benitez, K., & Malin, B. (2010). Evaluating re-identification risks with respect to the HIPAA privacy rule. *Journal of the American Medical Informatics Association, 17*(2), 169–77. https://doi.org/10.1136/jamia.2009.000026

Bierer, B.E., Li, R., Barnes, M., & Sim, I. (2016). A global, neutral platform for sharing trial data. *New England Journal of Medicine, 374*(25), 2411–13. https://doi.org/10.1056/NEJMp1605348

Boon, W., & Moors, E. (2008). Exploring emerging technologies using metaphors: A study of orphan drugs and pharmacogenomics. *Social Science & Medicine, 66*(9), 1915–27. https://doi.org/10.1016/j.socscimed.2008.01.012

Brown, I., Brown, L., & Korff, D. (2010). Using NHS patient data for research without consent. *Law, Innovation & Technology, 2*(2), 219–58. https://doi.org/10.5235/175799610794046186

Bruckner, T. (2017). *Clinical trial transparency: A guide for policy makers.* Report prepared by TranspariMED in close consultation with Cochrane, the Collaboration for Research Integrity and Transparency (CRIT), and Transparency International's Pharmaceuticals and Healthcare Programme (PHP). Retrieved from https://docs.wixstatic.com/ugd/01f35d_def0082121a648529220e1d56df4b50a.pdf

Budin-Ljøsne, I., Teare, H.J.A., Kaye, J., Beck, S., Bentzen, H.B., Caenazzo, L., … Mascalzoni, D. (2017). Dynamic consent: A potential solution to some of the challenges of modern biomedical research. *BMC Medical Ethics, 18*, 4. https://doi.org/10.1186/s12910-016-0162-9

Canadian Institutes of Health Research (CIHR). (2002). *Secondary use of personal information in health research: Case studies, November 2002.* Ottawa, ON: Public Works and Government Services Canada. Retrieved from https://cihr-irsc.gc.ca/e/1475.html

Canadian Organization for Rare Disorders (CORD). (2005). Canada's orphan drug policy: Learning from the best. Retrieved from https://www.raredisorders.ca/content/uploads/CanadaOrphanDPFinal-copy.pdf

Caulfield, T., & Kaye, J. (2009). Broad consent in biobanking: Reflections on seemingly insurmountable dilemmas. *Medical Law International, 10*(2), 85–100. https://doi.org/10.1177/096853320901000201

Cavoukian, A., & El Emam, K. (2011). *Dispelling the myths surrounding de-identification: Anonymization remains a strong tool for protecting privacy.* Retrieved from https://www.ipc.on.ca/wp-content/uploads/2016/11/anonymization.pdf

Chen, D.T., Worrall, B.B., Brown, R.D., Brott, T.G., Kissela, B.M., Olson, T.S., … Meschia, J.F. (2005). The impact of privacy protections on recruitment in a multicenter stroke genetics study. *Neurology, 64*(4), 721–4. https://doi.org/10.1212/01.WNL.0000152042.07414.CC

Clinical Study Data Request. (2020a). Our mission. Retrieved from https://www.clinicalstudydatarequest.com/

Clinical Study Data Request. (2020b). Sponsor specific details: Bayer. Retrieved from https://www.clinicalstudydatarequest.com/Study-Sponsors/Study-Sponsors-Bayer.aspx

Collier, R. (2011). Bye, bye blockbusters, hello niche busters. *Canadian Medical Association Journal, 183*(11), E697–8. https://doi.org/10.1503/cmaj.109-3874

Coté, T.R., Xu, K., & Pariser, A.R. (2010). Accelerating orphan drug development. *Nature Reviews Drug Discovery, 9*(12), 901–2. https://doi.org/10.1038/nrd3340

Council of Canadian Academies Expert Panel on Timely Access to Health and Social Data for Health Research and Health System Innovation. (2015). *Accessing health and health-related data in Canada*. Ottawa, ON: Council of Canadian Academies Expert Panel. Retrieved from https://cca-reports.ca/reports/accessing-health-and-health-related-data-in-canada/

Darrow, J.J., Avorn, J., & Kesselheim, A.S. (2014). New FDA breakthrough-drug category – Implications for patients. *New England Journal of Medicine, 370,* 1252–8. https://doi.org/10.1056/NEJMhle1311493

Dolgin, E. (2010). Big pharma moves from "blockbusters" to "niche busters." *Nature Medicine, 16,* 837. https://doi.org/10.1038/nm0810-837a

Dupont, A.G., & Van Wilder, P.B. (2011). Access to orphan drugs despite poor quality of clinical evidence. *British Journal of Clinical Pharmacology, 71*(4), 488–96. https://doi.org/10.1111/j.1365-2125.2010.03877.x

Eichler, H-G., Pignatti, F., Flamion, B., Leufkens, H., & Breckenridge, A. (2008). Balancing early market access to new drugs with the need for benefit/risk data: A mounting dilemma. *Nature Reviews Drug Discover, 7*(10), 818–26. https://doi.org/10.1038/nrd2664

El Emam, K. (2013). *Guide to the de-identification of personal health information.* Boca Raton, FL: CRC Press.

El Emam, K. (2018, 25 January). Exploratory discussion with the authors.

El Emam, K., Jonker, E., Sams, S., Neri, E., Neisa, A., Gao, T., & Chowdhury, S. (2007). *Pan-Canadian de-identification guidelines for personal health information.* Ottawa, ON: CHEO Research Institute.

European Commission. (2016, 19 April; updated 29 October 2020). *The European Cloud Initiative.* Retrieved from https://ec.europa.eu/digital-single-market/en/european-cloud-initiative

European Federation of Pharmaceutical Industries and Associations (EFPIA) & Pharmaceutical Research and Manufacturers of America (PhRMA). (2013, 24 July). EFPIA and PhRMA release joint principles for responsible clinical trial data sharing to benefit patients. Press release. Retrieved from https://www.efpia.eu/news-events/the-efpia-view/statements-press-releases/130724-efpia-and-phrma-release-joint-principles-for-responsible-clinical-trial-data-sharing-to-benefit-patients/

European Medicines Agency (EMA). (2021a). *Background to clinical data publication policy.* Retrieved from https://www.ema.europa.eu/en/human-regulatory/marketing-authorisation/clinical-data-publication/background-clinical-data-publication-policy

European Medicines Agency (EMA). (2021b). *Human regulatory: Clinical trial data publication.* Retrieved from https://www.ema.europa.eu/en/human-regulatory/marketing-authorisation/clinical-data-publication

Fletcher, B., Gheorghe, A., Moore, D., Wilson, S., & Damery, S. (2012). Improving the recruitment activity of clinicians in randomised controlled trials: A systematic review. *BMJ Open, 2*(1), e000496. https://doi.org/10.1136 /bmjopen-2011-000496

Forrest, M. (2017, 17 Oct). Canada gives "kiss of death" to planned policy for rare-disease drugs. *National Post.* Retrieved from https://nationalpost.com /news/politics/health-canada-gives-kiss-of-death-to-planned-policy-for-rare -disease-drugs

Garrison, N.A., Sathe, N.A., Matheny Antommaria, A.H., Holm, I.A., Sanderson, S.C., Smith, M.E., ... Clayton, E.W. (2016). A systematic literature review of individuals' perspectives on broad consent and data sharing in the United States. *Genetics in Medicine, 18*(7), 663–71. https://doi.org/10.1038 /gim.2015.138

Geelen, E., Horstman, K., Marcelis, C.L.M., Doevendans, P.A., & Van Hoyweghen, I. (2012). Unravelling fears of genetic discrimination: An exploratory study of Dutch HCM families in an era of genetic non-discrimination acts. *European Journal of Human Genetics, 20*(10), 1018–23. https://doi.org/10.1038/ejhg .2012.53

Genetic and Rare Diseases Information Center (GARD). (2017). FAQs about rare diseases. Retrieved from https://rarediseases.info.nih.gov/diseases /pages/31/faqs-about-rare-diseases

Genomics England. (n.d.). *About Genomics England.* Retrieved from https://www .genomicsengland.co.uk/about-genomics-england/

Gertz, R. (2008). Withdrawing from participating in a biobank – A comparative study. *European Journal of Health Law, 15*(4), 381. https://doi.org/10.1163 /157180908X338269

Gibson, S.G., & Lemmens, T. (2014). Niche markets and evidence assessment in transition: A critical review of proposed drug reforms. *Medical Law Review, 22*(2), 200–20. https://doi.org/10.1093/medlaw/fwu005

Gibson, S.G., & von Tigerstrom, B. (2015). Orphan drug incentives in the pharmacogenomic context: Policy responses in the US and Canada. *Journal of Law and the Biosciences, 2*(2), 263–91. https://doi.org/10.1093/jlb/lsv013

Government of Canada. (2019a). *Budget 2019: Budget plan.* Retrieved from https://www.budget.gc.ca/2019/docs/plan/toc-tdm-en.html

Government of Canada. (2019b). Regulations Amending the Food and Drug Regulations (Public Release of Clinical Information): SOR/2019-62. *Canada Gazette,* Part II, *153*(6). Retrieved from http://www.gazette.gc.ca/rp-pr/p2 /2019/2019-03-20/html/sor-dors62-eng.html

Government of Canada. (2019c). Regulations Amending the Medical Devices Regulations (Public Release of Clinical Information): SOR/2019-63. *Canada Gazette,* Part II, *153*(6). Retrieved from http://www.gazette.gc.ca/rp-pr/p2 /2019/2019-03-20/html/sor-dors63-eng.html

Gowans, H., Kanellopoulou, N., Hawkins, N., Curren, L., Melham, J., Kaye, J., & Boddington, P. (2011). Consent forms in genomics: The difference between law and practice. *European Journal of Health Law, 18*(5), 491–519. https://doi .org/10.1163/157180911X598744

Hansson, M.G. (2009). Ethics and biobanks. *British Journal of Cancer, 100*(1), 8–12. https://doi.org/10.1038/sj.bjc.6604795

Hansson, M.G. (2012). Where should we draw the line between quality of care and other ethical concerns related to medical registries and biobanks? *Theoretical Medicine and Bioethics, 33*(4), 313–23. https://doi.org/10.1007 /s11017-012-9229-x

Harding, R. (2018, 24 January). Exploratory discussion with the authors.

Health Canada. (2012). *An orphan drug framework for Canada.* News Release, 3 October 2012. Mentioned in House of Commons, Canada. (2013). *HESA Committee Report: Technological Innovation in Health Care – Report of the Standing Committee on Health,* 41st Parliament, First Session (p. 37). Retrieved from https://www.ourcommons.ca/Content/Committee/411/HESA/Reports /RP6221741/hesarp14/hesarp14-e.pdf

Herder, M., & Lemmens, T. (2015a, 27 October). Diclectin data: Testing Canada's new pharmaceutical transparency law. *BMJ Opinion.* Retrieved from https://blogs.bmj.com/bmj/2015/10/27/diclectin-data-testing-canadas -new-pharmaceutical-transparency-law/

Herder, M., & Lemmens, T. (2015b, 9 November). Testing Canada's new pharmaceutical transparency law. *Impact Ethics.* Retrieved from https:// impactethics.ca/2015/11/09/testing-canadas-new-pharmaceutical -transparency-law/

Hill, M.D., & Buchan, A.M. (2001). Methodology for the Canadian Activase for Stroke Effectiveness Study (CASES). *Canadian Journal of Neurological Science, 28*(3), 232–8. https://doi.org/10.1017/S0317167100001384

Hirschler, B. (2013, 30 April). *Europe's regulator digs in for drug data fight. Reuters.* Retrieved from https://www.reuters.com/article/idUSBRE93T0KU20130430

Institute of Medicine. (2015a). Access to clinical trial data: Governance. In Institute of Medicine, *Sharing clinical trial data: Maximizing benefits, minimizing risk* (pp. 139–61). Washington, DC: National Academies Press. Retrieved from https://www.nap.edu/read/18998/chapter/7

Institute of Medicine. (2015b). *Sharing clinical trial data: Maximizing benefits, minimizing risk.* Washington, DC: National Academies Press.

Katzan, I.L., Furlan, A.J., Lloyd, L.E., Frank, J.I., Harper, D.L., Hinchey, J.A., ... Sila, C.A. (2000). Use of tissue-type plasminogen activator for acute ischemic stroke: The Cleveland area experience. *JAMA, 283*(9), 1151–8. https://doi .org/10.1001/jama.283.9.1151

Kaye, J. (2012). The tension between data sharing and the protection of privacy in genomics research. *Annual Review of Genomics & Human Genetics, 13*, 415–31. https://doi.org/10.1146/annurev-genom-082410-101454

Kaye, J., Whitely, E.A., Lund, D., Morrison, M., Teare, H., & Melham, K. (2015). Dynamic consent: A patient interface for twenty-first century research networks. *European Journal of Human Genetics, 23*(2), 141–6. https://doi.org/10.1038/ejhg .2014.71

Kesselheim, A.S., & Treasure, C.L. (2017). Biomarker-defined subsets of common diseases: Policy and economic implications of Orphan Drug Act coverage. *PloS Medicine, 14*(1), e1002190. https://doi.org/10.1371/journal .pmed.1002190

Kesselheim, A.S., Wang, B., Franklin, J.M., & Darrow, J.J. (2015). Trends in utilization of FDA expedited drug development and approval programs, 1987–2014: Cohort study. *BMJ, 351*, h4633. https://doi.org/10.1136/bmj.h4633

Kesselheim, A.S., Woloshin, S., Eddings, W., Franklin, J.M., Ross, K.M., & Schwartz, L.M. (2016). Physicians' knowledge about FDA approval standards and perceptions of the "breakthrough therapy" designation. *JAMA, 315*(14), 1516–18. https://doi.org/10.1001/jama.2015.16984

Krishnamurti, T., Woloshin, S., Schwartz, L.M., & Fischhoff, B. (2015). A randomized trial testing US Food and Drug Administration "breakthrough" language. *JAMA Internal Medicine, 175*(11), 1856–8. https://doi.org/10.1001 /jamainternmed.2015.5355

Krleža-Jerić, K. (2018, 29 January). Exploratory discussion with the authors.

Krleža-Jerić, K., Chan, A.-W., Dickersin, K., Sim, I., Grimshaw, J., & Gluud, C. (2005). Principles for international registration of protocol information and results from human trials of health related interventions: Ottawa statement (Part 1). *BMJ, 330*, 956. https://doi.org/10.1136/bmj.330.7497.956

Krleža-Jerić, K., Gabelica, M., Banzi, R., Krnić-Martinić, M., Pulido, B., Mahmić-Kaknjo, M., ... Hrgović, I. (2016). IMPACT Observatory: Tracking the evolution of clinical trial data sharing and research integrity. *Biochemia Medica, 26*(3), 308–7. https://doi.org/10.11613/bm.2016.035

Krleža-Jeriç, K., Lemmens, T., Reveiz, L., Cuervo, L.G., & Bero, L.A. (2011). Prospective registration and results disclosure of clinical trials in the Americas: A roadmap toward transparency. *Pan American Journal of Public Health, 30*(1), 87–96.

Lapham, E.V., Kozma, C., & Weiss, J.O. (1996). Genetic discrimination: Perspectives of consumers. *Science, 274*(5287), 621–4. https://doi.org/10.1126 /science.274.5287.621

Lemmens, T. (2013). Pharmaceutical knowledge governance: A human rights perspective. *Journal of Law, Medicine & Ethics, 41*(1), 163–84. https://doi.org /10.1111/jlme.12012

Lemmens, T., Mahadevia Ghimire, K., Rafferty, E., Krleža-Jerić, K., Lee, J.Y., Vacaflor, C.H., & Ringkamp, G. (2020). *Balancing the privacy right of research participants with the public interest in access to clinical drug trials data in the context of rare diseases.* Report, funded by the Office of the Privacy Commissioner of Canada. (*Transparency Report*). Toronto: University of Toronto. Retrieved from https://library.law.utoronto.ca/privacy-access-drug-trials-data

Lemmens, T., & Vacaflor, C.H. (2018) Clinical trials transparency in the Americas: The need to coordinate regulatory spheres. *BMJ, 362*, k2493. https://doi.org /10.1136/bmj.k2493

Lexchin, J. (2012). New drugs and safety: What happened to new active substances approved between 1985 and 2010? *Arch Internal Medicine, 172*(21), 1680–1. https://doi.org/10.1001/archinternmed.2012.4444

Lexchin, J. (2015). Health Canada's use of its priority review process for new drugs: A cohort study. *BMJ Open, 5*(5), e006816. https://doi.org/10.1136 /bmjopen-2014-006816

Lexchin, J., Doshi, P., Graham, J.E., Herder, M., Jefferson, T., Lemmens, T., ... Stewart, I. (2017, 19 May). Response to Health Canada on release of clinical data. Joint Letter. Retrieved from https://haiweb.org/publication/13057/

Lin, D.H., Lucas, E., Murimi, I.B., Kolodny, A., & Alexander, G.C. (2017). Financial conflicts of interest and the Centers for Disease Control and Prevention's 2016 Guideline for Prescribing Opioids for Chronic Pain. *JAMA Internal Medicine, 177*(3), 427–8. https://doi.org/10.1001/jamainternmed .2016.8471

Loorand-Stiver, L., Cowling, T., & Perras, C., for the Canadian Agency for Drugs and Technologies in Health (CADTH). (2016). CADTH environmental scan: Drugs for rare diseases: Evolving trends in regulatory and health technology assessment perspectives. Project no. ES0300-000. Retrieved from https:// www.cadth.ca/sites/default/files/pdf/ES0300_Rare_Disease_Drugs_e.pdf

Lowrance, W.W. (2003). Learning from experience: Privacy and the secondary use of data in health research. *Journal of Health Services Research & Policy, 8*(1, suppl.), 2–7. https://doi.org/10.1258/135581903766468800

MacLeod, A. (2012, 8 September). *Research stopped by ministry might have cut big pharma profits. The Tyee.* Retrieved from https://thetyee.ca/News/2012/09 /08/BC-Pharma-Research/

Marešová, P., Mohelská, H., & Kuča, K. (2015). Cooperation policy of rare diseases in the European Union. *Procedia – Social and Behavioral Sciences, 171*, 1302–8. https://doi.org/10.1016/j.sbspro.2015.01.245

Mariner, W.K. (2009). Toward an architecture of health law. *American Journal of Law & Medicine, 35*(1), 67–87. https://doi.org/10.1177/009885880903500102

Mascalzoni, D., Paradiso, A., & Hansson, M. (2014). Rare disease research: Breaking the privacy barrier. *Applied & Translational Genomics, 3*(2), 23–9. https://doi.org/10.1016/j.atg.2014.04.003

McCabe, C., Tsuchiya, A., Claxton, K., & Raftery, J. (2006). Orphan drugs revisited. *Quarterly Journal of Medicine, 99*(5), 341–5. https://doi.org/10.1093 /qjmed/hcl033

McCormack, P., Kole, A., Gainotti, S., Mascalzoni, D., Molster, C., Lochmüller, H., & Woods, S. (2016). "You should at least ask." The expectations, hopes and fears of rare disease patients on large-scale data and biomaterial sharing for genomics research. *European Journal of Human Genetics, 24*(10), 1403–8. https://doi.org/10.1038/ejhg.2016.30

Melnikova, I. (2012). Rare diseases and orphan drugs. *Nature Reviews Drug Discovery, 11*(4), 267–8. https://doi.org/10.1038/nrd3654

Menon, D., Clark, D., & Stafinski, T. (2015). Reimbursement of drugs for rare diseases through the public healthcare system in Canada: Where are we now? *Healthcare Policy, 11*(1), 15–32. https://doi.org/10.12927/hcpol.2015.24360

Minssen, T., Neethu, R., & Bogers, M. (2019). Clinical trial data transparency and GDPR compliance: Implications for data sharing and open innovation. In K. Sideri & G. Dutfield (Eds.), *Openness, intellectual property and science policy in the age of data driven medicine.* (Special issue of *Science and Public Policy*). Retrieved from https://papers.ssrn.com/sol3/papers.cfm?abstract _id=3413035

Mintzes, B., Lexchin, J., & Quintano, A.S. (2015). Clinical trial transparency: Many gains but access to evidence for new medicines remains imperfect. *British Medical Bulletin, 116*(1), 43–53. https://doi.org/10.1093/bmb/ldv042

Moore, T.J., & Furberg, C.D. (2014). Development times, clinical testing, postmarket follow-up, and safety risks for the new drugs approved by the US Food and Drug Administration: The class of 2008. *JAMA Internal Medicine, 174*(1), 90–5. https://doi.org/10.1001/jamainternmed.2013.11813

Moynihan, R., & Bero, L. (2017). Toward a healthier patient voice: More independence, less industry funding. *JAMA Internal Medicine, 177*(3), 350–1. https://doi.org/10.1001/jamainternmed.2016.9179

Nelson, G.S. (2015). Practical implications of sharing data: A primer on data privacy, anonymization, and de-identification. Paper 1884-2015, ThotWave Technologies, Chapel Hill, NC. Retrieved from https://support.sas.com /resources/papers/proceedings15/1884-2015.pdf

Nisen, P., & Rockhold, F. (2013). Access to patient-level data from GlaxoSmithKline clinical trials. *New England Journal of Medicine, 369*, 475–8. https://doi.org/10.1056/NEJMsr1302541

Ohm, P. (2010). Broken promises of privacy: Responding to the surprising failure of anonymization. *UCLA Law Review, 57*, 1701–77. Retrieved from https:// www.uclalawreview.org/pdf/57-6-3.pdf

Ohmann, C., Banzi, R., Canham, S., Battaglia, S., Matei, M., Ariyo, C., ... Demotes-Mainard, J. (2017). Sharing and reuse of individual participant data from clinical trials: Principles and recommendations. *BMJ Open, 7*(12), e018647. https://doi.org/10.1136/bmjopen-2017-018647

Owen, A.J., Spinks, J., Meehan, A., Robb, R., Hardy, M., & Kwasha, D. (2008). A new model to evaluate the long-term cost effectiveness of orphan and highly specialised drugs following listing on the Australian Pharmaceutical Benefits Scheme: The Bosentan Patient Registry. *Journal of Medical Economics, 11*(2), 235–43. https://doi.org/10.3111/13696990802034525

Peddicord, D., Waldo, A.B., Boutin, M., Grande, T., & Gutierrez, L. (2010). A proposal to protect privacy of health information while accelerating comparative effectiveness research. *Health Affairs, 29*(11), 2082–90. https://doi.org/10.1377/hlthaff.2010.0635

Picavet, E., Cassiman, D., Hollak, C.E., Maertens, J.A., & Simoens, S. (2013). Clinical evidence for orphan medicinal products – A cause for concern. *Orphanet Journal of Rare Diseases, 8*(1), 164. https://doi.org/10.1186/1750-1172-8-164

Ploem, M.C. (2006). Towards an appropriate privacy regime for medical data research. *European Journal of Health Law, 13*(1), 41–63. https://doi.org/10.1163/157180906777036319

President's Council of Advisors on Science and Technology (US). (2012). Report to the President on propelling innovation in drug discovery, development, and evaluation. Washington DC. Retrieved from https://permanent.fdlp.gov/gpo32081/pcast-fda-final.pdf

Rasi, G., (2013, 29 April). Clinical data: Time for new approach. *Financial Times.* Retrieved from https://www.ft.com/content/5c769724-adcb-11e2-82b8-00144feabdc0

Rawson, N.S., & Adams, J. (2018, 2 Mar). RE: Access to new drugs for rare disorders in Canada. *CMAJ.* Retrieved from https://www.cmaj.ca/content/re-access-new-drugs-rare-disorders-canada

Roberts, E.A., Herder, M., & Hollis, A. (2015). Fair pricing of "old" orphan drugs: Considerations for Canada's orphan drug policy. *CMAJ, 187*(6), 422–5. https://doi.org/10.1503/cmaj.140308

Rockhold, F., Nisen, P., & Freeman, A. (2016). Data sharing at a crossroads. *New England Journal of Medicine, 375*(12), 1115–17. https://doi.org/10.1056/nejmp1608086

Rockoff, J.D. (2013, 30 January). Drug makers see profit potential in rare diseases. *Wall Street Journal.* Retrieved from https://www.wsj.com/articles/SB10001424127887323926104578273900197322758

Rubinstein, I.S., & Hartzog, W. (2016). Anonymization and risk. *Washington Law Review, 91*(2), 703–60. Retrieved from https://www.law.uw.edu/wlr/print-edition/print-edition/vol-91/2/anonymization-and-risk

Sardana, D., Zhu, C., Zhang, M., Gudivada, R.C., Yang, L., & Jegga, A.G. (2011). Drug repositioning for orphan diseases. *Briefings in Bioinformatics, 12*(4), 346–56. https://doi.org/10.1093/bib/bbr021

Sheehan, M. (2011). Can broad consent be informed consent? *Public Health Ethics, 4*(3), 226–35. https://doi.org/10.1093/phe/phr020

Silverman, E. (2018, 10 January). *Parents accuse companies of stealing medical data from their very sick children. StatNews.* Retrieved from https://www.statnews.com/pharmalot/2018/01/10/sucampo-lawsuit-twins-rare-disease/

So, D., Joly, Y., & Knoppers, B.M. (2013) Clinical trial transparency and orphan drug development: Recent trends in data sharing by the pharmaceutical industry. *Public Health Genomics, 16*(6), 322–35. https://doi.org/10.1159/000355941

Solove, D.J. (2013). Privacy self-management and the consent dilemma. *Harvard Law Review, 126*(7), 1880–1903. Retrieved from https://papers.ssrn.com/sol3/papers.cfm?abstract_id=2171018

Song, P.P., Gao, J.J., Inagaki, Y., & Tang, W. (2012). Rare diseases, orphan drugs, and their regulation in Asia: Current status and future perspectives. *Intractable & Rare Diseases Research, 1*(1), 3–9. https://doi.org/10.5582/irdr.2012.v1.1.3

Strom, B.L., Buyse, M., Hughes, J., & Knoppers, B.M. (2014). Data Sharing, Year 1 – Access to data from industry-sponsored clinical trials. *New England Journal of Medicine, 371*(22), 2052–4. https://doi.org/10.1056/NEJMp1411794

Taichman, D.B., Backus, J., Baethge, C., Bauchner, H., de Leeuw, P.W., Drazen, J.M., … Wu, S. (2016). Sharing clinical trial data: A proposal from the international committee of medical journal editors. *JAMA, 315*(5), 467–8. https://doi.org/10.1001/jama.2015.18164

Tambuyzer, E. (2010). Towards a framework for personalized healthcare: Lessons learned from the field of rare diseases. *Personalized Medicine, 7*(5), 569–86. https://doi.org/10.2217/pme.10.52

Taylor, J., & Denegri, S. (2017). Industry links with patient organisations. *BMJ, 356*, j1251. https://doi.org/10.1136/bmj.j1251

Trusheim, M.R., Berndt, E.R., & Douglas, F.L. (2007). Stratified medicine: Strategic and economic implications of combining drugs and clinical biomarkers. *Nature Reviews Drug Discovery, 6*(4), 287–93. https://doi.org/10.1038/nrd2251

Tu, J.V., Willison, D.J., Silver, F.L., Fang, J., Richards, J.A., Laupacis, A., & Kapral, M.K. (2004). Impracticability of informed consent in the registry of the Canadian Stroke Network. *New England Journal of Medicine, 350*, 1414–21. https://doi.org/10.1056/NEJMsa031697

Wendler, D. (2006). One-time general consent for research on biological samples. *BMJ, 332*(7540), 544–7. https://doi.org/10.1136/bmj.332.7540.544

Woodcock, J. (2007). The prospects for "personalized medicine" in drug development and drug therapy. *Clinical Pharmacology & Therapeutics, 81*(2), 164–9. https://doi.org/10.1038/sj.clpt.6100063

World Health Organization (WHO). (2017). Joint statement on public disclosure of results from clinical trials. Retrieved from https://www.who.int/news/item/18-05-2017-joint-statement-on-registration

World Medical Association (WMA). (2018). WMA Declaration of Helsinki – Ethical principles for medical research involving human subjects. Retrieved

from https://www.wma.net/policies-post/wma-declaration-of-helsinki-ethical
-principles-for-medical-research-involving-human-subjects/

Wu, F.T. (2013). Defining privacy and utility in data sets. *University of Colorado Law Review, 84,* 1117–77. Retrieved from https://papers.ssrn.com/sol3/papers.cfm?abstract_id=2031808

Yakowitz, J. (2011). Tragedy of the data commons. *Harvard Journal of Law & Technology, 25*(1), 1. Retrieved f rom http://jolt.law.harvard.edu/articles/pdf/v25/25HarvJLTech1.pdf

Yale University Open Data Access (YODA) Project. (n.d.). *Welcome to the YODA Project.* Retrieved from https://yoda.yale.edu/welcome-yoda-project

10 The European Registration of the Pandemic Influenza Vaccine Pandemrix: A Case Study of the Consequences of Poor Clinical Data Transparency

TOM JEFFERSON

It is easy to forget the lessons of the not-so-distant past, and especially so in an environment of fear and turmoil. The following account should make us think hard about the vital need for transparency in light of the COVID-19 pandemic. In the mid-1990s, several outbreaks of influenza H5N1, often originating in Asian "wet markets," began a new narrative over pandemics that crested in the H1N1 pandemic in 2009. An integral part of this account is the development of vaccines to address the spread of pandemics. But in a heightened environment where the political imperative to "find a solution" encourages the rapid development of vaccines and antivirals, careful consideration of the full safety implications of new compounds can be undermined. To ensure that we are not put in a position to have to re-learn recent lessons, this chapter explains why transparency in the development of new vaccines is essential. The source material for this chapter is partly declassified litigation documents and partly regulatory documents obtained by the author from the European regulator, the European Medicines Agency (EMA), prior to his involvement as an expert witness in the litigation (which was ultimately settled out of court).

Rapid gains towards greater transparency in clinical research were made in the early part of this decade thanks mainly to a series of effects by activists and the Nordic Cochrane Centre (see chapter three of this volume). In 2010, the centre was instrumental in convincing the European Ombudsman to support access to EMA holdings of clinical study reports. This access was quickly exploited by the Cochrane Acute Respiratory Infections Group, who delivered a review on antivirals for influenza based only on regulatory material. The review showed the extent of reporting bias in journal publications of antiviral trials and documented a whopping 60 per cent publication bias. Access to regulatory material led the same review team to change the conclusions of earlier versions of the review. Subsequent damage limitation exercises by the pharmaceutical industry were very effective in blurring the facts, taking over the reporting bias agenda, and setting up several trial data access sources through which industry was able to control the release of data while giving the image of transparency.

These very successful efforts were aided by activists and their initiatives, which gave the impression that the reporting bias question had been tackled effectively, if not solved. The niche question surrounding use of participant level data was allowed to slow down and sidetrack the main issue of accessing clinical study reports and other parts of the common technical document (that is, the industry standardized structure for submitting marketing authorization applications). In addition, Cochrane, as a corporate entity, failed to pursue the initial impetus, thereby conceding the initiative to industry. This narrative is mainly based on documents released by the EMA after a Freedom of Information (FOI) request. It is a case study illustrating the way in which a major public health initiative was launched, leading to rare but serious side effects *that could have been identified had existing data been made available earlier.* It also highlights the political context within which decisions about transparency are made. In the case of vaccines, high levels of vaccine scepticism make public health authorities hesitant about admitting to potentially serious, if rare, adverse events. Barriers to transparency, in this case, arguably serve the interests not only of the industry itself but also of public health authorities.

In September 2009, at the height of the influenza pandemic, the monovalent adjuvanted pandemic influenza vaccine Pandemrix developed by GlaxoSmithKline (GSK) was registered by the EMA. Registration followed an emergency procedure to rapidly introduce vaccines to prevent pandemic influenza by allowing a variation in the required content: from preregistered vaccines containing a non-pandemic virus to pandemic vaccines with a "novel" pandemic influenza virus. The pre-approval process was based on trials with serological surrogate outcomes of dubious significance and was underpowered to detect important rare harms. In short, Pandemrix was registered in the absence of sufficient data. When the first pharmacovigilance data became available at the end of 2009, signals of high toxicity including deaths and miscarriages were ignored and only emerged through litigation. Pandemrix was later associated with narcolepsy. Despite the EMA changing the registration procedures for pandemic influenza vaccines, these have not substantially altered the evidence requirements. In 2009, a culture of secrecy and lack of transparency allowed the registration and vaccination of an untested product in healthy people.

This chapter begins by examining the narrative through which the 2009 influenza pandemic unfolded. The World Health Organization (WHO) declared the influenza outbreak a pandemic on 11 June 2009, thereby activating regulatory procedures and preparations set out in the previous decade. These preparations had been predicated on a series of assumptions that were considered scientifically rock solid and were based on a developing influenza pandemic narrative. This chapter will summarize this pandemic narrative and describe the regulatory pathway expressly established for the pandemic emergency registration of influenza vaccines. It will show how Pandemrix was licensed in the complete absence of direct data of its clinical properties. I will also examine some of the consequences of this action and the role of public health bodies and of industry. Finally, the chapter will briefly examine regulatory vaccine changes since the 2009 influenza pandemic and address the issues raised by the Pandemrix affair in the context of pharmaceutical data transparency.

The Influenza Pandemic Narrative

In the decade preceding 2009, WHO documents included the following definition: "An influenza pandemic occurs when a new influenza virus appears against which the human population has no immunity, resulting in several simultaneous epidemics worldwide with enormous numbers of deaths and illness" (Doshi, 2011a). The influenza pandemic narrative has its origins in the 1997 Hong Kong outbreak, when an influenza viral strain known as H5N1, hitherto thought not to be pathogenic for humans, caused several deaths and went on to cause sporadic deaths in the Far and Middle East in contexts of deprivation (Doshi, 2011b).

Despite the definition undergoing several changes, it was the cornerstone of WHO policy and decision-making during the years leading up to the 2009 pandemic. It appeared on the WHO's Pandemic Preparedness home page for over six years. A detailed and documented account of the origins and changes undergone by the definition (and some of its assumptions), or "description-definition," as the WHO called it after 2009, is available (Doshi, 2011a). The WHO's definition includes several assumptions that were considered fact. The first is the inevitability and cyclical nature of an influenza pandemic, despite the well-known capriciousness of influenza and its manifestations. The second is the severity of the infection with very high numbers of dead and ill: this assumption was grounded on historical accounts of the so-called Spanish flu of 1918–19. The third is its rapid and simultaneous global spread. The fourth is the appearance of a distinctly new influenza virus type, against which humanity has little or no natural immunity. Although none of these assumptions were fulfilled (at least in their entirety) in the 2009 pandemic, what matters here is the effects of the supine acceptance of this pervasive narrative on the manufacture and registration of what were regarded as the cornerstones of prevention or amelioration of the pandemic: influenza vaccines. The narrative's emphasis on the sense of *urgency* and its corollary of *preparedness* provided the rationale for the introduction of a vaccine regulatory pathway set up specifically for an impending influenza pandemic. The production of pandemic influenza vaccines is not fundamentally different from that of "seasonal" influenza vaccines. This process is a well-established one, based on the capture of the annual viral changes with subsequent yearly production of new vaccines containing antigens with the latest configuration. However, because the time involved in the production of an antigenically different vaccine from that of a previous "season" is upwards of six months, any preparedness planning aimed at a pandemic should entail the saving of time: the deployment of the pandemic vaccine as quickly as possible.

The Regulatory Pathway for Pandemic Influenza Vaccines: The 2004 Guideline

Two EMA guidelines, the first appearing in 2004 (European Medicines Agency [EMA], 2004), provided the legal basis for registering a pandemic vaccine in the European Union. The procedure takes into account two distinct periods of pandemic influenza vaccine development and evidence generation, which it calls "interpandemic" and "intrapandemic" periods. The key time-saving idea involved the preparation, submission, and evaluation of a "core pandemic dossier" on a pre-pandemic vaccine (or "mock-up") during the "interpandemic period" (the interlude when only so-called seasonal influenza viruses circulate), followed by a pandemic influenza "variation application" once a pandemic was declared by the WHO and a pandemic viral strain was identified. When the composition of the pandemic vaccine was finalized, a variation in (viral) strain content was applied for, and the vaccine was fast-tracked through the pre-approved core dossier, completing the transition between mock-up (or pre-pandemic) and pandemic vaccine. The advantage of such a procedure is that, if the pre-pandemic vaccine is similar to the final product, some supporting evidence would be already available, thus expediting registration, production, and distribution of the vaccine.

The underlying time pressure came from the emergence of a "novel" pandemic viral strain. This strain would not be the same as that circulating before the pandemic, as implied by the WHO's definition of influenza

Figure 10.1. Procedure for Authorization of Mock-Up and Pandemic Vaccines in Europe Using the Centralized Procedure

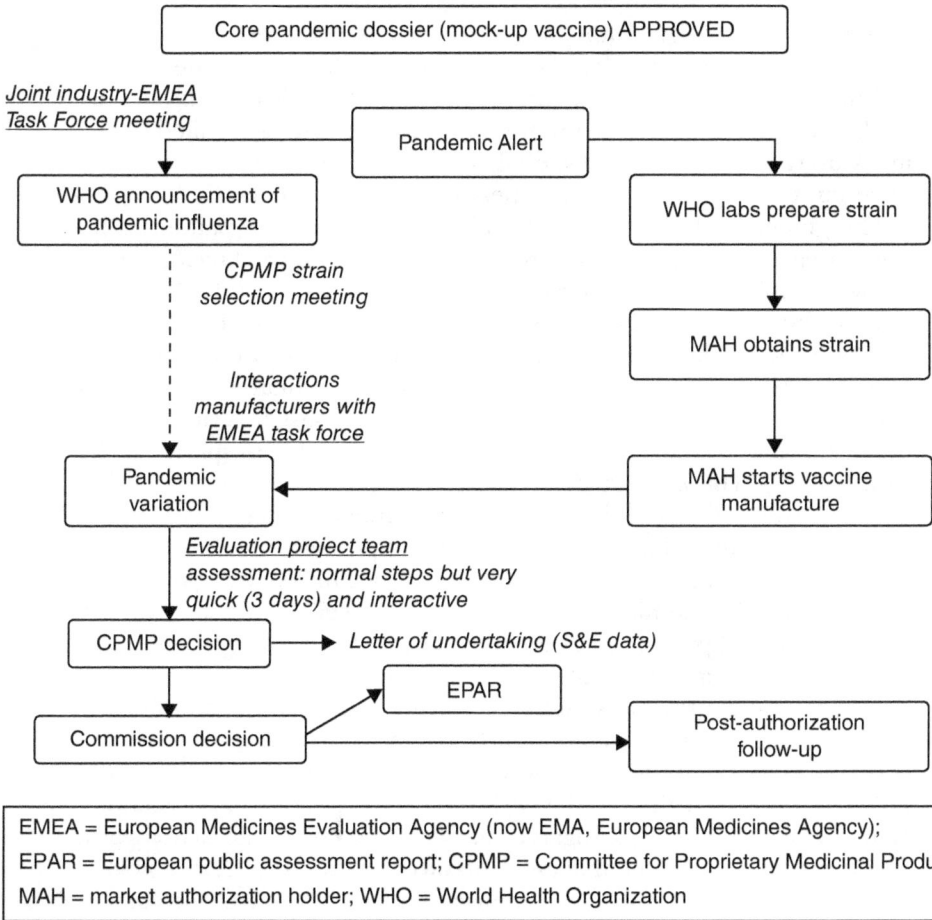

EMEA = European Medicines Evaluation Agency (now EMA, European Medicines Agency);
EPAR = European public assessment report; CPMP = Committee for Proprietary Medicinal Products;
MAH = market authorization holder; WHO = World Health Organization

Source: Adapted from EMEA/CPMP/VEG/4986/031.

pandemic. A novel strain would mean catastrophic vulnerability of the unprotected population. The EMA 2004 guideline indicates that the average assessment of the variation application takes two to three days, further saving time. The procedure includes a post-authorization follow-up to accumulate immunogenicity, effectiveness, and safety data from use of the pandemic vaccine in the field. The phases are summarized in Figure 10.1, which is adapted from the 2004 EMEA (now EMA) guideline (EMA, 2004).

The Regulatory Pathway for Pandemic Influenza Vaccines: The 2008 Guideline

The second EMA guideline, based on the WHO's 2007 guidelines (World Health Organization [WHO], 2007), adds greater detail, listing non-clinical and clinical safety and immunological requirements (EMA, 2008a). However, the immunological criteria to be fulfilled by any mock-up vaccine listed in the core dossier seem to reflect a fundamental uncertainty about the satisfactory performance of a mock-up.

The guideline details the differential characteristics of pandemic influenza viruses compared to seasonal viruses: different clinical course, higher complications and mortality rates, different age distribution, high rate of infectivity, and a waved pattern of incidence. The characteristics are reflected in the WHO's pandemic definition. Because of these differences, the immunological criteria applied to annual influenza vaccine licensing (such as assessment of antibody response to a viral antigen called haemagglutinin or HA) would not apply to this trespasser strain (EMA, 1997). The EMA guideline suggests recourse to literature review and the results of non-clinical data (such as animal models) to obtain information on the immunological correlates of protection. A "correlate of protection" is a standardized, reproducible procedure yielding outcomes or indicators of immunity (such as antibodies or cell activation) that reliably predict field protection from an infectious agent. The guideline also suggests collecting further information on the full characteristics of the immune response such as serum-neutralizing antibodies, neuraminidase antibody, and cell-mediated immunity, "although these responses are still of unknown relevance to protection" (EMA, 2008a, p. 12). The inter- and intra-laboratory variations in the performance of these assays are acknowledged. The EMA guideline suggests that, "with no other criteria to suggest at present, it is anticipated that mock-up vaccines should at least be able to elicit sufficient immunological responses to meet all three of the current standards set for vaccine in adults and older adults >60 years" (p. 12).

For safety, the EMA (2008a, p. 13) guideline stipulates that "the database should be sufficient to detect adverse reactions or events at a frequency of approximately 1%." For the pandemic variation application, the guideline stipulates that "provided ... the mock-up and final pandemic vaccines are similar other than in vaccine virus and the dose schedule is unchanged, the final pandemic vaccine may be approved for use by means of a variation that addresses only the quality issues and without the provision of clinical data" (p. 14). Finally, there is a requirement for post-approval commitment of pharmacovigilance and accrual of further safety as agreed in a pharmacovigilance or risk management plan and for field effectiveness data.

Adjuvants

The EMA 2005 Guideline on Adjuvants in Vaccines for Human Use (EMA, 2005) sits chronologically between the two regulatory guidelines. It defines adjuvants as substances of various nature that are added to vaccines to enhance immunogenicity. The guideline was relevant to all adjuvants and not specifically to those included in pandemic influenza vaccines. However, the adding of adjuvants to vaccines may pose problems in addition to potential immunogenicity benefits.

The EMA 2005 guideline remarks that "any increase in the rates and/or severity of adverse reactions as a consequence of the presence of an adjuvant in a vaccine is of concern. Therefore, the risk associated with the adjuvant must be outweighed by the potential benefit conferred by enhancement of the immune response" (p. 14). The EMA 2008 guideline also suggests that "if applicable, special consideration should be given to the control of the extemporaneous mixing of antigen and adjuvant to ensure a consistent preparation" (EMA, 2008a, p. 7). However, adjuvants are not regulated or registered separately from the vaccine (that is, their clinical effects in humans are not assessed separately). The reasons for this decision are unclear, but one explanation could be that regulators do not consider adjuvants to be active ingredients (EMA, 2005). This stance seems odd in the light of two further points. First, it is generally recognized that the mode of action of adjuvants is not always known or not fully understood, and animal models that can predict safety and efficacy of an adjuvant-antigen combination are not available (Krause, 2014). These limitations are shared by the 2008 US National Vaccine Advisory Committee (NVAC) report *Dose Optimization Strategies for Vaccines: The Role of Adjuvants and New Technologies*. The NVAC states: "Antigen/adjuvant combination is vaccine specific and no data are available currently that would allow an extrapolation to another antigen or even to the same formulation given by a different route" (Dekker, Gordon, & Klein, 2008). This view was still held in 2013, when the WHO warned that "an adjuvant-mediated enhancement of the immune response to one vaccine antigen, as a rule, cannot be extrapolated to the enhancement of the immune response to another antigen" (WHO, 2013, p. 20). Second, the WHO in its 2007 guideline stated that "because of the inherent variability in the assay systems used to measure immune responses, it is unwise to directly compare results from different studies" (WHO, 2007, p. 124). The EMA 2005 guideline also stresses the uncertainties of novel adjuvant use: "Unpredictability of adjuvant effects in humans results from a complex interplay between such factors as route of administration, antigen dose and the nature of the antigen. For this reason, a final safety evaluation of the newly developed vaccine formulation can only be conducted on the basis of clinical trials" (EMA, 2005, p. 5).

Table 10.1. Content of GSK's Vaccine Mock-Up and Pandemrix Vaccines

Components and quantity / 0.5 ml dose	H5N1 mock-up	H1N1 Pandemrix
Active ingredients		
Fractions of inactivated split virions	A/Vietnam/1194/2004 3.75 micrograms haemagglutinin or A/Indonesia/5/2005	A/California/7/2009 (H1.N1) v-like virus 3.75 micrograms haemagglutinin
AS03 adjuvant		
Squalene	10.86 milligrams	10.69 milligrams
DL-tocopherol	11.86 milligrams	11.86 milligrams
Polysorbate 80	4.85 milligrams	4.86 milligrams
Excipients		
Polysorbate (Tween 80)	>28.75 micrograms	NK
Octoxynol 10 (Triton X100)	3.75 micrograms (not listed in Q-pan content)	NK
Thiomersal	5 micrograms	5 micrograms
Sodium chloride	3.7 micrograms	NK
Disodium phosphate	0.51 micrograms	Disodium hydrogen phosphate (concentration NK)
Potassium dihydrogen phosphate	0.13 micrograms	NK
Potassium chloride	0.09 micrograms	NK
Magnesium chloride	0.012 micrograms (not listed in Q-pan content)	NK
Water for injections	0.5 millilitres	NK
Residuals from the manufacturing process		
	Formaldehyde, ovalbumin, sucrose, and sodium deoxycholate	Formaldehyde, ovalbumin, sucrose, and sodium deoxycholate

Sources: Dekker et al., 2008; WHO, 2013; EMA, n.d.; GlaxoSmithKline, 2007a, 2007b.
Note: NK = not known

Pandemrix was created by the mixing of the Adjuvant System AS03 with the H1N1 antigens (Table 10.1). For harms, the EMA 2005 guideline on adjuvants advises:

> The safety data [available] should allow for estimation of, with a reasonable degree of precision, the likely rates of reactions that may be expected based on the known properties of the adjuvant(s) and antigen(s). In some cases,

it may be appropriate that the data focus on immune mediated reactions. In all instances, the risk-benefit relationship for the modified product [with a modified adjuvant content because of safety or other concerns] should be at least as favourable as for the existing product. (EMA, 2005, p. 18)

The WHO guideline recommends proof of concept and in vitro testing studies prior to testing an adjuvant as part of a vaccine, but in all guidelines, adjuvant testing stops well short of placebo-controlled clinical trials (WHO, 2007; EMA, 2005; WHO, 2013). Precursor H5N1 vaccines had undergone in vitro and animal testing during their development (EMA, n.d.)

In summary, the emergency registration procedure was based on *presumed similarities* between precursor and pandemic vaccines. Adjuvants in pandemic vaccines, like all other adjuvants, had never been tested in trials against an inert substance in humans.

The Pandemrix Testing Program at Mock-Up and Licensed Product Stage

The mock-up and Pandemrix testing program reconstruction is based on two formerly confidential GSK regulatory documents released by the EMA following an FOI request (GlaxoSmithKline, 2007a, 2007b) and one available from the web (GlaxoSmithKline, 2007c). All three documents are part of the common technical document (CTD), the industry standard format for regulatory submissions. Searches on the GSK trial register and clinical trials.gov were also conducted to cross-reference each study. As well, four other regulatory documents reporting product characteristics and the EMA's assessments of the product were consulted (EMA, 2008b, 2009a, 2009c, 2010).

The EMA recommended the registration of GSK's Pandemrix (H1N1 AS03 adjuvanted monovalent vaccine) and Novartis's Focetria on 25 September 2009 (EMA, 2010, 2009b). Although the EMA states that the authorization was based on mock-up data from over 6,000 individuals, it also states that preliminary data would not be available for some months. The GSK mock-up H5N1 program consisted of nine studies run from 2004 and 2011 (Table 10.2). By the autumn of 2009, 8,938 subjects had been enrolled in completed trials, none aged nine to eighteen at the time of the presentation of the variation application from the H5N1 to the H1N1 AS03-adjuvanted vaccine. The largest post-authorization safety study (PASS UK – NCT00996853) was carried out mainly in adults: 47.7 per cent were aged over sixty, but only 0.4 per cent were aged less than two. The study did not report results until May 2011 (Table 10.2). At the time of Pandemrix registration, one study of Pandemrix had just commenced (number 9 in Table 10.2).

Table 10.2. GSK Vaccines Mock-Up H5N1-Containing Program from 2004 and 2011 and Initial H1N1-Containing Program from 2009

Serial	Study ID	Title	Design/ Objectives	Product tested	Enrolled/ Planned	Population	Start/ Completion dates	Sources
1.	NCT00319098 H5N1-008 (107064)	A Phase III, observer-blind, randomized study to evaluate the safety and immunogenicity of 1 and 2 administrations of pandemic monovalent (H5N1) influenza vaccine (adjuvanted split virus formulation) in adults aged 18 years and older	RCT Phase III/ S&I	– MIV H5N1 Spilt – Fluarix (1st dose) – Placebo (2nd dose)	5,052, 5,075 Safety 3,802, 1,269	Healthy >18	May 2006/ Jan. 2007	CTD, CSR, GSK website
2.	NCT00309634 H5N1-007 (106750)	Observer-blind monocentric study in adults aged between 18 and 60 years to evaluate reactogenicity and immunogenicity of 1 and 2 administrations of pandemic monovalent influenza vaccines administered at different antigen doses and adjuvanted or not	RCT Phase I/ S&I	– MV H5N1 Spilt + AS03	400	Healthy >18–60	Mar. 2006/ Oct. 2008	CTD, CSR, GSK website
3.	NCT00449670 H5N1-002 (109630)	Assess consistency of immunogenicity of GlaxoSmithKline Biologicals' pandemic influenza vaccine (GSK1562902A) in adults	RCT Phase III/ S&I	– MIV H5N1 Split – different concentrations of AS03 – Fluarix	1,206	18–60	Mar. 2007/ June 2007	CTD, CSR, GSK website

#	Study ID	Objective	Design	Intervention	N	Population	Dates	Source
4.	NCT00502593 H5N1-009 (107066)	A Phase II, randomized, open, controlled study to evaluate the safety and immunogenicity of different formulations of a pandemic influenza vaccine candidate (split virus formulation adjuvanted with AS03) given following a two-administration schedule (21 days apart) in children between 3 and 9 years of age	Open RCT Phase II, staggered design/S&I	– MIV H5N1 Split with diff concentrations of AS03 – Fluarix	138	3–9 year olds	July 2007/ Dec. 2009	CTD, CSR, GSK website
5.	NCT00397215 H5N1-010 (108251)	Evaluate immunogenicity & safety of a single or double dose of the pandemic influenza candidate vaccine (GSK1562902A) given following a two-administration schedule (21 days apart) in adults over 60 years of age	Open RCT Phase II/S&I	– MIV H5N1 Split with diff concentrations of AS03 Single vs double dose	480/437	Adults >60	Nov. 2006/ Sept. 2007	CTD, CSR, GSK website
6.	NCT00430521 H5N1-012 (107495)	Reactogenicity and immunogenicity study of GlaxoSmithKline Biologicals' pandemic influenza vaccine (GSK1119711A) administered according to different vaccination schedules	Open RCT Phase II/S&I	– MIV H5N1 Split with diff concentrations of AS03	512	Healthy 18–60	Feb. 2007/ Oct. 2008	CTD, CSR, GSK website

(Continued)

Table 10.2. (Continued)

Serial	Study ID	Title	Design/ Objectives	Product tested	Enrolled/ Planned	Population	Start/ Completion dates	Sources
7.	NCT00506350 H5N1-015 (109817)	Evaluate the reactogenicity & immunogenicity of 1 or 2 booster administrations of an influenza pandemic candidate vaccine (GSK1562902A) in primed adults aged between 19 and 61 years	Open non-randomized Phase II/I	– MIV H5N1 Spilt with diff concentrations of AS03	350	Healthy 19–61	Aug. 2007/ Oct. 2009	CTD, CSR, GSK website
8.	NCT00812981 (111954)	Non-inferiority study of GSK Biologicals' pandemic influenza vaccine 1562902A	RCT Phase III/ S&I	– Non-inferiority of H5N1 GSK1562902A + thiomersal	320	18–59	Nov. 2008/ June 2009	CTD, CSR, GSK website
9.	113462 (NCT00971321)	Safety and immunogenicity study of GSK Biologicals' pandemic influenza candidate vaccine (GSK2340272A) in children aged 6 to 35 months	RCT open Phase II/S&I	– H1N1 Pandemrix different schedules	157	6–35 months	Sept. 2009/ Nov. 2010	CTD, CSR, GSK website

No.	Study ID	Description	Design	Objective	N	Age	Dates	Sources
10.	106378 (NCT00309647)	A partially blind multi-centric study in adults aged between 18 and 60 years designed to evaluate the reactogenicity and immunogenicity of 1 and 2 doses of pandemic monovalent (H5N1) influenza vaccines (whole virus formulation) administered at different doses and adjuvanted or not	RCT partial blind, Phase I/S&I	– H5N1 different composition & schedules	400	18–60	Mar. 2006/ Nov. 2006	CTD, CSR, GSK website
11.	111756 (NCT00742885)	Immunogenicity and safety of GSK Biologicals' (pre-) pandemic influenza candidate vaccine GSK 1557484A	Non-randomized open Phase II/S&I	– H5N1 Pandemrix different age groups	100	20–64	Sept. 2008/ Mar. 2009	CTD, CSR, GSK website
12.	113585 (NCT00996853)	Post-authorization safety study (PASS) of GlaxoSmithKline Biologicals' pandemic influenza vaccine (GSK2340272A) in the United Kingdom (UK)	Cohort Phase IV/S	GlaxoSmithKline Biologicals' pandemic influenza vaccine (GSK2340272A) in the United Kingdom (UK)	9,206	1–97	Oct. 2009/ April 2011	CTD, CSR, GSK website

Notes: CSR = clinical study report; CTD = common technical document; RCT = randomized controlled trial; S&I = safety and immunogenicity

At the time of registration, GSK's application was also supported by six months' worth of data from mock-up trial H5N1-009 (NCT00502593) testing the effects of different vaccines doses in 138 children aged three to nine compared to Fluarix (GSK's trivalent non-adjuvanted seasonal influenza vaccine). Like all trials in the study program, H5N1-009 tested immune response and adverse events. At the six months' follow-up, the children given a higher dose had a significantly better antibody response than those given half dose, and greater in turn than those given Fluarix, who nevertheless seroconverted because of natural exposure to seasonal influenza. So the increased response by mock-up recipients is likely due to the effect of the adjuvant, given the non-circulation of wild type H5N1 viruses.

The Pandemrix Roll Out

Soon after registration, large quantities of pre-ordered Pandemrix were delivered and rolled out. One estimate points to 30 million doses of Pandemrix being used in children with variable coverage (1 per cent to 74 per cent) in the European Union during 2009–10. Advance purchasing agreements (APAs) now in the public domain all lay the legal and financial liability for any problems with all pandemic vaccines on governments, except in the case of procurement of a clearly defective vaccine.

An interesting feature of the German contract (for the procurement of 8,430,000 doses of Pandemrix manufactured in GSK's plant in Dresden) is the contractual separation of the antigen and adjuvants, and consequent different purchasing arrangements, including price. Antigens and adjuvant were produced in separate GSK plants and boxed separately. Thus Pandemrix did not de facto exist until reconstituted prior to administration.

In August 2010, the first cases of cataplexy and narcolepsy in children were reported, chiefly from Scandinavian countries (Canelle, Dewé, Innis, & van der Most, 2016; Nohynek et al., 2012; Heier et al., 2013; European Centre for Disease Prevention and Control [ECDC], 2012). Narcolepsy is an incurable neurological disease that causes alteration of the sleep-wake cycles. Lack of muscle control (cataplexy) is often an associated feature. Subsequently, the association between Pandemrix (manufactured in Dresden and known as D-Pan) and narcolepsy was confirmed by several observational studies and reviews of the evidence (ECDC, 2012; Stowe et al., 2016; Dauvilliers et al., 2013; O'Flanagan et al., 2014; Vaarala et al., 2014). Interest turned to the differences between the two GSK pandemic vaccines: D-Pan and Arepanrix manufactured in Quebec (Q-Pan). Arepanrix had similar composition as Pandemrix but no increased risk of narcolepsy (Canelle et al., 2016). The role of the antigenic component, environmental factors, and the manufacturing process in the two plants (Vaarala et al., 2014; Ahmed, Schur, MacDonald, & Steinman, 2014) have also been investigated. Despite the interest, the causes of narcolepsy today remain elusive, although autoimmunity is thought to play a role in its genesis. Its occurrence is rare, but devastating to the victim and family. The contention that Pandemrix was associated with narcolepsy only in Scandinavia because of genetic susceptibility is not supported by reports of cases in the United Kingdom, Ireland, and France.

Data-Free Registration in an Impending Doom Scenario

The H1N1 program consisted of fourteen studies, all commenced in September 2009 or afterwards, so that, at registration, no direct evidence of the effects of Pandemrix was available. In part, this timing was due to the "impending doom scenario" of hysteria surrounding the H1N1 pandemic and industry pressure (see later discussion). By the beginning of September 2009, however, there were signs that the threat was not as dire as predicted (Doshi, 2009), and registration of an untested vaccine for mass use in healthy persons should have induced caution. An FOI request to the European Commission sheds some light on the role played by industry in the registration process.

On 2 July, the European Vaccine Manufacturers (EVM) wrote to the vice president of the European Commission to elicit the Commission's support to expedite the approval of pandemic vaccines. This action was necessary, as the EMA was challenging the agreed data requirements, arguing that the pandemic was still considered of moderate severity. The EVM complained that delay in implementing pre-agreed regulatory steps would delay the roll out of the vaccine and protection of citizens. There does not seem to have been a written response to the EVM letter. Thus the EMA in early July 2009 had doubts as to the severity of the influenza pandemic and was requesting more data to fulfil its statutory obligations in what did not appear to be an emergency.

The carefully contrived narrative of excess deaths (compared to annual seasonal influenza) and changes to the various definitions and interpretations of the term "pandemic," even before the 2009 events were over, have been described by Doshi (2010). The point of interest in the case of registration of pandemic influenza vaccines is the notion of an impending dreadful global event that could be prevented or ameliorated by deploying vast quantities of influenza vaccines hurriedly produced and registered following pre-agreed rules to save time.

Unknown Benefits, Questionable Generalizability, and Underestimated Toxicity

During assessment of the mock-up, no benefits could be quantified as there was no H5N1 viral circulation in Europe. By the definition of the time, the pandemic virus would be novel, against which there was little or no immunity in the population. With no knowledge of what was coming and with the urgency impelled by the doomsday scenario, regulators used serological surrogates (antibodies) as correlates of field protection against influenza, that is, markers of effectiveness, to kick start production of the vaccines. This practice was a standard procedure at the time for seasonal influenza vaccines. However, regulators themselves were unsure of the significance of the antibody response surrogate used as a proxy for field effectiveness estimation. These doubts are supported by the observed modest field performance of seasonal vaccines, registered yearly using the same surrogates of effectiveness (Jefferson, Smith et al., 2005; Jefferson, Rivetti et al., 2005; Jefferson, 2006; Thomas, Jefferson, Demicheli, & Rivetti, 2006). None of these doubts were allowed to interfere with the juggernaut unleashed by the pandemic declaration. As Alcabes (2009, p. 294) wrote: "We are supposed to be prepared for a pandemic of some kind of influenza because the flu watchers, the people who make a living out of studying the virus and who need to attract continued grant funding to keep studying it, must persuade the funding agencies of the urgency of fighting a coming plague."

In such a situation, extreme attention should have been paid to toxicity, but the denominators of the trials in the pre-approval dossiers were inadequate to detect rare but serious adverse events, and Pandemrix trials did not start until September 2009 at the earliest. A further underlying problem was the already-mentioned generalization from a vaccine with one antigen and an adjuvant with unclear properties in humans to a different vaccine with different antigens and the same adjuvant. These limits were well known to regulators and to manufacturers, who demanded watertight liability exemption clauses in the APAs.

The rarity of narcolepsy, the relatively long latency in the development or reporting of narcolepsy,[1] the retreat of the influenza pandemic from front-line news, the swift financial settlement of litigation by Nordic countries, and the contractual impunity of manufacturers kept attention away from a crucial aspect of the whole matter. Perhaps the biggest barrier of all to knowing what really happened is the secrecy of the government-industry complex. A legal affidavit filed in 2017 in an Irish court during the course of litigation in a case of narcolepsy contains details of periodic reports of vaccine vigilance events made by GSK

Table 10.3. Comparison of Harms Reported in Pandemrix Recipients versus Arepanrix Recipients as at 28 December 2009 with Effect Estimates (with 95% confidence intervals)*

Events	Pandemrix		Arepanrix and non-adjuvanted vaccine		Effects estimate
	Events	Rate	Events	Rate	Odds Ratio [M-H, Fixed, 95% CI]
Cumulative	12,180	320.5	584	43.4	5.87 [5.40, 6.37] (p < .0001)
SAE	3,280	86.3	108	8.0	8.54 [7.05, 10.35] (p < .0001)
Deaths	107	2.8	6	0.4	5.02 [2.20, 11.41] (p < .0001)
Anaphylaxis	264	6.9	47	3.4	15.80 [11.58, 21.55] (p < .0001)
Facial palsy	35	0.9	2	0.1	4.92 [1.18, 20.46] (p < .0001)
GBS	28	0.7	4	0.2	1.97 [0.69, 5.61] (p = .21)
Encephalitis	7	0.1	0	0	4.22 [0.24, 73.87] (p = .32)
Demyelination	18	0.4	0	0	10.41 [0.63, 172.68] (p = .10)
Convulsions	214	5.6	7	0.5	8.60 [4.05, 18.25] (p < .0001)
Neuritis	11	0.2	0	0	6.47 [0.38, 109.77] (p = .20)
Vasculitis	21	0.5	0	0	12.09 [0.73, 199.65] (p = .08)
Stillbirth^	8	132.2	0	0	13.91 [0.80, 241.02] (p = .03)
Abortion spontaneous^	30	495.8	0	0	49.93 [3.05, 816.61] (p < .0001)
Vaccines failure	18	0.4	0	0	10.41 [0.63, 172.68] (p = .10)

Source: GSK, H1N1 Enhanced Safety Review, contained in Affidavit by Gillian O'Connor, filed in the High Court, Dublin, 28 June 2017.
Notes: AE = adverse event; CI = confidence interval; GBS = Guillain-Barre syndrome; M-H = Mantel-Haenzel; SAE = serious adverse event
* Rates of AEs are per million doses administered by vaccine.
^ Denominator (doses administered) estimated from GSK report dated 2 December 2009.

to Irish authorities in the months following the worldwide start of the 2009 Pandemrix vaccination campaigns. It is difficult to believe that such reports were not copied as part of the condition for vaccine registration to the EMA and all other governments that had invested in Pandemrix. The monthly reports compare selected events in recipients of D-Pan, Q-Pan, and an unspecified non-adjuvanted pandemic vaccine. Denominators or exposure events are estimated from the administered doses of vaccines, also reported by GSK. This provides the opportunity to compare rates of events. Table 10.3 reconstructs event rates and calculates odds ratios with cumulative data available at the end of 2009 that has never before been seen in public.

All odd ratios are high and in excess of the point estimate threshold of 2, with some strikingly different in comparisons between the two vaccines. Pandemrix manufactured in Dresden was associated with a higher cumulative rate of harms, serious adverse events, deaths, anaphylaxis, facial palsy, convulsions, and miscarriages compared to Quebec-manufactured Arepanrix and another unidentified non-adjuvanted vaccine. Data for these indicators of rare but serious toxicity were available from the end of October 2009, and should have led to immediate action by the competent authorities, either switching to a less toxic pandemic or seasonal influenza vaccine or halting the program. None of this happened, and the failure and inadequacy of influenza vaccine regulation and surveillance has only come to light because of litigation from the victims.

None of the harms would have been detected by the 1 per cent threshold indicated by the EMA (2008a), and the gap in the trial program for group 9–18 is unexplained. The evidence shows the inadequacy of WHO guidance, EMA regulation, and ethics of the public health authorities recommending Pandemrix.

Vaccines to be administered to millions of healthy people cannot be tested in a few hundred people using an analogy logic in which regulators themselves and the academic community showed little confidence. Nor is it acceptable that important public health information comes to light only because of persistent academic enquiry or litigation. This secrecy is another reflection of the close ties between manufacturers, governments, and regulators preventing democratic debate.

In response to the *BMJ*'s Peter Doshi reporting the story in the autumn of 2018 (Doshi, 2018), the EMA's Peter Arlett stated: "[Pandemrix] … was authorised in the European Union (EU) on 29 September 2009 to immunize citizens against the H1N1 pandemic influenza strain. Information from clinical trials in more than 6,000 subjects was assessed as part of an extensive review of the vaccine's safety profile before its authorisation, and the outcome of the assessment is available on the EMA website" (Arlett, 2018). As readers of this article now know, the product was completely untested in its combination of novel antigens (H1N1) and adjuvant (AS03) at the time of licensing. Arlett's claim is playing on the public lack of awareness of the facts. Arlett goes on to state that "potential signals of possible new safety issues were promptly reviewed using all the available information. At the time, these evaluations indicated that the overall benefit-risk profile of Pandemrix remained favourable" (Arlett, 2018).

Yet the EMA appears not to have taken any action on the 2009 GSK reports, and it is wholly unclear what benefit Arlett refers to, given that all trials used surrogate outcomes of dubious significance and that Pandemrix achieved very low coverage in European countries where it was used. Arlett and the EMA call into question the validity of comparing the data from the GSK reports because of differences in surveillance and reporting of the same vaccines. Although details are scarce, had the program been halted, we may have had fewer cases of narcolepsy, more transparency and honesty, and, arguably, ultimately less vaccine hesitancy. As another respondent (David Healy) remarked: "Studies of vaccine hesitancy should include company and regulatory behaviour in their remit, but likely never will" (Healy, 2018). Such is the cost of secrecy.

Conclusion

Modest field results have led the EMA to make changes to the registration procedures of seasonal, pre-pandemic, and pandemic influenza vaccines in 2014 (EMA, 2016). The new system is still based on surrogate outcomes but requires a direct comparison with demonstration of non-inferiority of antibody response (immunogenicity) by a candidate seasonal influenza vaccine compared to an established one. This provision is a clear nod to industry, as such trials are smaller and far less expensive than field trials (where the outcomes are real: that is, cases and complications of influenza). They are also far less risky, as the unpredictable circulation of influenza is not a factor. An extensive review of the use and meaning of such surrogates has challenged the science at the basis of current use of serological outcomes as correlates of immunity (Ward et al., 2018). There is a likelihood that the continued emphasis on serologic outcomes would skew any "outcome" in favour of vaccines producing higher antibody responses (such as adjuvanted vaccines). This bias in turn raises the possibility of a higher rate of harms, but the Pandemrix 2009 story reveals a disregard for possible harms by governments that does not bode well for the future and for institutional credibility in this matter.

In addition, the use of surrogate outcomes of unclear clinical significance is compounded by the problems with the non-inferiority design of trials. Such designs cannot prove superiority (or equivalence, especially in biologics) with serological outcomes compared to an unstable comparator, which itself has only been tested using serological outcomes. The candidate vaccine may actually be worse than its established comparator, but would we know?

For pandemic vaccines, the mock-up (now called "pandemic preparedness vaccine") still requires pre-approval of a vaccine that is as similar as possible to the candidate pandemic vaccine with several different sets of antigens and dosages. The EMA emphasizes data collection in healthy adults aged eighteen or older. The EMA has recently called for a six-month consultation on a draft guideline on clinical evaluation of vaccines that is meant to replace both the 2007 new vaccines and 2005 adjuvants guidelines. In the parts that are relevant to influenza vaccines, the reliance on non-inferiority designs and serological outcomes remains unchanged (EMA, 2018).

The partly serendipitous circumstances of the rapid gains made a decade ago conceal the slow rate of overall progress made in accessing regulatory material around the world. The FDA is ponderously and conservatively considering release of limited material in select circumstances, whereas the few in-depth studies of the use of regulatory and internal documents were mainly by-products of litigation. As the Pandemrix example shows, the public should expect that whatever material is used at the societal level is fully documented and those responsible for its development are held to account.

NOTE

1 In one case control study, 68 per cent of cases took up to 180 days from exposure to Pandemrix to develop narcolepsy (O'Flanagan et al., 2014).

REFERENCES

Ahmed, S.S., Schur, P.H., MacDonald, N.E., & Steinman, L. (2014). Narcolepsy, 2009 A(H1N1) pandemic influenza, and pandemic influenza vaccinations: What is known and unknown about the neurological disorder, the role for 600 autoimmunity, and vaccine adjuvants. *Journal of Autoimmunity, 50*, 1–11. https://doi.org/10.1016/j.jaut.2014.01.033

Alcabes, P. (2009). *Dread: How fear and fantasy have fueled epidemics from the black death to the avian flu.* New York, NY: Public Affairs.

Arlett, P. (2018, 26 September). Re: Pandemrix vaccine: Why was the public not told of early warning signs? Rapid responses. Retrieved from https://www.bmj.com/content/362/bmj.k3948/rapid-responses

Canelle, Q., Dewé, W., Innis, B.L., & van der Most, R. (2016). Evaluation of potential immunogenicity differences between *Pandemrix*™ and *Arepanrix*™. *Human Vaccines & Immunotherapeutics, 12*(9), 2289–98, https://doi.org/10.1080/21645515.2016.1168954

Dauvilliers, Y., Arnulf, I., Lecendreux, M., Charley, M.C., Franco, P., Drouot, X., … Pariente, A. (2013). Increased risk of narcolepsy in children and adults after pandemic H1N1 vaccination in France. *Brain, 136*(8), 2486–96. https://doi.org/10.1093/brain/awt187

Dekker, C., Gordon, L., & Klein, J. (2008). *Dose optimization strategies for vaccines: The role of adjuvants and new technologies.* Report (with recommendations) approved at the 6 February 2008 American National Vaccine Advisory Committee (NVAC) Meeting. Washington, DC: Health and Human Services.

Doshi, P. (2009). Calibrated response to emerging infections. *BMJ, 339*, b3471. https://doi.org/10.1136/bmj.b3471

Doshi, P. (2010). Pandemic influenza: Severity must be taken into account. *Journal of Infectious Diseases, 201*(9), 1444–5. https://doi.org/10.1086/651701

Doshi, P. (2011a). The elusive definition of pandemic influenza. *Bulletin of the World Health Organization, 89*, 532–8. https://doi.org/10.2471/BLT.11.086173

Doshi, P. (2011b). *Influenza: A study of contemporary medical politics.* Doctoral dissertation, MIT. Retrieved from https://dspace.mit.edu/handle/1721.1/69811

Doshi, P. (2018). Pandemrix vaccine: Why was the public not told of early warning signs? *BMJ, 362*, k3948. https://doi.org/10.1136/bmj.k3948

European Centre for Disease Prevention and Control (ECDC). (2012). *Narcolepsy in association with pandemic influenza vaccination – A multi-country European epidemiological investigation.* Stockholm: ECDC. Retrieved from https://www.ecdc.europa.eu/en/publications-data/narcolepsy-association -pandemic-influenza-vaccination-multi-country-european

European Medicines Agency (EMA), Committee for Proprietary Medical Products (CPMP). (1997, 12 March). Note for guidance on harmonisation of requirements for influenza vaccines. CPMP/BWP/214/96. Retrieved from https://www.ema.europa.eu/en/documents/scientific-guideline/note -guidance-harmonisation-requirements-influenza-vaccines_en.pdf

European Medicines Agency (EMA), Committee for Proprietary Medical Products (CPMP). (2004, 5 April). Guideline on submission of marketing authorisation applications for pandemic influenza vaccines through the centralised procedure. EMEA/CPMP/VEG/4986/03. Retrieved from https://www.ema.europa.eu/en /documents/scientific-guideline/guideline-submission-marketing-authorisation -applications-pandemic-influenza-vaccines-through_en.pdf

European Medicines Agency (EMA), Committee for Medicinal Products for Human Use (CHMP). (2005, 20 January). Guideline on adjuvants in vaccines for human use. EMEA/CHMP/VEG/134716/2004. Retrieved from https:// www.ema.europa.eu/en/documents/scientific-guideline/guideline-adjuvants -vaccines-human-use-see-also-explanatory-note_en.pdf

European Medicines Agency (EMA), Committee for Medicinal Products for Human Use (CHMP). (2008a, 18 December). Guideline on dossier structure and content for pandemic influenza vaccine marketing authorisation application (Revision). EMEA/CPMP/VEG/4717/2003-Rev. 1. Retrieved from https://www.ema.europa.eu/en/documents/scientific-guideline/guideline -dossier-structure-content-pandemic-influenza-vaccine-marketing-authorisation -application_en.pdf

European Medicines Agency (EMA), Committee for Proprietary Medical
    Products (CPMP). (2008b). Assessment report for pandemic influenza
    vaccine (H5N1) (split virion, inactivated, adjuvanted) GlaxoSmithKline
    biologicals. A/VietNam/1194/2004 NIBRG-14. EMEA/H/C/1206. Retrieved
    from https://www.ema.europa.eu/en/documents/assessment-report
    /pandemic-influenza-vaccine-h5n1-split-virion-inactivated-adjuvanted
    -glaxosmithkline-biologicals-epar_en.pdf
European Medicines Agency (EMA), Committee for Medicinal Products
    for Human Use (CHMP). (2009a, 23 July). Core summary of product
    characteristics for pandemic influenza vaccines. EMEA/CHMP/VWP/193031/
    2004 Rev-1. Retrieved from https://www.ema.europa.eu/en/documents
    /scientific-guideline/core-summary-product-characteristics-pandemic
    -influenza-vaccines-superseded_en.pdf
European Medicines Agency (EMA), Committee for Medicinal Products for
    Human Use (CHMP). (2009b, 24 September). CHMP assessment report for
    Focetria. EMEA/H/C/710. Retrieved from https://www.ema.europa.eu/en
    /documents/assessment-report/focetria-epar-assessment-report_en.pdf
European Medicines Agency (EMA), Committee for Proprietary Medical
    Products (CPMP). (2009c, 22 October). Variation assessment report.
    Invented name/Name: Pandemrix. International non-proprietary name/
    Common name: pandemic influenza vaccine (H1N1) (split virion, inactivated,
    adjuvanted) a/california/7/2009 (H1N1)v like strain (X-179A). Type II
    Variation: EMEA/H/C/000832/II/0019. EMEA/CHMP/667130/2009.
    Retrieved from https://www.ema.europa.eu/en/documents/variation-report
    /pandemrix-h-c-832-ii-0019-epar-assessment-report-variation_en.pdf
European Medicines Agency EMA), Committee for Proprietary Medical Products
    (CPMP). (2010, 24 June). Assessment report for the re-assessment of the specific
    obligations and the benefit/risk profile. Invented name/Name: Pandemrix.
    International non-proprietary name/Common name: Pandemic influenza
    vaccine (H1N1) (split virion, inactivated, adjuvanted) A/California/7/2009
    (H1N1)v like strain (X-179A). Authorised under exceptional circumstances
    EMEA/H/C/832/SW/41. EMEA/CHMP/508065/2010. Retrieved from https://
    www.ema.europa.eu/en/documents/variation-report/pandemrix-h-c-832-sw
    -0041-epar-assessment-report-variation_en.pdf
European Medicine Agency (EMA). (2016, 21 July). Guideline on influenza
    vaccines: Non-clinical and clinical module. EMA/CHMP/VWP/457259/2014.
    Retrieved from https://www.ema.europa.eu/en/documents/scientific
    -guideline/influenza-vaccines-non-clinical-clinical-module_en.pdf
European Medicines Agency (EMA). (2018, 26 April). Updated rules for
    clinical development of vaccines. Retrieved from https://www.ema.europa.eu
    /en/news/updated-rules-clinical-development-vaccines

European Medicines Agency (EMA). (n.d.). Annex I to Pandemrix EPAR – Summary of product characteristics. Retrieved from https://www.ema .europa.eu/en/documents/product-information/pandemrix-epar-product -information_en.pdf

GlaxoSmithKline (GSK). (2007a). AS03 Adjuvanted H5N1 Vaccine (for pandemic use). Common Technical Document (CTD). Module 5, Volume 1. Obtained through a Freedom of Information request.

GlaxoSmithKline (GSK). (2007b). AS03 Adjuvanted H5N1 Vaccine (for pandemic use). Common Technical Document (CTD). Module 2, Section 2.5. Clinical Overview. Obtained through a Freedom of Information request.

GlaxoSmithKline (GSK). (2007c). AS03 Adjuvanted H5N1 Vaccine (for pandemic use). Common Technical Document (CTD). Module 2, Section 2.6: Nonclinical written and tabulated summary. Retrieved from https://www .mhlw.go.jp/shingi/2010/01/dl/s0115-7l.pdf

Healy, D. (2018, 27 September). Re: Pandemrix vaccine: Why was the public not told of early warning signs? Rapid responses. Retrieved from https://www .bmj.com/content/362/bmj.k3948/rr-9

Heier, M.S., Gautvik, K.M., Wannag, E., Bronder, K.H., Midtlyng, E., Kamaleri, Y., & Storsaeter, J. (2013). Incidence of narcolepsy in Norwegian children and adolescents after vaccination against H1N1 influenza A. *Sleep Medicine*, *14*(9), 867–71. https://doi.org/10.1016/j.sleep.2013.03.020

Jefferson, T.O. (2006). Influenza vaccination: Policy versus evidence. *BMJ*, *333*(7574), 912–15. https://doi.org/10.1136/bmj.38995.531701.80

Jefferson, T., Rivetti, D., Rivetti, A., Rudin, M., Di Pietrantonj, C., & Demicheli, V. (2005). Efficacy and effectiveness of influenza vaccines in the elderly: A systematic review. *Lancet*, *366*(9492), 1165–74. https://doi.org/10.1016 /S0140-6736(05)67339-4

Jefferson, T., Smith, S., Demicheli, V., Harnden, A., Rivetti, A., & Di Pietrantonj, C. (2005). Assessment of the efficacy and effectiveness of influenza vaccines in healthy children: Systematic review. *Lancet*, *365*(9461), 773–80. https:// doi.org/10.1016/S0140-6736(05)17984-7

Krause, P. (2014). Update on vaccine regulation: Considerations for adjuvanted vaccines. Presented at the CMC Strategy Forum, Europe, 5 May, 2014. Retrieved from https://cdn.ymaws.com/www.casss.org/resource/resmgr/CMC _Euro_Speaker_Slides/2014_CMCE_KrausePhil.pdf

Nohynek, H., Jokinen, J., Partinen, M., Vaarala, O., Kirjavainen, T., Sundman, J., … Kilpi, T. (2012). AS03 Adjuvanted AH1N1 vaccine associated with an abrupt increase in the incidence of childhood narcolepsy in Finland. *PLoS ONE*, *7*(3), e33536. https://doi.org/10.1371/journal.pone.0033536

O'Flanagan, D., Barret, A.S., Foley, M., Cotter, S., Bonner, C., Crowe, C., … Purcell, E. (2014). Investigation of an association between onset of narcolepsy and vaccination with pandemic influenza vaccine, Ireland, April 2009–December 2010. *Eurosurveillance, 19*(17), pii=20789. https://doi.org/10.2807/1560-7917.ES2014.19.17.20789

Stowe, J., Andrews, N., Kosky, C., Dennis, G., Eriksson, S., Hall, A., ... Miller, E. (2016). Risk of narcolepsy after AS03 adjuvanted pandemic A/H1N1 2009 influenza vaccine in adults: A case-coverage study in England. *Sleep, 39*(5), 1051–7. https://doi.org/10.5665/sleep.5752

Thomas, R.E., Jefferson, T.O., Demicheli, V., & Rivetti, D. (2006). Influenza vaccination for health-care workers who work with elderly people in institutions: A systematic review. *Lancet Infectious Diseases, 6*(5), 273–9. https://doi.org/10.1016/S1473-3099(06)70462-5

Vaarala, O., Vuorela, A., Partinen, M., Baumann, M., Freitag, T.L., Meri, S., ... Kilpi, T. (2014). Antigenic differences between AS03 adjuvanted influenza A (H1N1) pandemic vaccines: Implications for Pandemrix-associated narcolepsy risk. *PLoS ONE, 9*(12), e114361. https://doi.org/10.1371/journal.pone.0114361

Ward, B.J., Pillet, S., Charland, N., Trepanier, S., Couillard, J., & Landry, N. (2018). The establishment of surrogates and correlates of protection: Useful tools for the licensure of effective influenza vaccines? *Human Vaccines & Immunotherapeutics, 14*(3), 647–56. https://doi.org/10.1080/21645515.2017.1413518

World Health Organization (WHO), Expert Committee on Biological Standardization. (2007). Guidelines on regulatory preparedness for human pandemic influenza vaccines (Adopted 2007). Annex 2 to the Fifty-eighth report. Retrieved from https://www.who.int/biologicals/vaccines/Annex_2_WHO_TRS_963-3.pdf

World Health Organization (WHO). (2013). *Guidelines on the nonclinical evaluation of vaccine adjuvants and adjuvanted vaccines.* Retrieved from https://www.who.int/biologicals/areas/vaccines/ADJUVANTS_Post_ECBS_edited_clean_Guidelines_NCE_Adjuvant_Final_17122013_WEB.pdf

11 The Road Forward: How Researchers Can Sustain an Ethical and Transparent Health System

RITA BANZI

Is a health research regime based upon open and transparent data merely an aspirational ideal? Or, conversely, does a sustainable and ethical health system *require* transparency? Many chapters in this volume have identified entrenched power dynamics that hamper and frustrate the attempt to achieve a more open system. Some of these accounts suggest a certain disheartening inevitability in the ability of vested interests to impede progress on this front. This chapter provides a more optimistic outlook drawn from the literature and from the experience of the Mario Negri Institute for Pharmacological Research. From patients to experimental models – at the cellular and molecular level – and back to patients, the institute conducts research to improve people's health and well-being (Light & Maturo, 2015; Mario Negri Institute, 2019). It conducts clinical studies in several medical areas, sponsored by itself or other entities (mainly collaborative clinical groups or academic centres). The Mario Negri Institute (n.d.) may play different roles (sponsor, partner, or service provider), but, irrespective of its role and the source of funding, any clinical study involving the institute must be registered and report its results.

The Basics: Register and Monitor

Trial registration has become the standard (at least for drug studies) for over twenty years, since the Food and Drug Administration Modernization Act was issued in the United States in 1997 (Government of the United States, 1997). The information to be reported in the registry was intended for a wide audience, including individuals with serious or life-threatening diseases or conditions, members of the public, health-care providers, and researchers. When the major medical journals started asking for prospective registration of trials as a prerequisite to study publication (De Angelis et al., 2004), there was considerable resistance on the part of academic researchers, even where the pharmaceutical industry itself articulated its support for the principle of transparency (Scherer & Trelle, 2008). At that time, GlaxoSmithKline was in the midst of a major lawsuit in the United States for the concealment of negative trial results for the antidepressant paroxetine (Dyer, 2004). By promoting transparency to save their reputations, pharmaceutical companies proposed using their own registries, rather than the institutional ones, and attempted to weaken the minimum requirements for trial registration regarding the amount of detail to be disclosed (Krleža-Jerić, 2005). In the end, they accepted the requirements proposed by the World Health Organization (WHO) to adhere (at least partly) to the existing regulations, often with better compliance than academic researchers (Zarin, Tse, Williams, & Rajakannan, 2017; Law, Kawasumi, & Morgan, 2011).

Besides encouraging trial registration in well-known international registries, the Mario Negri Institute has run its own registry since 2011, collecting data on all studies where the institute's researchers are involved as coordinators or collaborators, including observational studies. The registry aims to increase transparency and accessibility of information and to stimulate research collaboration among researchers. Members of the public who may be interested in gathering general information on the studies carried out by the institute, or patients who wish to become a participant, can access the registry website as well.

Establishing a registry is only the first important step towards ensuring the institute's goal of transparency. The registry was recently assessed, as any "intervention" should be after its implementation (Pandolfini & Bonati, 2018). Information on the experience of users, both internally and externally, and monitoring the completeness and quality of the data uploaded, as well as adherence to registration requirements, represent the bases for future revisions designed to increase the registry's usefulness and impact. Any initiative that aims to monitor compliance with transparency requirements is to be welcomed as a tool to create a virtuous cycle and further improve reporting rates. Reporting performance may encourage organizations to prioritize results reporting in general or to highlight technical inconsistencies that may have contributed to partial reporting and, more generally, to the difficulties faced by researchers. Monitoring compliance with reporting requirements, done internally by the institution itself (or by third parties such as the eu.trialstracker.net initiative), is as important as the establishment of such requirements. This work will particularly support academic researchers, who are sometimes unaware of changing requirements and are often subject to less structured processes and operating procedures, to track their compliance. We simply need to learn from our mistakes and improve day by day.

Openness: The Essence of Public-Oriented Research

Millions of scientific papers are published every year, and almost 2 *trillion* US dollars are invested annually in research (UNESCO Institute for Statistics, n.d.). Given the increase of warnings for research misconduct and the level of waste of resources, however, it appears that the enterprise is not working properly. This failure largely applies to health research, discrediting participant and patient contributions. Why is health research not satisfying expectations? The reasons are many, of course, but surely part of the problem is due to the lack of ability or willingness to respond to the *real* needs of patients and health systems, the lack of collaboration, and the refusal to share ideas and data. While walking the corridors of the Mario Negri Institute, I often hear the words "research is an expression of care." Without disregarding the importance of basic research, which may fuel important scientific knowledge, *public*-oriented research should address the needs of citizens and society. As Alessandro Liberati pointed out:

> If we want more relevant information to become available, a new research governance strategy is needed. Left to themselves, researchers cannot be expected to address the current mismatch. Researchers are trapped by their own internal competing interests – professional and academic – which lead them to compete for pharmaceutical industry funding. (Liberati, 2011)

Better research governance would help, but it should operate in a system where one does not have to continually debate whether the results of publicly funded research should be publicly available, or whether the data underlying the findings should be maximized and shared with a wider public to create a "knowledge society" of better-informed citizens. This attitude should be part of the core business of any researcher, especially those working for, and funded by, public sources. The downstream (long-term) effect of such an attitude would be that the germ of openness could permeate any research project, irrespective of the funding sources. As a positive side effect, there would be the creation of a savvier generation of researchers, able to detect vested interests and aware of their impact on research independence, for which transparency is a pillar. These efforts may cumulatively represent a gradual bottom-up shift towards the adoption of a culture that embraces transparency and replication, contributing to the creation of a model in which openness is the expected norm (Institute for Science, Ethics and Innovation, 2009; Graham & Jones, 2016).

Plan to Be Transparent from the Beginning

A complete and fair reporting of clinical studies includes information on trial registration, details on hypotheses and methods (protocol), and the results – ideally both aggregate and individual participant data – that include possible harms of the interventions. It should be one of the main operating principles of any research project. Along with framing a relevant research question and applying the most robust methodology, making all the necessary information available is the best way to maximize the impact of studies. Clinical studies, especially randomized trials, are the bases of informed decision-making. Any scientist involved in clinical research should know that reporting results, thereby making science more credible and accessible, is part of their job responsibilities. Although several problems regarding information management in clinical trials continue to pose serious risks to optimal patient care, there has been real progress towards more transparency in health research in the last decades.

There is still an issue with compliance in academic institutions, as reported by TranspariMED, a research driven initiative aimed to "end" distortion in medicine (TranspariMED, n.d.; All Trials, n.d.). Academics may be worried about their ideas getting scooped, being accused of pursuing irrelevant hypotheses, or applying wrong methods; or they may simply ignore the requirement that they should register their trials (Reveiz, Krleža-Jerić, Chan, & De Aguiar, 2007). Although academic researchers supported trial registration in general, their reluctance became apparent when it came to disclosing study details. According to a survey of academic researchers running investigator-initiated clinical studies in 2006, the disclosure of details regarding planned subgroup analyses, sample size calculation, and planned methods of analysis was barely tolerated. Sharing key study documents, such as the study protocol and financial agreements, was quite taboo (Scherer & Trelle, 2008). At the present time, the discussion has shifted towards what academic organizations should do to support trial registration and reporting, especially as evidence suggests that these organizations are unprepared to meet such requirements. Often they perform worse than industry in registering trials prospectively. The publication of study results is steadily increasing, although there is still much to do to improve the discoverability of results and link together all the sources of information about a given study. Many clinical trials conducted by academic organizations are still not published, and according to a survey of academic organizations in the United States, less than half have institutional registration or a policy on reporting results (Mayo-Wilson et al., 2018). The same may be true in Europe, so there is a constant need to reinforce the requirement that all trials be registered and published.

What, then, should be done to address this issue? First, researchers need to be aware of the problems of biased reporting and understand that their work is complete only when the research community and the public can read, fully understand, and apply the results of their experiments. Second, researchers have to be supported by specific tools and guidelines. Reporting guidelines are the most extraordinary example of how researchers have produced useful resources for researchers. To cite a famous line from the Italian movie *Palombella Rossa*, directed by Nanni Moretti, "*Chi parla male, pensa male e vive male, bisogna trovare le parole giuste: le parole sono importanti*" ("Those who speak badly, think badly and live badly. We must find the right words: words are important"). Reporting guidelines are not a snobbish mannerism but rather an instrument that researchers should know how to handle as well as they do a microscope or a stethoscope. Third, clinical researchers should be trained in methodology and have at least some basic data management skills, which is currently not always the case. Publication and data sharing plans should be prepared early in the development of any clinical project to avoid late-stage issues. These activities cannot be fully delegated to technical roles, such as those of the data manager or statisticians; they should be embedded in the core curriculum of any good clinical researcher, as methods, ethics, and relevance are all linked together in research.

Beyond Trial Registration and Result Publication

I will use a personal experience to illustrate the way that thinking about access to clinical trial data has shifted over time. In 2015, I had the opportunity to give a speech on the Institute of Medicine's report concerning clinical trial sharing. While preparing the speech, I did not fully understand that data sharing in health research was becoming a vital, if controversial, topic in the medical literature. I was deeply involved in the activities of the European Clinical Research Infrastructure Network (ECRIN) at that time. ECRIN (n.d.) is a not-for-profit intergovernmental organization that supports the conducting of multinational clinical trials in Europe. Through a headquarters based in Paris that connects people across Europe, ECRIN provides its services to those conducting clinical studies, delineating a series of basic criteria for relevance, rigour, and transparency. These include study registration and the publication of results, irrespective of findings, as well as a commitment to make raw anonymized data sets available to the scientific community upon request. The latter criterion had been introduced some years before, prompted by the passionate plea of one member of the ECRIN Scientific Board, who was wisely anticipating the current intense discussion on data sharing. I had up to that point been teaching a very basic concept of data analyses using a real data set published by Vickers and collaborators as an appendix of a 2004 *BMJ* paper (Vickers et al., 2004). I was familiar with collaborative groups who were pooling data from several clinical trials, testing interventions on breast cancers and producing more reliable estimates of the effects in specific subgroups of women or exploring a given set of prognostic factors (Nuffield Department of Population Health, n.d.). And I knew that it was quite common for groups at the Mario Negri Institute to share their clinical trials data with other researchers when asked to do so.

Under the guise of preparing that speech, I committed myself to maintaining a comprehensive paper library of the literature on data sharing in health research, which is very much a full-time job. Almost every week, the main medical journals publish viewpoints, editorials, and, occasionally, some interesting empirical analyses on barriers and incentives, perceptions on benefits and risks of sharing health data, and reasons (or excuses) for not sharing. Social science journals publish articles on the ethical aspects of sharing and on the legal implications surrounding privacy and the boundaries of consent. Technical issues on data standardization and coding, de-identification, and so on populate the information technology journals. More slowly than in other research areas, the consensus that data sharing is an inseparable part of the research process was starting to catch on. In time, the discussion shifted to *how to make data sharing happen*, rather than simply whether or not to share data. Everyone who submits research for the public good should expect that they will be asked to make their data available for examination and re-analysis. Implementation of data sharing may be perceived as complicated, costly, and onerous. Without trust between researchers and the communities they serve, this perception is certainly true. Who should access what, when, under which conditions, to what end, following which procedure, managed by whom, under which jurisdictions? I experienced this complexity in a project called CORBEL aimed at developing principles and recommendations on sharing data from clinical trials.[1] The multidisciplinary group ended up with a list of fifty recommendations (Ohmann et al., 2017). That number may appear considerable, but it was probably not enough to cover all the caveats that may be relevant in data sharing. We run the risk of being overwhelmed by procedural issues and throwing the baby out with the bathwater, deciding to share data only when all the steps are clearly defined and agreed. To borrow Voltaire's words, "*le mieux est l'ennemi du bien*" ("perfection is the enemy of the good"). Nonetheless, the change in perspective, even from 2015 when I began thinking deeply about data sharing, to the present has been considerable.

Data Sharing: A Worthwhile Value

The willingness to share data should be an inherent component of academic research (especially publicly funded research). In essence, clinical researchers should look at health needs and orient pharmaceutical research to this end rather than (for example) simply trying to promote the drug they are developing. This outlook would facilitate a kind of research that goes beyond its own bubble of development, aimed not only at maximizing patent and publication but also at promoting collaboration and open access. Researchers should also investigate clinical strategies to better address the questions that matter to doctors and patients rather than serve only the demands of drug development by recruiting participants into studies that others design and coordinate. Practising doctors may then become leaders of the study team, rather than simply participant brokers, and can in this way help to improve the standard of care for their patients (Montori, 2017). Under a framework of trust in the research community, with the capacity to promote good use (and limit and report misuse), data sharing can contribute to the advancement of science and medicine. The scientific community might then recapture its perceived image as a self-regulating and ethically open entity, a role that has been fading in the eyes of the public over the past decades (Saltelli & Funtowicz, 2017; Ravetz & Saltelli, 2015; Baker, 2016).

Several examples of effective data sharing from academic clinical studies have developed largely through the spontaneous collaboration of groups and networking among academic centres. Perhaps my best example is the series of *Gruppo Italiano per lo Studio della Sopravvivenza nell'Infarto Miocardico* (GISSI) trials, coordinated by the Mario Negri Institute since the mid-1980s (Tognoni, Franzosi, & Garattini, 2018). The GISSI output contributed significantly to optimizing the treatment of myocardial infarction, showing, among other results, that thrombolytic therapy was able to reduce mortality and that the early use of ACE-inhibitors can furtherly improve the survival after an infarction. Besides providing answers to relevant clinical questions in a pragmatic, fast, and relatively inexpensive way, the GISSI trials established a model for embedding patient and public health–oriented research into the Italian National Health Service.

This series of trials represented the first nationwide experience of *true* effectiveness research, a research nested within practice. Moreover, it created one of the most exceptional research teams in the cardiovascular field, which attracted numerous international collaborations. The GISSI 1 trial, published in 1986, collected data on more than 11,000 patients. It represents a priceless source of information to investigate further questions, optimize the conditions for use of intravenous streptokinase, explore determinants of mortality, and determine the populations most likely to benefit from the treatment. Secondary analyses were done by members of the network, as well as by other researchers both within and outside of Italy. Some validation studies published in 2018 are still using data collected in the 1990s by the GISSI trials. In at least one case, data were even accessible to pursue a hypothesis not fully endorsed by the GISSI coordinators. Bertele' and collaborators questioned the methodological and ethical soundness of equivalence and non-inferiority trials using the data from the GISSI 1 study (Bertele', Angelici, Barlera, & Garattini, 2008). They provocatively showed that, by applying the hypothesis of an equivalence trial comparing saruplase and streptokinase, one may demonstrate that patients who did not undergo the thrombolysis approach in the GISSI trial had a similar death rate as those who were given streptokinase. In other words, the reasoning challenged the assumption of the effectiveness of an established treatment (thrombolysis) simply because it identified that the starting hypothesis was fallacious.

Maria Grazia Franzosi, former head of the cardiovascular department at the Mario Negri Institute and one of the lead researchers of the GISSI studies, explained that the governance of data access has been always simple (M.G. Franzosi, personal communication, 4 December 2018). Any researcher with a research question may contact the institute's Scientific Committee and gain access to the relevant part of the databases. Analyses are usually – but not necessarily – conducted together with one or more GISSI researchers to effect broader collaborations. In this way, GISSI researchers themselves have gained prestige, increased their impact, and created valuable links with other researchers. It also prompted academic researchers and clinicians to pay attention to data quality and management in order to allow other researchers to make sense of them and reduce possible misunderstanding or misuse.

For the members of the GISSI network, it was an obvious side product of their efforts and a logical consequence of their work. The broad cultural atmosphere during the 1980s and 1990s was nourished through collaborative dialogue across independent research groups. It was the age of the first megatrials, enthusiasm for evidence-based medicine, and research methodology. Such collaborations were not fully free of occasional conflicts, but they were usually focused on real unmet public health needs. One may argue that this vision, which cynics perceive as idealistic and naïve, is not feasible anymore given the highly competitive and conflicted research landscape that has emerged in the last twenty years. There is substance to this claim: the market is so dominant that threats to this ethos are constant. However, disillusionment should just be the first step in reflecting on the direction taken by health research. Several observers have argued that evidence-based medicine has been hijacked (Ioannidis, 2016). Researchers' reluctance to take unpopular positions, scepticism about novelties, and worries about technicalities are among the reasons for this failure.

But disillusionment can also be the catalyst for change. A shift towards a system of high-quality, transparent, shared research addressing relevant questions is possible and should take its inspiration from our past. According to Guido Bertolini, former coordinator of the *Gruppo Italiano per la Valutazione degli Interventi in Terapia Intensiva* (GiViTI) network, this shift should be informed by the idea that such a system is both achievable and desirable – a sort of "banality of good" (G. Bertolini, personal communication, 28 November 2018). We recently discussed how the GiViTI network is planning to share the data it collects from over 250 intensive care units in Italy. Bertolini recalled the ultimate goal of the GiViTI initiative: the improvement of the quality of care for critically ill people and the creation of an appropriate environment to promote better clinical research in such a complex field of medicine. In this context, expanding the use of data through new queries on the database or new research projects is inevitable. A patient admitted to an intensive care unit is often unable to provide any consent to the use of their data for research. The patient is often not even able to say yes or no to any medical intervention. Without going into detail regarding the delicate discussion around obtaining consent in emergency situations to use data for research purposes, it is useful to consider consent, however defined, as a gift. "Gifts are never truly free," argued Marcel Mauss; they are most often linked to reciprocal exchange (Mauss, 2002, p. 143). Researchers should be grateful for this generosity – one of the building blocks of their professional advancement – and do everything possible to honour this collective good that serves to benefit present and future people in similar situations.

Data sharing should be part of the core business of networks of this kind, but to work properly it must be embedded in a fully open environment. Data represent a power centre. Opening access to these data diffuses this power and diminishes the capacity of vested interests to manipulate the data to their advantage. Once the information is in the public domain, its exploitation is under the responsibility of the users and, by ensuring transparency in each stage, the research community and the public have an adequate tool to identify incorrect use. A commercial partner may have access to the GiViTI data at the same time as everyone else does. This policy is intended to guarantee the absence of any preferential relationship for one or more companies.

Both the GISSI's and GiViTI's experiences rest on the assumption that data belong to the network, which applies to every cooperative clinical research experience promoted by the Mario Negri Institute. The networks, in turn, are an expression of the National Health Service taking the configuration of the Italian cardiologic units (then) and the Italian intensive care units (now). Any threat to this assumption has the potential to undermine the whole endeavour. For instance, the commercialization of health, which is creeping into countries where a public health service based on universal coverage, social financing, and non-discriminatory access to the health-care services is a flagship, may hamper this view. If the assumption is that data do not belong to the public but to a private owner who should maximize profits rather than cures, then data sharing has no future. One way to tackle this risk is to shift from a model where data sharing and transparency in general are left to the goodwill of researchers to more structured initiatives. This shift is not simply a mannerism of idealistic researchers but, rather, a good system for the entire scientific community. Only by letting researchers swim in transparent seas can we achieve this goal.

Incentives and Environment Matter

If researchers do not embrace the ethical and cultural benefit of transparency and data sharing, incentives can facilitate behavioural change. An open access environment will promote those researchers who have the suitable characteristics to evolve: those who are more prone to share their ideas and data to improve knowledge, quality of care, and research. This strategy is, in other words, a new application of the Darwinian evolution of the species: from *homo occulens* (the man who conceals) to *homo praebens* (the man who discloses). The drivers of this process may have idealized norms, such as universalism, communality, disinterestedness, and organized scepticism, as per Merton's original ideals about science (Merton, 1973). Of course, altruism and curiosity are to be nurtured. However, given the human nature of researchers, we should not underestimate the value of concrete areas where other incentives work better: money and ambition. In this way, funding and career promotion are the two levers that should be pursued.

At present, several funders are engaged in the discussion about the promotion of open access. Broadly speaking, open access refers to the practice of providing online (and reusable) access to scientific information that is free of charge to the user. In the context of research and development, open access to scientific information comprises two main categories: peer-reviewed scientific publications (primarily research articles published in academic journals) and scientific research data (data underlying publications and/or unpublished data sets or raw data).

Concerning publications, several relevant initiatives that may improve data openness have recently been launched in Europe. The European Commission, the main researcher funder in Europe, supported the shift towards making research findings available free of charge for readers (see chapter three of this volume). The Commission requires publication of scientific output in open access journals; funds ad hoc projects on innovative approaches to release and disseminate research results (and measure their impact); and encourages member states to put publicly funded research results in the public domain. Even more ambitious is the announcement made by a group of twelve European research funding agencies in 2018. They plan to make mandatory, from 2021, the immediate publication of research findings in open access journals or platforms for all researchers receiving funds from European public bodies (cOALition S, 2020). Unfortunately, neither major Italian health research bodies nor universities have taken a position on this initiative at present. The plan does not accept a "hybrid" model of publishing; it requires funders to monitor compliance, and it sanctions non-compliance. It will be interesting to follow the impact of this plan on the scientific journal business model, as partially happened when the Bill & Melinda Gates Foundation (2020) adopted a similar approach. Similar initiatives have been promoted in Canada by the major federal granting agencies that promote and support research, the Canadian Institutes of Health Research, the Natural Sciences and Engineering Research Council of Canada, and the Social Sciences and Humanities Research Council of Canada. As publicly funded organizations, these agencies promote the widespread and barrier-free access to research data and knowledge. The European Open Science Policy Platform set actionable recommendations concerning eight aspects, including rewards and incentives, new indicators and metrics, scholarly communication, European Open Science Cloud, FAIR Data, research integrity, skills and education, and citizen science (European Commission, n.d.).

General statements and recommendations may be useful, even if they appear too generic to have an impact. Their lay translation is simple: an exhortation that funders should support, enforce, and monitor (1) prior registration of research; (2) open access to methods and protocols; (3) publication and dissemination of results; (4) complete and accurate reporting, for example, via the use of reporting guidelines; and (5) reuse of data by other researchers. An analysis of eleven international funding agencies published in 2017 found that all of the agencies required registration of clinical trials before recruitment of patients, while the registration of other study designs or the publication of protocols was required less often. Only six of the eleven funding agencies explicitly required publication of full reports of the research they had funded. At the time of the analysis, none of the funders had a comprehensive strategy to make full data sets available for further analyses (Nasser et al., 2017).

The corollary to the action implemented by funders is that academia too should reward scientists who are transparent and share their data and methodologies. In a competitive environment such as the research field, scientists' behaviour is guided by the reasonable desire for recognition and career advancement. Researchers know this mechanism well; they should be reassured that transparency will provide them advantages and abandon the idea that sharing protocols or data is like offering ammunition to competitors. Some years ago, during a meeting about clinical trial data sharing organized by the *New England Journal of Medicine* (2017) in the United States, I realized that the public has little understanding concerning either the importance of publications for researchers or the existence of disincentives to data sharing. Though all the members of the discussion panel embraced the principles of transparency, some academic trialists appeared reluctant to share participant-level data. They questioned its value and timing, and emphasized the need to have exclusive access to data to incentivize research. The debate collapsed into the appropriate length for an "exclusivity period" to allow front-line manuscripts to be completed. The patient representative at that panel, who had participated in multiple cancer trials, broke the diatribe. I was expecting her reprimand to be along the lines of "C'mon guys – be serious. People like me don't have time to wait for a paper to be published in an international journal. If data are useful to answer questions that matter to me and people with similar conditions, you must release them *now*." What she actually said (in a much softer way) was something like "I now feel even more strongly that data should be shared, the sooner the better, and in as much detail as possible." Notably, however, the *first* thing she said was: "My apologies – I just didn't realize your personal careers depend so much on journal publications." This woman had a metastatic cancer, and yet she felt pity for the pressures facing academic trialists with stellar h-index. Given the enormous physical, emotional, and financial toll of cancer, one might expect researchers to promote the free and open exchange of information. Rather than disseminating knowledge to improve the lives of those who, like this patient, are facing immediate and acute adversity, the objective of publishing results has been to further the careers of researchers.

To change their behaviour, researchers should be given incentives to publish open access, receiving appropriate acknowledgment and academic rewards when other researchers use "their" shared information to advance knowledge. Universities and research institutes could preferentially hire, promote, or tenure those who are champions of transparency. While some countries, as noted earlier, are moving in this direction, more widespread progress is uneven. An exemplary case emerged in 2016 in Italy. The commissions, which select scholars suitable to become professors in the Italian universities, have made public the evaluation criteria that they propose to adopt. While the criteria focused on publication or participation in editorial committees of national and international journals, one commission explicitly excluded open access journals. Talented researchers saw their open access publications excluded by the evaluation.

Data generators and data users should be collaborators rather than antagonists. Scientists are concerned that the data they have painstakingly gathered will be "scooped," or that someone will challenge their conclusions with a new analysis. Open access and data sharing are often perceived as a zero-sum game in which those who produce the original data lose if others perform further analyses. To the contrary, data generators and data users belong to the same species: each can be both, one day playing one role, another day the other. Investigators reusing data should apply the same level of transparency, meaning that they should make their results available and share their own data analyses. Trust is the crux of the matter (Packer, 2018).

Finally, we should fight those incentives that are against openness, such as the expectations that academic centres or research organizations must commercially exploit their results. Commercialization is not *necessarily* antithetical to openness; but when profits are tied to exclusionary data it often is. The boundary between scientific and applied research has blurred. There is increasing attention on patent research results and on extracting as much value as possible from intellectual property. While there might be several science areas where technology transfer is advisable, there is growing evidence that the pressure to commercialize is directly or indirectly associated with adverse impacts (Caulfield & Ogbogu, 2015). This pressure results in science hype, premature implementation or translation of research, research policy conflicts, confusion and concealment of information, and data withholding. Moreover, patenting is a costly activity; the evidence of a link between university research and economic growth is tenuous at best. Researchers should be aware of the risks any public-private partnership creates. However, they cannot be left alone in the assessment of these risks, which often take the form of legal technicalities in draft agreements. Universities and research organizations should give them tools to understand and identify the benefits and risks of these collaborations (for example, ethical codes and structured risk analyses). Public funding bodies and charities who advocate for industry partnerships should monitor how those projects manage knowledge dissemination and access to data.

Some years ago, the Mario Negri Institute withdrew from a clinical project funded by the European Commission under the framework of the public-private scheme of the Innovative Medicines Initiative because the commercial partner wanted to control to whom the data could be disclosed and why, as well as what could be published and when. The clinical investigators involved in the project were not even allowed access to the data. For an institute that does not patent its discoveries and publishes all information for the benefit of the scientific community, patients, and the public, this deal was unacceptable. The Mario Negri Institute lost a considerable amount of money by quitting that project, and – considering the hard times we are facing – it was a substantial sacrifice. "However," commented the then director, Silvio Garattini, "we could not renounce our principles and betray the trust of people who support our research" (Garattini, Bertele', & Bertolini, 2013).

Conclusion

There is much room for improvement in medical research openness. Researchers should take the lead, as they are in the unique position of being the ones who *generate* information and are also among the most important *users* of that information. Researchers are not locked in their laboratories. Clinical researchers are often doctors treating patients; sometimes they (or their family members) become patients and research participants themselves. They sit on guideline development panels and journal editorial boards; they review articles and funding applications; sometimes they advise public bodies or even have political roles. They write books, blogs, and tweets. They are teachers too, with the responsibility of creating better future generations of doctors and scientists. Taking the lead does not mean they should work alone. They can only succeed if they encourage the participation of others and do not see their interests as more important than the interests of others who benefit from their research. The scientific community and the public should become shareholders in a model where the benefits of research and innovation remain open to them in the form of services and knowledge. Clinical data are public goods because they belong not only to trial participants, researchers, and medical staff but also to the taxpayers who fund most of the investigations, infrastructure, and facilities included in clinical research (Banzi, Bertele', & Garattini, 2014).

The venture is tough, but researchers, especially those working in the public field, are used to risk and often have a strong sense of duty and sacrifice. They can be reassured by acknowledging that small advancements may have major impact, as in the case of trial registries or reporting guidelines.

Transparency must be a prerequisite for funding and publishing. We arguably need *better* research rather than *more* research (Altman, 1994). Better research means collaboration: sharing ideas and data. In addition to the usual benefit of bringing new expertise and ideas to a scientific paper, co-authoring with a diverse group of colleagues helps disseminate research findings more widely. Researchers could participate in the creation of better infrastructure to enable transparency, openness, and sharing. They should also put their expertise into making data truly "fair": FAIR is an incisive acronym that stands for "Findable, Accessible, Interoperable, and Reusable" (Wilkinson et al., 2016). More structured initiatives to facilitate data sharing and data reuse have the advantage of increasing the visibility and discoverability of studies and data sets, and make the process of accessing data more accountable, reproducible, and transparent. These guarantees could also temper some of the reluctance of investigators and, to some extent, of study participants, to buy into this system. Political indecisiveness, the weaknesses of researchers, and the interests of individuals cannot stop the transition that has, in any case, begun.

NOTE

1 For information on the Coordinated Research Infrastructures Building Enduring Life-science Services (CORBEL), see the CORBEL website, https://www.corbel-project.eu/home.html.

REFERENCES

All Trials, All Trials Registered | All Results Reported [Home page]. (n.d.). Retrieved from https://www.alltrials.net/

Altman, D.G. (1994). The scandal of poor medical research. *BMJ, 308*(6924), 283–4. https://doi.org/10.1136/bmj.308.6924.283

Baker, M. (2016). 1,500 scientists lift the lid on reproducibility: Survey sheds light on the "crisis" rocking research. *Nature, 533*(7604), 452–4. https://doi.org/10.1038/533452a

Banzi, R., Bertele', V., & Garattini, S. (2014). EMA's transparency seems to be opaque. *Lancet, 384*(9957), 1847. https://doi.org/10.1016/S0140 -6736(14)62241-8

Bertele', V., Angelici, L., Barlera, S., & Garattini, S. (2008). Thrombolysis or nothing for acute myocardial infarction? It's all the same! *British Journal of Clinical Pharmacology, 65*(6), 955–8. https://doi.org/10.1111/j.1365-2125.2008.03125.x

Bill & Melinda Gates Foundation. (2020). How we work: Bill & Melinda Gates Foundation open access policy. Retrieved from https://www.gatesfoundation .org/How-We-Work/General-Information/Open-Access-Policy

Caulfield, T., & Ogbogu, U. (2015). The commercialization of university-based research: Balancing risks and benefits. *BMC Medical Ethics, 16,* 70. https:// doi.org/10.1186/s12910-015-0064-2

cOALition S. (2020). Plan S: Making full and immediate Open Access a reality. Retrieved from https://www.coalition-s.org/

De Angelis, C.D., Drazen, J.M., Frizelle, F.A., Haug, C., Hoey, J., Horton, R., ... Van Der Weyden, M.B. (2004) Clinical trial registration: A statement from the International Committee of Medical Journal Editors. *JAMA, 292*(11), 1363–4. https://doi.org/10.1001/jama.292.11.1363

Dyer, O. (2004). GlaxoSmithKline faces US lawsuit over concealment of trial results. *BMJ, 328*(7453), 1395. https://doi.org/10.1136/bmj.328.7453.1395

European Clinical Research Infrastructure Network (ECRIN). (n.d.). Facilitating clinical research [home page]. Retrieved from https://ecrin.org/

European Commission. (n.d.). Open science. Retrieved from https://ec.europa .eu/research/openscience/index.cfm?pg=open-science-policy-platform

Garattini, S., Bertele', V., & Bertolini, G. (2013). A failed attempt at collaboration. *BMJ, 347,* f5354. https://doi.org/10.1136/bmj.f5354

Government of the United States. (1997). Food and Drug Administration Modernization Act of 1997. Retrieved from https://www.govinfo.gov/content /pkg/PLAW-105publ115/pdf/PLAW-105publ115.pdf

Graham, J.E., & Jones, M. (2016). Just evidence: Opening health knowledge to a parliament of evidence. In B.H. MacDonald, S.S. Soomai, E.M. De Santo, & P.G. Wells (Eds.), *Science, Information, and Policy Interface for Effective Coastal and Ocean Management* (pp. 325–49). Boca Raton, FL: CRC Press.

Institute for Science, Ethics and Innovation (ISEI), The University of Manchester. (2009). *Who owns science? The Manchester Manifesto.* Retrieved from http://www.isei.manchester.ac.uk/TheManchesterManifesto.pdf

Ioannidis, J.P.A. (2016). Evidence-based medicine has been hijacked: A report to David Sackett. *Journal of Clinical Epidemiology, 73,* 82–6. https://doi.org /10.1016/j.jclinepi.2016.02.012

Krleža-Jerić, K. (2005). Clinical trial registration: The differing views of industry, the WHO, and the Ottawa Group. *PLoS Medicine, 2*(11), e378. https://doi.org /10.1371/journal.pmed.0020378

Law, M.R., Kawasumi, Y., & Morgan, S.G. (2011). Despite law, fewer than one in eight completed studies of drugs and biologics are reported on time on ClinicalTrials.gov. *Health Affairs*), *30*(12), 2338–45. https://doi.org/10.1377/hlthaff.2011.0172

Liberati, A. (2011). Need to realign patient-oriented and commercial and academic research. *Lancet*, *378*(9805), 1777–8. https://doi.org/10.1016/S0140-6736(11)61772-8

Light, D.W., & Maturo, A.F. (2015). *Good Pharma: The public-health model of the Mario Negri Institute.* Basingstoke, UK: Palgrave Macmillan.

Mario Negri Institute of Pharmacological Research. (2019). Manifesto: Contributing to defending health and human life. Retrieved from https://www.marionegri.it/eng/manifesto

Mario Negri Institute of Pharmacological Research. (n.d.). Clinical studies at the Mario Negri. Retrieved from https://registro.marionegri.it/index.php?type=12

Mauss, M. (2002). *Saggio sul dono Saggio sul dono. Forma e motivo dello scambio nelle società arcaiche* [*An essay on the gift: The form and reason of exchange in archaic societies*]. Trans. F. Zannino. Piccola Biblioteca Einaudi Ns. (Original work, *Essai sur le don. Forme et raison de l'échange dans les sociétés archaïques*, published in *Année Sociologique*, seconde série, 1923–1924)

Mayo-Wilson, E., Heyward, J., Keyes, A., Reynolds, J., White, S., Atri, N., ... Ford, D.E. (2018). Clinical trial registration and reporting: A survey of academic organizations in the United States. *BMC Medicine*, *16*, 60. https://doi.org/10.1186/s12916-018-1042-6

Merton, R.K. (1973). *The sociology of science: Theoretical and empirical investigations.* Chicago, IL: University of Chicago Press.

Montori, V. (2017). *Why we revolt: A patient revolution for careful and kind care.* Rochester, MN: The Patient Revolution.

Nasser, M., Clarke, M., Chalmers, I., Brurberg, K.G., Nykvist, H., Lund, H., & Glasziou, P. (2017). What are funders doing to minimize waste in research. *Lancet*, *389*(10073), 1006–7. https://doi.org/10.1016/S0140-6736(17)30657-8

New England Journal of Medicine (NEJM). (2017). *Aligning incentives for sharing clinical trial data.* Web event held on 3–4 April 2017. Retrieved from https://challenge.nejm.org/pages/free-web-event

Nuffield Department of Population Health, Clinical Trial Service Unit & Epidemiological Studies Unit (CTSU). (n.d.). The Early Breast Cancer Trialists' Collaborative Group (EBCTCG). Retrieved from https://www.ctsu.ox.ac.uk/research/ebctcg

Ohmann, C., Banzi, R., Canham, S., Battaglia, S., Matei, M., Ariyo, C., ... Demotes-Mainard, J. (2017). Sharing and reuse of individual participant data from clinical trials: Principles and recommendations. *BMJ Open*, *7*(12), e018647. https://doi.org/10.1136/bmjopen-2017-018647

Packer, M. (2018). Data sharing in medical research. *BMJ*, *360*, k510. https://doi.org/10.1136/bmj.k510

Pandolfini, C., & Bonati, M. (2018). An audit to evaluate an institute's lead researchers' knowledge of trial registries and to investigate adherence to data transparency issues in an Italian research institute registry. *Trials*, *19*, 509. https://doi.org/10.1186/s13063-018-2910-2

Ravetz. J., & Saltelli, A. (2015). The future of public trust in science. *Nature*, *524*, 161. https://doi.org/10.1038/524161d

Reveiz, L., Krleža-Jerić, K., Chan, A.-W., & De Aguiar, S. (2007). Do trialists endorse clinical trial registration? Survey of a PubMed sample. *Trials*, *8*, 30. https://doi.org/10.1186/1745-6215-8-30

Saltelli, A., & Funtowicz, S. (2017). What is science's crisis really about? *Future*, *91*, 5–11. https://doi.org/10.1016/j.futures.2017.05.010

Scherer, M., & Trelle, S. (2008). Opinions on registering trial details: A survey of academic researchers. *BMC Health Services Research*, *8*, 18. https://doi.org/10.1186/1472-6963-8-18

Tognoni, G., Franzosi, M.G., & Garattini, S. (2018). Embedding patient- and public health-oriented research in a national health service: The GISSI experience. *JLL Bulletin: Commentaries on the history of treatment evaluation.* Retrieved from https://www.jameslindlibrary.org/articles/embedding -patient-and-public-health-oriented-research-in-a-national-health-service-the -gissi-experience/

TraspariMED. (n.d.). TrapariMED works to end evidence distortion in medicine [home page]. Retrieved from https://www.transparimed.org/about

UNESCO Institute for Statistics. (n.d.). How much does your country invest in R&D. Retrieved from http://uis.unesco.org/apps/visualisations/research -and-development-spending/

Vickers, A.J., Rees, R.W., Zollman, C.E., McCarney, R., Smith, C.M., Ellis, N., … Van Haselen, R. (2004). Acupuncture for chronic headache in primary care: Large, pragmatic, randomised trial. *BMJ*, *328*, 744. https://doi.org/10.1136 /bmj.38029.421863.EB

Wilkinson, M.D., Dumontier, M. Aalbersberg, I.J., Appleton, G., Axton, M., Baak, A., … Mons, B. (2016). The FAIR Guiding Principles for scientific data management and stewardship. *Scientific Data*, *3*, 160018. https://doi.org /10.1038/sdata.2016.18

Zarin, D.A., Tse, T., Williams, R.J., & Rajakannan, T. (2017). Update on trial registration 11 years after the ICMJE policy was established. *New England Journal of Medicine*, *376*(4), 383–91. https://doi.org/10.1056/NEJMsr1601330

12 Conclusion

KATHERINE FIERLBECK, JANICE GRAHAM,
AND MATTHEW HERDER

This volume addresses two discrete but tightly interwoven themes. The first sets out the value of transparency in pharmaceutical regulation per se. The second takes a more longitudinal perspective and asks whether substantive progress is being made in the achievement of transparency in this sector. On this question, contributors to this volume express both optimism and (slightly more emphatically) pessimism. To the extent that the evaluation of progress has been positive, contributors have identified why and how these successes have arisen; to the extent that the evaluation of progress towards greater transparency has been less than favourable, they have tried to identify the dynamics that obstruct it.

The contributors attend to the processes and mechanisms established to provide transparency in the regulatory standards for pharmaceuticals in Canada, the European Union, and the United States. They uncover the gaps and provide insights to reflect on the facilitators of, and barriers to, greater transparency, including the processes and mechanisms that legitimize pharmaceutical regulation. The task of policy-makers is to build relevant programs and strategies that fit with practical contexts and values. The work of the clinical and social researchers contributing to this volume, by contrast, has been to study what is underneath the fault lines of structure and function, and to unpack and critically examine the political, cultural, legal, and technical contexts that might explain the disjuncture between rhetoric and practice. They have attended to the dynamics and pragmatics of data, guidelines, regulations, and legislation, refracted by the political processes in their respective jurisdictions. These dynamics, as we have seen, are driven by both the pragmatic interests and the unconscious assumptions of a wide range of actors.

Individuals seldom make decisions independent of context – rather, decisions are often influenced by interests, values, and emotions as well as data, directives, guidelines, and policies. This part of the real world is too often overlooked or dismissed: when written down and authoritatively stamped, the stuff of evidence is used as guidance for "rational" or evidence-based, or evidence-*informed*, decision-making. But the specifics related to the underlying reasons for selecting particular kinds of evidence, as well as the role of opinions, common sense, ideology, and competing interests of experts, peers, and local advisors in defining the evidence, are largely neglected. Our contributors have challenged the claims of validity and reliability of our best evidence-based research practices and cast scepticism on the rhetoric of full disclosure of conflicts of interest. Confidence cannot always be assured, either in the safety and efficacy of reported study results or in the quality of the decisions made. The power of the pharmaceutical industry that sponsors and controls the results of most clinical trials gives them the upper hand in defining what gets counted as "relevant evidence." This control can include the way the study is designed, the manner in which data are gathered, the kinds of metrics that are used, the outcomes that are measured (and those that are ignored), the determination of therapeutic advantage, and so on. Together, the chapters in this volume provide a detailed account of a process to open up the regulatory black box, to make transparent the evaluation of the pipeline, beginning in the lab and advancing through animal and clinical trials to the manufacturing processes, regulatory approval decision-making, and active ongoing surveillance and monitoring.

The Movement Towards Transparency

Why is transparency important in pharmaceutical policy? Unlike many other consumer products, pharmaceutical products have considerable impact upon individual well-being, and as such, public safety requires regulatory oversight. Yet, the nature of this regulatory oversight is often hampered by the quality of data submitted that may be compromised by conflicts of interest, constrained by review timelines, and limited by underfunding. It may also be impeded by conflicting political goals when pharmaceutical policy is viewed as a means of achieving the objectives of both health policy and industrial policy (Vandergrift & Kanavos, 1997). Transparency is in this way an essential component of accountability for an industry whose products can be both beneficial (Gilead's Sovaldi) or catastrophic (Purdue's OxyContin).

Regulation might well be considered a silent but salient mediator of science and politics. Before the innovative products of science reach the public, they must meet regulatory standards regarding safety, efficacy, and quality. After a product is authorized for use in humans, it is widely understood as continuing to meet the standards of safety and effectiveness in both more particular and broader populations than those in which the pivotal clinical trial research was conducted, and for which the initial authorization for approval was granted. Citizens in civil society expect due diligence in the scientific evaluatory process and trust that the health products they are prescribed meet these standards. For the most part, the public are unaware of the gaps between evidence collected in clinical study populations and that which is discovered through use in the wider population until serious adverse events – multiple deaths or morbidities – provoke them into awareness.

Notwithstanding the trail of adverse events, industry advocates (and some portion of the public and clinical science communities) regard present regulatory systems as too onerous, charging that their bureaucracy delays market access for useful products and thwarts research by making investment costs prohibitive. Other constituents argue, conversely, that regulation has already become too flexible, that an intimate relationship fostered between industry and government has rendered the regulatory system ineffective, and that public safety is thereby compromised.

In Canada, for example, drugs are the fastest growing health expenditure, second only to hospitals (28.3 per cent) and representing 15.7 per cent of the 2018 health budget (Canadian Institute for Health Information, 2018, p. 4). Nonetheless, government regulators at Health Canada have not seen proportionate increases in their operating budgets over the years to handle the submissions or the monitoring of the approved drugs and vaccines afterwards. The Marketed Health Product Directorate at Health Canada was established in 2004, with insufficient funding to meet the mandate of post-marketing product surveillance and monitoring, as mentioned in Gagnon, Herder, Graham, Fierlbeck, and Danyliuk (chapter 5 of this volume), and at the same time as the Public Health Agency of Canada was created; these two important new departments added to an already limited budget line for public health safety and protection. Armed with these fiscal limitations, Health Canada then secured the discretion to set user fees, paid by industry sponsors with the expectation of receiving regulatory reviews within a set time frame (Health Canada, 2019). In the United States, by contrast, where the existence of user fees has motivated concerns of regulatory capture, fees are set by Congress.

Transparency – its absence, how to incorporate it into practice, and whether openness in one area might cast a shadow over another – has long been a site of tension in Canada. In the 1990s, the Canadian Science Advisory Board recommended new standards of access to information at all stages of the drug review process to enhance transparency and public confidence. Following an international trend for new public management models, in 1995 the Health Protection Branch established the Therapeutic Products Program and, in 2000, was divided into three branches: for environment, for population and disease control, and for health products and food. Some have argued that "protection" indeed went out the window in the flurry for risk management rather than technical risk assessment. Health promotion rather than protection became the business of government, with the Throne Speech of 2002 signposting that "the government will move forward with a smart regulation strategy to ... promote health and sustainability, to contribute to innovation and economic growth, and to reduce the administrative burden on business ... It will speed up the regulatory process for drug approvals to ensure that Canadians have faster access to the safe drugs they need" (Government of Canada, 2002). It was clear that the actions being addressed for greater transparency were coming from industry rather than from public watchdogs.

In 2003, the Health Products and Food Branch introduced a series of new policies to look "*beyond regulation*" to operate as a timely, transparent, innovative, and sustainable regulator. The Therapeutic Access Strategy provided funds to hire more clinical and scientific evaluators to address the backlog of submissions that had grown with government cuts due to the retrenchment in the 1990s. More policy analysts were also hired to streamline and speed up drug approval and harmonize standards, especially between Canada and the United States, for international competitive advantage. That policy shift towards increased transparency created an avenue for co-author Graham to access Health Canada's regulatory authority in order to study regulatory practices in Health Canada during the early stages of the transparency turn. Still, she was required to obtain approval from industry itself via the industry umbrella organization Research-Based Pharmaceutical Development (Rx&D), the precursor of Innovative Medicines Canada, before Health Canada permitted her access to follow their evaluation process, negotiations, and decision-making surrounding regulatory approval of biologic submissions. Health Canada's Therapeutic Access Strategy was intended to provide the organizational tools and structures for more public accountability. The need for both accountability and additional resources were critical since, as Lexchin (chapter seven of this volume) reminds us, the Canadian Association of Journalists had presented Health Canada in 2004 with its "Code of Silence" award. The Therapeutic Access Strategy succeeded in making the government look more transparent, although their planned "smart regulation" policy had counterintuitively called for *deregulation*, contrary to what would reasonably be expected from a public regulator. The term "smart regulation" was quietly retired after criticism (Graham,

2005) and sanitized in the Blueprint for Renewal (2006) and the Strategic Plan (2007) into the Progressive Licensing Framework (2008), which maps to the lifecycle management and adaptive pathways that promote faster access (Davis, Lexchin, Jefferson, Gøtzsche, & McKee, 2016).

While openness and accountability were a central tenet of Health Canada's regulatory modernization project during the first decade of the twenty-first century, it is difficult to determine whether the construction of transparency was a genuine effort to open up pharmaceutical information to independent reviewers or an instrument to divert risks and responsibilities to the public (Graham & Jones, 2010). For example, Lexchin, in chapter seven of this volume and elsewhere (Habibi & Lexchin, 2014), and others (Graham & Nuttall, 2013) have found much to critique in the Summary Basis of Decision documents, as well as in the safety of drugs approved under the priority review process and in the presumed "novelty" of "new drugs" that are heavily weighted by supplementary (secondary, derivative) products. More recent research has sought to clarify the contributions of various actors in the research and development process, in effect using transparency to interrogate the assumptions that tend to drive conversations about pharmaceutical innovation and regulatory standards (Graham, 2019; Herder, Graham, & Gold, 2020).

Likewise, the narrative of the trajectory towards (and away from) greater transparency in the pharmaceutical sector in the United States and the European Union shows patterns of advancement and retrenchment. Given that these shifts in direction are the result of concerted human agency, it is useful to summarize the observations of contributors gleaned from broad historical surveys and focused case studies alike.

What Lessons Can We Learn from the Past Two Decades?

To understand why particular policies are implemented (or defeated), it is, as Greer and colleagues (2017) write, important to ascertain what shapes political options: what variables determine the strategic landscapes and political techniques that can influence policy-making? Health policy analysis, the authors argue, generally tends to be politically unsophisticated; policy exponents have a strong tendency to assume that enlightened health policies depend on some inchoate form of "'political will' that can overcome inertia and industry lobbying" (p. 42). To better understand policies and outcomes, they explain, "we need a more sophisticated understanding of political systems and institutions that shape the political processes and conditions for policy adoption" (p. 42). In evaluating the recent history of regulatory transparency in the pharmaceutical sector, how can we explain why some jurisdictions were successful on certain fronts, while other jurisdictions or strategies were not? And how can we use this information to think about future strategic campaigns towards greater transparency? Together, the contributors to this volume highlight four discrete factors that are analytically useful, both to understand the resistance to greater transparency and to consider what kinds of strategies can be employed to achieve it. The first is the set of structures and institutions in which policy debates are situated. These features are more static (or "sticky," as policy theorists write) and generally constrain – though occasionally facilitate – policy change. The second is the set of political actors who are generally responsible for more dynamic policy shifts and the ways in which they organize to achieve these goals. The third factor is ideational construction (or "constructivism"), which focuses on the way in which ideas can be used to shape support for, or resistance to, policy change. The ability to discern temporal opportunities – and the capacity to take advantage of them – is the final factor that is identified in this analysis.

Structures and Institutions

"Political institutions," note Greer, Bekker, Azzopardi-Muscat, and McKee (2018, p. 5), "shape the receptiveness of governments to different political initiatives and the sustainability of different policies." These institutions are often themselves the product of power struggles and political settlements (Campbell, 2004; Béland, 2019). The most important structural variable determining the nature of transparency policies across the three jurisdictions examined in this volume is the nature of the legal framework in each system. In the first instance, each jurisdiction's ability to achieve greater transparency is dependent upon the legal context within which pharmaceutical regulation is situated. As Davis, Mulinari, and Jefferson in chapter three; McCarthy and Ross in chapter four; and Gagnon, Herder, Graham, Fierlbeck, and Danyliuk in chapter five describe in this volume, the starting point for pharmaceutical transparency was the way in which the legal structures in each jurisdiction facilitated public access to information in general terms. In the case of the European Union, as Davis, Mulinari, and Jefferson observe, "Article 15 of the Treaty on the Function of the European Union, in conjunction with Regulation 1049/2001 (the so-called 'Transparency Regulation'), granted the public a right to access European Parliament, Council, and Commission documents." It was this broader statutory authority – which itself had no specific reference to pharmaceuticals – that led to more specific requirements pertaining to public access of information held by the European Medicines Agency (EMA). Another institutional feature of the European Union (that has no parallel in either the United States or Canada) is the existence of the Ombudsman, which, as Davis, Mulinari, and Jefferson again describe, played a pivotal role in pushing the European Union to implement greater transparency provisions.

In the United States, by contrast, much disclosure of industry practices occurred through civil and criminal litigation. Nonetheless, as McCarthy and Ross explain, pharmaceutical transparency in the United States was facilitated by the 1966 Freedom of Information Act; this same act – implemented against much opposition – also clearly defined the restrictions on access to pharmaceutical information (particularly in the broad interpretation of "confidential commercial information"). Canada's inertia on transparency can also be understood with reference to its own (even less stringent) Access to Information Act, which did not require any disclosure of clinical data. Nonetheless, the subsequent enactment of the Canadian Charter of Rights and Freedoms ultimately facilitated a challenge to Health Canada in 2018 with reference to the right to freedom of expression. Likewise, the particular nature of the federal structure itself can determine the scope for transparency: in Canada, for example, the devolution of responsibility for the provision (though not regulation) of pharmaceuticals to the provinces meant that they were not subject to the federal transparency statute, as McCarthy and Ross note.

Other pertinent institutional variables include international trade agreements and the structure of academic research. Canada's experience with the original Canada–United States Free Trade Agreement in 1987 illustrated the way in which access to trade required a willingness to reinforce intellectual property rights to clinical data. The utilization of trade policy as a means of weakening transparency can also be seen in the negotiations over the Transatlantic Trade and Investment Partnership (TTIP) and the Trans-Pacific Partnership (TPP) (Jarman, 2014). And yet, as Banzi (chapter eleven of this volume) cautions, impediments to accessing scientific data are not the sole purview of the pharmaceutical industry. By uncritically supporting a system of academic research in which openness and collaboration is devalued, researchers themselves reinforce barriers to greater transparency.

The first concluding observation, then, is that those wanting to achieve greater transparency within the pharmaceutical sector must understand the particular institutional context within which policy change is attempted. What kinds of access to data, for example, does a legal system protect or prevent? How do international treaties and agreements influence disclosure of data? How does the structure of governance mechanisms impede or facilitate access to information? As McCarthy and Ross note, the particular distribution of authority established by Canada's federal system, where public drug formulary listings made at the provincial level are not subject to federal access to information legislation, has posed limits to what can be achieved through federal legislation. One could perhaps also argue, with Fritz Scharpf, that the very nature of European law incorporates a "constitutional asymmetry" towards market-oriented policy-making (and thus the protection of confidential commercial information), given that the concept of the common market was the raison d'être for the establishment of the original European Economic Community (Scharpf, 2010; Permanand & Mossialos, 2005). Nonetheless, while determining the parameters for action, institutions are not destiny. Regardless of whether the European Union exhibits a constitutional bias towards market-oriented policy, the agency of numerous political actors, as Davis, Mulinari, and Jefferson observe, was able to make a substantial impact upon the provision of pharmaceutical transparency within the EMA.

Structural-institutional theories are useful in explaining the way in which transparency initiatives have been implemented. These kinds of explanations are also helpful in highlighting the kinds of barriers that obdurately remain despite ongoing calls for greater "political will" to implement greater transparency. But structural explanations are less useful in explaining political *change* – and particularly policy successes. That is why it is also important to identify the causal mechanisms leading to policy transformation (Tuohy, 2018).

Advocacy and Organization

Who are the agents of political change? Löblová (2018, p. 7) identifies the role of epistemic communities, or "groups of experts with a common policy goal derived from their shared knowledge," in discussions of pharmaceutical policy. These communities can, if they are able to mobilize effectively, form advocacy coalitions that help them "to identify potential allies and establish mechanisms or sustainable political influence" (Brooks, 2018, p. 11). As Davis, Mulinari, and Jefferson explain in some detail in chapter three, it was the consolidation of numerous advocacy groups across twelve European member states to form the Medicines in Europe Forum (MiEF) in the early 2000s that facilitated a concerted effort to place pharmaceutical transparency on the political agenda: "Through its early advocacy activities between 2002 and 2004, while the complex European co-decision procedure unfolded, the MiEF gained an important understanding of and insights into the orientation of the

Commission and complex legislative processes, as well as valuable experience in engaging with the formal institutions of the supranational European Union." In this way, transparency became a central focus for MiEF and resulted in a petition to the EU Parliament in 2002. Within two years, the European Union adopted Regulation 726/2004 and Directive 2004/27/EC, establishing a key treaty base for the expansion of data transparency. While the EMA interpreted its obligations to disclose information "extremely narrowly," MiEF members such as Prescrire, Health Action International, and the Nordic Cochrane Collaboration focused on sustained campaigns for greater access to EMA data, culminating in Access Policy 0043 in 2010.

Likewise, as Gagnon and colleagues point out in chapter five, Canada's revision to the Food and Drugs Act – Vanessa's Law – did not originally focus on transparency; it was the concerted efforts of a number of well-placed advocates working in tandem that put transparency on the legislative agenda when the window of opportunity for policy reform opened. McCarthy and Ross in chapter four and Gagnon and colleagues detail the enduring persistence of academic and clinician-initiated advocacy since the 2000s, which employed processes to attain and then publicly disclose clinical trial data in Canada, culminating in a landmark ruling that Health Canada was unreasonable in denying disclosure of clinical trial data to an independent researcher in July 2018, contrary to the spirit of Vanessa's Law.

The second lesson, then, is that establishing networks of key advocacy stakeholders is imperative in developing the capacity to frame policy problems and to offer viable solutions. The theoretical iteration of this observation is known as the "advocacy coalition framework." These coalitions are comprised of interest group leaders, researchers, policy-makers, and others "who share a particular belief system – i.e. a set of basic values, causal assumptions, and problem perceptions – and who show a non-trivial degree of coordinated activity over time" (Sabatier, 1988, p. 139). These coalitions inhabit policy subsystems, and when they work in concert, they are able to exert considerable influence on defining problems, suggesting solutions, and shaping long-term policy objectives. Rather than social movements that arise in response to single issues, advocacy coalitions are formed within broader epistemic communities that remain relatively stable over long periods of time. Academic researchers, especially in highly technically specific fields, are often key actors within advocacy coalitions. Those coalitions that are able to constructively learn from each other generally tend to be the most successful (Jenkins-Smith & Sabatier, 1993).

Framing, Narratives, and Bounded Rationality

The rise of "evidence-based policy-making" – loosely based on the "evidence-based medicine" movement – holds that giving better evidence to decision-makers will result in better policies. Yet, this approach fails to acknowledge that "policymakers have too many problems to pay attention to, too many solutions to consider, and too many choices to make, based on more information than they can process" (Cairney, 2016, p. 27). In consequence, they develop cognitive shortcuts to determine which items will be placed on the political agenda, how problems are conceptualized, and what solutions are seen as appropriate. In this volume, for example, Persaud in chapter six notes how information can fail to make an impact, not because it is obscured but rather because it must compete with an abundance of existing information. New data that contradicts existing data encounters a Proteus effect, in which the initial release of information seems to have a much greater effect than the release of subsequent information on the same issue. Health-care providers have little time to sift through multiple and conflicting sources of information, while health-care users are unsurprisingly intimidated by the preponderance of often contrary sources of information. New information must also be filtered through entrenched beliefs and practices, and is unlikely to receive a reflective reception.

If bounded rationality decreases the relevance of evidence in the decision-making process, it increases the import of the way in which ideas are presented. Agenda-setting is one example of the force of ideational construction. Agenda-setting is the ability of political actors to convince decision-makers that some issues are worthy of legislative attention, while others are not. Given a crowded political agenda allowing only a limited number of key issues to be debated, policy advocates work hard to place ideas – such as transparency – on the political agenda, while countervailing interests may work just as hard attempting to keep them off (Cairney, Heikkila, & Wood, 2019). Lexchin in chapter seven, for example, discusses the way in which Health Canada communicates information regarding regulation of the conduct of clinical trials, drug approvals, drug safety, and promotion. In these cases, the criteria for regulatory oversight are vague, the rationale for specific actions is not specified, or the evaluative mechanisms for these oversight functions are non-existent. In other words, regulatory mechanisms may be put into place, providing a sense that transparency mechanisms are performing their required functions, but if the public has no idea how (or whether) these mechanisms are working, then transparency issues fall far below other items on the political agenda where the deficiencies of other policies are clear and evident.

The third observation that the contributors to this volume offer is the need to be aware of the (often insidious) ways in which the framing of ideas and issues can be deployed to obtain political ends. Ideas are not necessarily benign; they can be "positioned as tools that can be constructed and deployed by interested policy actors as 'weapons of advocacy'" (Smith, 2014, p. 562; Weiss, 1989, p. 117). As Fierlbeck in chapter two describes, there are numerous ways in which discursive techniques can be employed in this manner. Ghimire and Lemmens in chapter nine, for example, challenge the presentation of a false binary choice – *either* strict protection of confidential commercial information *or* poor protection of patient data – and suggest that appropriate technical and legal mechanisms are available to mitigate fears of data breaches in clinical trial data for rare diseases. Gagnon in chapter eight provides a detailed explanation of the way in which "control of ideas, knowledge, habits of thought, and narratives have become central to how dominant corporations thrive." Similarly, Jefferson in chapter ten describes the development of a pandemic flu vaccine in 2009, showing how a narrative of fear can facilitate the diminution of rigour in the testing process. When public fears became stoked at the height of the H1N1 pandemic, argues Jefferson, less attention was paid to toxicity and to the fact that risks and liabilities resulting from this disregard of potential harms were absorbed by the public sector (and by the public themselves). It was the deliberate construction of a narrative based on "urgency" and the need for "preparedness," he argues, that made the hasty introduction of the vaccine seem both reasonable and justifiable.

Windows of Opportunity

The attempt in this volume to understand how transparency in the pharmaceutical sector has been achieved (or obstructed) over several decades and across three major jurisdictions also underscores the need to appreciate the temporal context of policy-making. Proponents of greater transparency may feel (with some justification) that the best time to insist on change is *now*, and may become discouraged or cynical when repeated attempts at achieving this goal fail. This is why a broader understanding of the policy process is useful. Policy implementation is a highly competitive process, and merit is only one reason some policies are adopted and others are not. As some of the contributions here illustrate exceptionally well, successful attempts at expanding transparency were the result of capturing brief windows of opportunity. As McCarthy and Ross document in chapter four, for example, it was the Watergate scandal in 1974 that provided the political impetus for the amendments to the US Freedom of Information Act (and the Sunshine Act) to be passed, facilitating the US Food and Drug Administration (FDA)'s release of summary-level data on drug submissions. Similarly, as Gagnon and colleagues write in chapter five, a strategic coalition of advocates were able to capitalize on the reforms to Canada's Food and Drugs Act in 2013 in order to push for greater clinical trial data transparency.

The fourth lesson is thus to be aware of the windows of opportunity that can facilitate the adoption of a policy direction that a government may have been resisting for some time. The ability to discern whether a window exists, and how best to capture it, is a critical talent, which is dissected in studies of policy entrepreneurship (for example, Baumgartner & Jones, 1993; Mintrom & Norman, 2009). Periods of political turbulence can be fertile ground for new policy formation. ("Never," quipped Obama's chief of staff, Rahm Emanuel, in 2008, "let a good crisis go to waste.") More problematic are instances where windows steadfastly refuse to open. Again, it is a matter of political judgement. As Davis, Mulinari, and Jefferson describe in chapter three, the transformation of the EMA from a laggard to a leader was not the product of a single event, but rather the cumulative result of steady political pressure exerted over a fairly lengthy period of time.

Politics

The final conclusion of this volume is perhaps the most obvious: the quest for greater transparency is not simply a matter of policy implementation; it is a battle for political dominance. From jostling for a line on the policy agenda, to framing what the problem actually is, to construction of what counts as evidence, and finally to development of a suitable solution, the policy realm, as Gagnon in chapter eight suggests, is an ideological battlefield. A corollary that follows is that highly political policy initiatives often *remain* highly political even when changes are implemented. Realization is followed by retrenchment.

The struggle for statutory change between MiEF and the organizations attempting to diminish regulatory standards (such as the European Federation of Pharmaceutical Industries and Associations, and the Pharmaceutical Research and Manufacturers of America), for example, is reflected both in the substantive changes to the regulatory landscape in the European Union and in structural shifts in the institutional framework of pharmaceutical regulation (including the transfer of jurisdiction over the EMA from the European Union's public health directorate, to its commerce and industry directorate, and back again to the health directorate). In 2019, the EU advocate general recommended that the

Court of Justice of the European Union (CJEU) find clinical trial data to be "presumptively confidential" when evaluating disclosure requests; in 2020, however, the CJEU unanimously rejected this position, ruling that clinical study reports did not contain confidential commercial information and were thus not covered by a general presumption of confidentiality.

Where to from Here?

Transparency in the pharmaceutical sphere is perhaps better understood as a process, or a site of policy contestation, rather than as a discrete end point. Contributors to this volume share a broad commitment to transparency, holding that improved access to clinical trial data for the purposes of independent scrutiny and, in turn, better decision-making (about which drugs to approve, prescribe, and consume) is, on balance, a good thing. But we also share a worry that transparency presents risks.

If data about the safety and efficacy of pharmaceuticals is made more transparent, whether to interested classes of researchers, health professionals, or the public more generally, it means little if too few take advantage of these data. Unless policy-makers, regulatory institutions, research funders, and others turn to the task of easing and supporting use of data, transparency can prove to be a pyrrhic victory. Worse, with time, transparency without use may work to erode the mission of pharmaceutical regulators by allowing regulators to offload the task of analysing the data, and deciding what to do, as the evidentiary profile of a given drug evolves.

This worry is what makes Banzi's contribution in chapter eleven to this volume so important and timely. What is needed now is a cultural change in the day-to-day practice of science and, even beyond what Banzi asks of researchers, corresponding changes in the institutional structures that support (and stand to benefit from) open pharmaceutical science and governance. Research funders must move beyond simple data sharing policies to policies that demand use of existing data or data that might be readily secured through new mechanisms such as Health Canada's public portal for clinical study reports. Organizations that sponsor systematic reviews must seize upon unpublished but now available data and build up the capacity of meta-researchers to locate and extract useful data from resources such as the FDA's Drugs@FDA.gov database. If a lifecycle approach to regulation is to be successful, then post-market active surveillance must be funded along with the big data systems for the ongoing analysis of safety and effectiveness throughout that lifecycle. And regulators must craft meaningful processes to allow outside researchers to fold new insights, derived from transparent data, into the regulatory decision-making process. Short of these cultural and institutional changes, any perceived gains in transparency in pharmaceutical governance may be both ephemeral and irrelevant.

REFERENCES

Baumgartner, F.R., & Jones, B.D. (1993). *Agendas and instability in American politics.* Chicago, IL: University of Chicago Press.

Béland, D. (2019). *How ideas and institutions shape the politics of public policy.* Cambridge, UK: Cambridge University Press.

Brooks, E. (2018). Using the Advocacy Coalition Framework to understand EU pharmaceutical policy. *European Journal of Public Health, 28*(S3), 11–14. https://doi.org/10.1093/eurpub/cky153

Cairney, P. (2016). *The politics of evidence-based policy making.* London, UK: Palgrave Macmillan.

Cairney, P., Heikkila, T., & Wood, M. (2019). *Making policy in a complex world.* Cambridge, UK: Cambridge University Press.

Campbell, J.L. (2004). *Institutional change and globalization.* Princeton, NJ: Princeton University Press.

Canadian Institute for Health Information (CIHI). (2018). *National health expenditure trends, 1975 to 2018.* Ottawa, ON: CIHI. Retrieved from https://secure.cihi.ca/free_products/NHEX-trends-narrative-report-2018-en-web.pdf

Coombes, R. (2019). European drug regulator fears return to days of data secrecy. *BMJ, 367,* l6133. https://doi.org/10.1136/bmj.l6133

Davis, C., Lexchin, J., Jefferson, T., Gøtzsche, P., & McKee, M. (2016). "Adaptive pathways" to drug authorization: Adapting to industry? *BMJ, 354,* i4437. https://doi.org/10.1136/bmj.i4437

Government of Canada. (2002). The Canada we want. Speech from the Throne to open the Second Session of the Thirty-Seventh Parliament of Canada, 30 September 2002. Retrieved from https://www.poltext.org/en/part-1-electronic-political-texts/canadian-throne-speeches

Graham, J.E. (2005). Smart regulation: Will the government's strategy work? *Canadian Medical Association Journal, 173*(12), 1469–70. https://doi.org/10.1503/cmaj.050424

Graham, J.E. (2019). Ebola vaccine innovation: A case study of pseudoscapes in global health. *Critical Public Health, 29*(4), 401–12. https://doi.org/10.1080/09581596.2019.1597966

Graham, J.E., & Jones, M. (2010). Rendre évident: Une approche symétrique de la réglementation des produits thérapeutiques [Determining evidence: A symmetrical approach to the regulation of therapeutic products]. *Sociologie et sociétés, 42*(2), 153–80. https://doi.org/10.7202/045360ar

Graham, J.E., & Nuttall, R. (2013). Faster access to new drugs: Fault lines between Health Canada's regulatory intent and industry innovation practices. *Ethics in Biology, Engineering & Medicine – An International Journal,* *4*(3), 231–9. https://doi.org/10.1615/EthicsBiologyEngMed.2014010771

Greer, S., Bekker, M.P.M., Azzopardi-Muscat, N., & McKee, M. (2018). Political analysis in public health: Middle-range concepts to make sense of the politics of health. *European Journal of Public Health, 28*(S3), 3–6. https://doi.org/10.1093/eurpub/cky159

Greer, S., Bekker, M., de Leeuw, E., Wismar, M., Helderman, J.-K., Ribeiro, S., & Stuckler, D. (2017). Policy, politics, and public health. *European Journal of Public Health, 27*(S4), 40–3. https://doi.org/10.1093/eurpub/ckx152

Habibi, R., & Lexchin, J. (2014). Quality and quantity of information in Summary Basis of Decision documents issued by Health Canada. *PLoS One, 9*(3), e92038. https://doi.org/10.1371/journal.pone.0092038

Health Canada. (2019). *Final report: Fees for drugs and medical devices.* Retrieved from https://www.canada.ca/en/health-canada/services/publications/drugs-health-products/fees-drugs-medical-devices.html

Herder, M., Graham, J.E., & Gold, R. (2020). From discovery to delivery: Public sector development of the rVSV-ZEBOV Ebola vaccine. *Journal of Law and the Biosciences,* Isz019. https://doi.org/10.1093/jlb/lsz019

Jarman, H. (2014). Public health and the Transatlantic Trade and Investment Partnership. *European Journal of Public Health, 24*(2), 181. https://doi.org/10.1093/eurpub/ckt201

Jenkins-Smith, H., & Sabatier, P., (Eds.). (1993). *Policy change and learning: An advocacy coalition approach.* Boulder, CO: Westview Press.

Löblová, O. (2018). Epistemic communities and experts in health policy-making. *European Journal of Public Health, 28*(S2), 7–10. https://doi.org/10.1093/eurpub/cky156

Mintrom, M., & Norman, P. (2009). Policy entrepreneurship and policy change. *Policy Studies Journal, 37*(4), 649–67. https://doi.org/10.1111/j.1541-0072.2009.00329.x

Permanand, G., & Mossialos, E. (2005). Constitutional asymmetry and pharmaceutical policy-making in the European Union. *Journal of European Public Policy, 12*(4), 687–709. https://doi.org/10.1080/13501760500160607

Sabatier, P.A. (1988). An advocacy coalition framework of policy change and the role of policy-oriented learning therein. *Policy Sciences, 21*(2/3), 129–68. https://doi.org/10.1007/BF00136406

Scharpf, F.W. (2010). The asymmetry of European integration, or why the EU cannot be a "social market" economy. *Socio-Economic Review, 8*(2), 211–50. https://doi.org/10.1093/ser/mwp031

Smith, K.E. (2014). The politics of ideas: The complex interplay of health inequalities research and policy. *Science and Public Policy, 41*(5), 561–74. https://doi.org/10.1093/scipol/sct085

Tuohy, C.H. (2018). *Remaking policy: Scale, pace, and political strategy in health care reform.* Toronto, ON: University of Toronto Press.

Vandergrift, M., & Kanavos, P. (1997). Health policy versus industrial policy in the pharmaceutical sector: The case of Canada. *Health Policy, 41*(3), 241–60. https://doi.org/10.1016/s0168-8510(97)00036-5

Weiss, J.A. (1989). The powers of problem definition. *Policy Science, 22,* 97–121. https://doi.org/10.1007/BF00141381

Contributors

Rita Banzi is a senior researcher, head of the Centre for Health Regulatory Policies at the Mario Negri Institute in Milan, Italy. Her research focuses primarily on drug regulatory policies, clinical studies, evidence synthesis methodology, and transparency in research. She collaborates with the European Clinical Research Infrastructure Network (ECRIN) and the Clinical Research Initiative for Global Health (CRIGH), and teaches in postgraduate training programs at the University of Milan.

Anna Danyliuk is a policy and program analyst at the Policy Innovation Hub in Cabinet Office within the Ontario Public Service.

Courtney Davis is a reader in the Department of Global Health and Social Medicine at King's College London, UK. Her research focuses on the intersections of science and technology policy, business regulation, and public health. She engages in empirically based, international comparative research investigating the sociopolitical, economic, cultural, and scientific factors underlying trends in regulation.

Katherine Fierlbeck is the McCulloch Professor of Political Science at Dalhousie University, with a cross-appointment as a professor of community health and epidemiology. She is the director of the Jean Monnet Network for Health Law and Politics. Fierlbeck focuses on the politics of health policy, with a particular interest in systems of governance and mechanisms of accountability.

Marc-André Gagnon is an associate professor at the School of Public Policy and Administration at Carleton University in Ottawa, Ontario. His research focuses on the political economy of the pharmaceutical sector, including business models, innovation policies, corporate influence over medical practices, and health and drug insurance regimes. He is a research fellow with the WHO Collaborating Centre for Governance, Transparency, and Accountability in the Pharmaceutical Sector.

Kanksha Mahadevia Ghimire is a legal practitioner and has worked in multiple countries. She has worked in premier law firms in India, the World Bank's Legal Vice Presidency, the United States, and the United Nations Office for Disaster Risk Reduction, Thailand, and has headed the legal team of a statutory regulator in Vanuatu. She is an adjunct faculty at the School of Law, University of the South Pacific, Vanuatu. She is a doctoral candidate at the Faculty of Law, University of Toronto. Her research explores mechanisms to improve regulation and governance.

Janice Graham is a medical anthropologist, professor of pediatrics (infectious diseases), university research professor, and director of the Technoscience and Regulation Research Unit at Dalhousie University. Graham studies the construction and legitimation of evidence for safety, efficacy, and trust in emerging therapeutics and vaccines in Canada, Europe, and Africa. She is interested in open data, regulation, public health, emergency response, and how public innovations are privatized.

Matthew Herder is the director of the Health Law Institute in the Schulich School of Law and an associate professor in the Department of Pharmacology in the Faculty of Medicine at Dalhousie University in Halifax, Nova Scotia. Herder's research focuses on biomedical innovation policy, with a particular emphasis on intellectual property rights and the regulation of biopharmaceutical interventions. He was appointed by federal cabinet as a member of the Patented Medicine Prices Review Board, Canada's national drug price regulator, in 2018, and became a member of the Royal Society of Canada's College of New Scholars, Artists and Scientists in 2019.

Tom Jefferson is a physician, researcher, and campaigner for access to randomized controlled trial data as well as Senior Associate Tutor in the Department of Continuing Education at the University of Oxford. He co-authored the Cochrane review solely based on regulatory data of neuraminidase inhibitors for preventing and treating influenza. This landmark study was added to the James Lind Library. He has finalized his suite of long-standing Cochrane influenza vaccine reviews and is currently working for the Oxford University Centre for Evidence-Based Medicine COVID-19 Evidence Service.

Trudo Lemmens is Professor and Scholl Chair in Health Law and Policy at the Faculty of Law of the University of Toronto, with cross-appointments in the Dalla Lana School of Public Health. His research focuses on the interaction of law, governance tools, and ethical norms and values in the context of health care, biomedical research, health product development, and knowledge production. He has been consulted by various national and international organizations, including the World Health Organization, and is currently a member of the Advisory Committee on Health Research of the Pan American Health Organization. He is also an associate member of the WHO Collaborating Centre for Governance, Transparency, and Accountability in the Pharmaceutical Sector.

Joel Lexchin is a professor emeritus in the School of Health Policy and Management at York University and an associate professor in the Faculty of Medicine at the University of Toronto, as well as an emergency physician at the University Health Network. His research and publications centre on pharmaceutical policy, drug regulation and promotion, pharmacosurveillance, research and development, as well as access to medications in developing countries. He is the author of four books on the pharmaceutical industry as well as the author or co-author of over 200 peer-reviewed articles. He is a fellow of the Canadian Academy of Health Sciences.

Margaret E. McCarthy is a public defender at Brooklyn Defender Services. She was previously the executive director of the Collaboration for Research Integrity and Transparency (CRIT) at Yale Law School, where her work focused on transparency and integrity in medical product regulation.

Shai Mulinari is an associate professor and senior lecturer at the Department of Sociology at Lund University in Lund, Sweden. He holds a PhD in medical sciences from Lund University. He undertakes research on pharmaceutical use and regulation, health and health-care inequalities, and pharmaceutical industry practices, regulation, and transparency.

Nav Persaud is the Canada Research Chair in Health Justice, associate professor in the University of Toronto's Department of Family and Community Medicine, and a staff physician at St. Michael's Hospital in Unity Health Toronto. He has led re-analyses of published clinical trials of a commonly used medication and a comparison of essential medicines used globally. He has also led several clinical trials.

Joseph S. Ross is a professor of medicine and of public health, a member of the Center for Outcomes Research and Evaluation (CORE) at the Yale-New Haven Hospital, and a co-director of the National Clinician Scholars program (NCSP) at Yale University. His research explores the use and delivery of higher quality care, pharmaceutical and medical device regulation, evidence development, post-market surveillance, and clinical adoption. He co-directs the Yale-Mayo Clinic Center for Excellence in Regulatory Science and Innovation (CERSI), the Yale Open Data Access (YODA) Project, and the Collaboration for Research Integrity and Transparency (CRIT) at Yale Law School.

Index

Figures and tables are indicated by page numbers in italics.

AbbVie, 80, 169
Abraham, J., 151
academic research, 82, 170, 244–5, 246–7, 249, 254–5
accelerated approval, 144
access, open, 252–4
access to information: Access to Information Act (ATIA; Canada, 1982), 100, 101–2, 108, 152, 267; clinical data and, 28–9, 64–5; Food and Drug Administration and, 29, 98–9, *99*, *100*, 100–1, 108–9; Freedom of Information Act (FOIA; US, 1966), 9, 97–9, 108–9, 267, 272; Health Canada and, *100*, 100–2, 103; Vanessa's Law (Protecting Canadians from Unsafe Drugs Act, 2014) and, 102–3
accountability, 7, 13–15, 52, 262
Acomplia (rimonabant), 69, 70
acquisitions and mergers, 172
adalimumab (Humira), 169
Addyi, 32
adjuvants, 225–7, 232, 238
ADM, 172
administrative and procedural oversight, *18*, 29–30

Adulteration Act (Canada, 1884), 96, 115
Adverse Event Reporting System (FAERS), 27–8
adverse events, 4, 25, 27–8, 29, 104, 108. *See also* Pandemrix
advertising, direct-to-consumer (DTCA), 150–1, 176. *See also* drug promotion
Advisory Committee Act (US, 1972), 98
advocacy and advocacy coalition framework, 268–9. *See also* patient (advocacy) organizations
Affordable Care Act (ACA; US, 2010), 31, 37, 38, 133
agenda-setting, 270
albuterol, 41
Alcabes, P., 234
Alexion Pharmaceuticals, 163
AllTrials campaign, 73, 74, 77, 197
Alves, Teresa, 75
American College of Cardiology, 35
American Heart Association, 35
American Medical Student Association (AMSA), 39, 40
American Society of Health-System Pharmacists, 44

antidepressants, 63–4, 129, 130,
    165–6, 244
anti-obesity drugs, 69–70
AO Spine North America, 141
Apotex, 167
approval. *See* drug approval
Arepanrix, 232–3, *235*, 236
Arlett, Peter, 236–7
Association of Medical Advertising
    Agencies, 149
Association of the British
    Pharmaceutical Industry (ABPI), 39
Aucoin, P., 14–15
Auditor General, of Canada, 140, 147
Austin, L.M., 201–2
Australia, 27, 33, 51, 186
Austria, 43
Avandia (rosiglitazone), 63–4, 167
Azzopardi-Muscat, N., 266

Baird, P.: *Report of the Committee of
    Inquiry on the Case Involving Dr.
    Nancy Olivieri* (with Thompson and
    Downie), 167
Baltic Partnership Agreement, 43
Bambauer, D.E., 194
Barbateskovic, M., 34
Barbour, Virginia, 75
Baron, R.B., 39
Baselga, José, 35
Bayer, 191
Bekker, M.P.M., 266
Belgium, 43
Bell, Leonard, 163
Beneluxa, 43
Bentham, Jeremy, 13
Bertele', V., 250
Bertolini, Guido, 251
Bill & Melinda Gates Foundation, 253
Bill C-17. *See* Vanessa's Law
    (Protecting Canadians from
    Unsafe Drugs Act, 2014)

Bill C-51 (Proposed Amendments to
    the Food and Drugs Act), 118
Bill C-52 (Proposed Consumer
    Product Safety Act), 118
biobanks, 199, 201
BioIndustry Association (BIA), 76
Biologics and Genetic Therapies
    Directorate (Canada), 119, 153
BIOTECanada, 150
Birkinshaw, P.J., 16
Blumenthal, Richard, 170
BMJ (formerly *British Medical
    Journal*), 40, 71–2, 73–4, 196
bounded rationality, 270
breakthrough therapies, 189, 190
Brigham and Women's Hospital: Multi-
    Regional Clinical Trials Center, 197
Bristol Myers Squibb, 33, 169
Bruser, D., 141
Bureau of Chemistry (US), 95–6

Cain, D.M., 52
California, 42
campaign financing, *19*, 30–1
Canada: approach to, 9; clinical trial
    registration and, 118–19; clinical
    trials database, 26; Constitution Act
    on health care, 115; drug spending
    in, 133; lobbying, 31–2; neoliberal
    relationship with industry, 151–2;
    open access and, 253; patient
    (advocacy) organizations, 33, 175;
    payments from industry to health-
    care providers, 39; pharmaceutical
    regulation historical background,
    95, 96, 97, 115–18, 119–20;
    structures, institutions, and
    transparency, 267; transparency
    overview, 263–5; Vigilance Adverse
    Reaction online database, 28. *See
    also* Health Canada; Health Canada,
    communications; Vanessa's Law

Canada–United States Free Trade
  Agreement (1987), 267
Canadian Agency for Drugs and
  Technologies in Health (CADTH),
  29
Canadian Association of Journalists,
  117, 153–4, 264
Canadian Association of Medical
  Publishers, 149–50
Canadian Blood Committee, 101
Canadian Broadcasting Corporation
  (CBC), 117
Canadian Generic Pharmaceutical
  Association, 150
Canadian Institutes of Health
  Research (CIHR), 118, 119, 193, 253
Canadian Medical Association Journal
  (CMAJ), 37
Canadian Network for Observational
  Drug Effect Studies (CNODES), 6
Canadian Proprietary Medicine Act
  (1908), 96
Canadian Science Advisory Board,
  263
capital accumulation, 162–4, 176
capture: about, 165; civil society
  capture, 174–5, 177; market
  capture, 171–3; media capture,
  173–4; professional capture, 167–8,
  176–7; regulatory capture, 170–1,
  177; scientific capture, 165–7, 176;
  technological capture, 168–70
career promotion, 254–5
Carpenter, D., 52, 165, 170
cartels, 172
cataplexy, 232
C.D. Howe Institute, 44
Center for Drug Evaluation and
  Research, 29
Center for Responsive Politics, 171
Centers for Disease Control and
  Prevention (CDC), 36

Centers for Medicare and Medicaid
  Services (CMS), 37–8
Central Eastern European and South
  Eastern Countries Initiative, 43
Chalmers, Iain, 71–2
Chandler, Alfred D., 168–9
Chirac, Pierre, 75
choice, construction of, 51
cholesterol, 36
cisapride (Prepulsid), 102, 120
Citizens United v. FEC (2010), 171
civil society capture, 174–5, 177
clientele pluralism, 116–17
clinical case report form (CRF), 22,
  23, 24, 25, 29
clinical guidelines, 35–7, 131, 132
ClinicalStudyDataRequest.com, 195
clinical study report (CSR), 24, 24–5,
  64
clinical trial data, 22–9; from
  academic research, 246–7,
  249; access issues, 28–9, 64–5;
  on adverse events, 25, 27–8,
  29; Australia, transparency in,
  51; civil society advocacy for
  transparency in EU, 67–8, 77–8,
  80, 219–20; clinical trial registries
  and, 25–6; components of,
  22–5, 23–4; Court of Justice of the
  European Union on, 28, 66, 80,
  273; European Medicines Agency
  and transparency, 7, 26–7, 28,
  65, 66–7, 68–71, 74–5, 80–1, 104,
  125, 146, 184, 196–7, 219–20, 272;
  Food and Drug Administration
  and transparency, 27, 65, 71;
  Health Canada and transparency,
  27, 28, 108, 114, 123–4, 124–5,
  152–3, 197–8; industry pushback
  against European Medicines
  Agency regulations, 78–80; for
  non-approved or withdrawn

pharmaceuticals, *17*, 27, 83n1, 108; privacy concerns, 184; problems from lack of transparency, 63–4; selective production of ignorance and, 166, 176; transparency and, 16, *17*, 26–7, 185, 246; transparency concerns and limitations, 80–3; value of data sharing, 249–52; Vanessa's Law and transparency, 27, 28, 102–3, 114, 121–3, 124, 197–8. *See also* privacy, and rare diseases

clinical trials: EU regulations, 75–7; importance of, 246; inspections of, 140–1; monitoring compliance, 244–5; Phase IV studies, 141–2; for rare diseases, 186, 188; registries, 6, 25–6, 118–19, 243–4

ClinicalTrials.gov, 26, 27, 119, 176, 197

Coca-Cola, 51

Cochrane Acute Respiratory Infections Group, 72–3, 82, 219–20

Cochrane Collaboration, 71–2, 73, 80, 196

collaboration: among researchers, 248, 250–1; industry agreements for, 172–3

commercialization, 252, 255–6

Committee for Medicinal Products for Human Use (CHMP), 66

communications. *See* Health Canada, communications

Confessore, N., 174

confidence, in government and medical profession, 133

confidential commercial (business) information: about, 4; Court of Justice of the European Union on, 28, 66, 80, 273; Food and Drug Administration and, 99; Health Canada and, 107, 123, 145, 152; structures, institutions, and

transparency, 267; terms of use agreements and, 204; Vanessa's Law and, 102–3, 121

conflicts of interest, 30–41; campaign financing, *19*, 30–1; definition, 30; drawbacks of transparency, 52; in drug promotion, 5–6; health media, 40–1; institutional membership, *20*, 35–7; journals, *19*, 33–5; lobbying, *19*, 31–2; medical education, *20*, 39–40; patient advocacy organizations, *19*, 32–3; payments to health-care providers, *20*, 37–9; professional conflicts of interest, 33; representational conflicts of interest, 30–3; transparency and, 16, *19–20*, 22

consent: dynamic consent, 200; informed consent, 198–202, 205

Consolidated Standards of Reporting Trials (CONSORT) group, 22

Constitution Act (Canada, 1982), 115

Consumer Health Products Canada, 150

consumers, 41–2, 51, 52, 147

Cooper, R., 34–5

CORBEL project, 197, 248–9

Cornyn, John, 170

Cosgrove, L., 36

Council of Canadian Academies Expert Panel, 193–4

Court of Justice of the European Union (CJEU), 28, 66, 80, 273

COVID-19 pandemic, 12, 219. *See also* H1N1 influenza pandemic and vaccine

cox-2 inhibitors, 63, 117

Crohn's and Colitis Canada, 33

dark money, 31

data. *See* clinical trial data

data sets, *23*, 24
data sharing websites, 27
Davis, C., 151
decision-making: contextual influences, 261–2; risk-based, 140; transparency, 65–6, 103, 108, 142–3
Declaration of Helsinki, 119, 196, 207n17
deferiprone, 167
Denmark, 38
Department of Health (Canada), 115
Department of Health and Human Services (US), 42
Department of Health and Welfare (Canada): Food and Drugs Division, 116. *See also* Health Protection Branch (Canada)
Diagnostic and Statistical Manual of Mental Disorders (DSM)-IV, 35–6
Diclectin, 28, 122
Dinan, W., 173
direct-to-consumer advertising (DTCA), 150–1, 176. *See also* drug promotion
"Dollars for Docs" (website), 38
Doshi, Peter, 25, 75, 80, 82, 122, 146, 197, 233
Doshi v. Attorney General of Canada (2018), 28, 103, 114, 122–3, 124, 197
Downie, J.: *Report of the Committee of Inquiry on the Case Involving Dr. Nancy Olivieri* (with Thompson and Baird), 167
doxylamine-pyridoxine, 129, 130–1
Dror, Y., 52
drug approval, 142–6; Notice of Compliance with conditions (NOC/c) and, 144; orphan drugs, 190; priority reviews, 143–4, 265; Summary Basis of Decision (SBD), 103, 117, 118, 142–3, 265;

Vanessa's Law and Health Canada's communication reforms, 144–6
drug licensing, 5, 81, 118
drug manufacturing facilities, inspections of, 147–8
drug prices, 6, *20–1*, 41–3, 172
drug promotion, 148–51; conflicts of interest in, 5–6; direct-to-consumer advertising, 150–1, 176; Innovative Medicines Canada and, 150; lack of regulatory oversight by Health Canada, 148–9; Pharmaceutical Advertising Advisory Board and, 30, 149–50; spending on, 167, 173, 176
drug safety, 146–8; communicating safety issues, 147; inspections of drug manufacturing facilities, 147–8; safety warnings, 146
Drug Shortage Program (DSP), 43–4
drug supply, *21*, 43–5
Dryad Digital Repository, 197
dynamic consent, 200

Economist, 172
education, medical, *20*, 39–40
Eisenberg, R.S., 170
El Emam, K., 80
electric common technical document (eCTD) format, 103, 104
Electronic Freedom of Information Act Amendments (US, 1996), 99
Emanuel, Rahm, 272
Energy East pipeline project, 159–60
EpiPens, 41
essential medicines lists, 134–6
EudraVigilance, 6, 27, 29
European Clinical Research Infrastructure Network (ECRIN), 196, 247–8
European Commission, 7, 67–8, 75–6, 79, 253. *See also* European Union

European Consumer Organisation
   (BEUC), 68
European Economic Area (EEA), 27
European Economic Community, 268
European Federation of
   Pharmaceutical Industries and
   Associations (EFPIA), 39, 78, 196,
   272
European Integrated Price
   Information Database (EURIPID), 6
European Medicines Agency (EMA):
   approach to, 8; clinical data for
   non-approved or withdrawn
   pharmaceuticals, 27, 83n1, 108;
   clinical data transparency and, 7,
   26–7, 28, 65, 66–7, 68–71, 74–5,
   80–1, 104, 125, 146, 184, 196–7,
   219–20, 272; decision-making
   process, access to, 65–6; drug
   supply and, 45; guidelines for
   adjuvants, 225–7; guidelines for
   influenza pandemic vaccines,
   222–3, 223, 224, 237–8; H1N1
   influenza vaccine and, 233, 236–7;
   industry pushback on transparency
   regulations, 78–80; jurisdiction
   over, 272; privacy concerns and,
   184; terms of use agreements and,
   203–4
European Network for Health
   Technology Assessment
   (EUnetHTA), 29
European Network of Centres for
   Pharmacoepidemiology and
   Pharmacovigilance (ENCePP), 6
European Open Science Cloud, 197
European Open Science Policy
   Platform, 253
European public assessment reports
   (EPARs), 66
European Public Health Alliance
   (EPHA), 68

European Union: approach to and
   conclusion, 8, 67, 82–3, 265; civil
   society advocacy for transparency,
   67–8, 77–8, 80, 268–9; clinical
   trial registries, 26; Clinical Trials
   Regulation, 75–7; drug pricing, 43;
   drug supply, 45; payments from
   industry to health-care providers,
   38–9; publication bias and
   "missing data" issues in journals,
   71–4; rare diseases, 186; structures,
   institutions, and transparency,
   266–7, 268. See also European
   Medicines Agency (EMA)
European Vaccine Manufacturers
   (EVM), 233
evidence, scientific, 3–4, 13
evidence-based policy-making, 270
expedited reviews: accelerated
   approval, 144; breakthrough
   therapies, 189, 190; fast-tracked
   reviews, 189, 190, 222; priority
   reviews, 143–4, 265; transparency
   and, 30

FAIR (Findable, Accessible,
   Interoperable, and Reusable) data,
   257
Fanon, Franz, 47
fast-tracked reviews, 189, 190, 222
FDA Safety and Innovation Act (US,
   2012), 44
Federal Election Commission (US), 30
Federal Trade Commission (US), 170
Figshare, 197
Figueras, J., 52
Finnish Medicines Agency (FIMEA), 81
Fluarix, 232
Focetria, 227
FOIA Improvement Act (US, 2016),
   99
FollowTheMoney.org, 30, 31

Food, Drug, and Cosmetic Act (US, 1938), 8, 96–7
Food and Drug Administration (FDA): access to information and, 29, 98–9, *99, 100,* 100–1, 108–9; Adverse Event Reporting System (FAERS), 27–8; clinical data for non-approved or withdrawn pharmaceuticals, 27, 83n1, 108; clinical data transparency and, 27, 65, 71; clinical trial registries and, 26; communications on clinical trial inspections, 140–1; comparison to Health Canada, 107–9; corporate influence on, 5; decision-making process, access to, 65, 103; Drug Shortage Program (DSP), 43–4; information requirements from industry, 103–4, 108; inspections of drug manufacturing facilities, 147–8; on orphan drugs, 189; pharmaceutical regulation historical background, 4–5, 95–7; on Prepulsid (cisapride), 120; transparency initiatives, 104, *105–6,* 106–7
Food and Drug Administration Amendments Act ((FDAAA) US, 2007), 72, 103, 197
Food and Drug Administration Modernization Act (US, 1997), 243
Food and Drugs Act (Canada, 1920), 96, 102, 115–16, 118, 148, 272
framing, 271
France, 38, 39
Franzosi, Maria Grazia, 250
Fraser Institute, 174
Freedom of Information Act (FOIA; US, 1966), 9, 97–9, 108–9, 267, 272

gabapentin, 63–4
Garattini, Silvio, 68, 256

Genentech, 175
genomic research, 187
Genomics England, 188
ghost-management: approach to, 10–11, 161, 271; capital accumulation and, 162–4, 176; civil society capture, 174–5, 177; market capture, 171–3; media capture, 173–4; pervasiveness of, 175–6; professional capture, 167–8, 176–7; regulatory capture, 170–1, 177; scientific capture, 165–7, 176; of social determinants of value, 160, 164–75; technological capture, 168–70; TransCanada Corporation's Energy East pipeline example, 159–60; transparency and, 176–7
ghostwriting, 165–6
GlaxoSmithKline, 166, 167, 175, 195, 220, 244. *See also* Pandemrix
Global Energy Balance Network, 51
Global South, 152
Godlee, Fiona, 75
Goldacre, Ben, 73, 74, 75, 77
Good Manufacturing Practices (GMP), 147
Gøtzsche, Peter, 34, 70, 75
Government in the Sunshine Act (US, 1976), 98, 272
Graham, Janice, 264
Greer, S.L., 52, 265, 266
Grundy, Q., 51
Gruppo Italiano per la Valutazione degli Interventi in Terapia Intensiva (GiViTI) network, 251–2
Gruppo Italiano per lo Studio della Sopravvivenza nell'Infarto Miocardico (GISSI) trials, 249–50, 252
guidelines, clinical, 35–7, 131, 132
guidelines, reporting, 247

Guidelines International Network
  (GIN), 37
Gupta, M., 34–5

H1N1 influenza pandemic and
  vaccine: adjuvants and, 225–7;
  adverse events from Pandemrix,
  232–3, *235*, 235–6, 238n1;
  approach to and conclusion,
  11–12, 219–21, 237–8; changes in
  registration process for vaccines
  and, 237–8; European Medicines
  Agency's guidelines for vaccines
  and, 222–3, *223*, 224; "impending
  doom scenario" and data-free
  registration, 220, 233; influenza
  pandemic narrative and, 221–2,
  271; Pandemrix roll out, 232;
  Pandemrix testing program,
  227, *228–31*, 232; problems from
  rushed development and lack of
  transparency, 234–7
H5N1 influenza, 219, 221, 234
Habibi, R., 51
Haivas, I., 35
Hansson, M.G., 199
Harkins, C., 164, 173–4
Hartzog, W., 194
Harvard University: Multi-Regional
  Clinical Trials Center, 197
Hayashi, Keiji, 73
Heads of Medicines Agencies
  (HMA), 45
Health Action International (HAI),
  68, 77, 269
Health Canada: access to information
  and, *100*, 100–2, 103; approach to,
  114–15; clientele pluralism and,
  116–17; clinical data transparency
  and, 27, 28, 108, 114, 123–4,
  124–5, 152–3, 197–8; commercial
  promotion of pharmaceuticals

and, 30; comparison to Food
  and Drug Agency, 107–9; drug
  pricing and, 43; drug supply
  and, 44; lobbying and, 32;
  neoliberal relationship with
  industry, 151–2; pharmaceutical
  regulation historical background,
  95, 96, 97, 115–18, 119–20; policy
  revision process and, 125; on
  Prepulsid (cisapride), 120; on
  rare diseases, 186; resource issues,
  263; terms of use agreements
  and, 203; thalidomide and, 116;
  transparency initiatives and issues,
  103, 107–8, 117–18, 184; user
  fees and, 263; Vanessa's Law and,
  102–3, 121–3
Health Canada, communications:
  approach to and conclusion,
  10, 139, 153–4, 270; clinical
  data and, 145–6, 152–3; clinical
  trial inspections and, 140–1;
  conduct of clinical trials and,
  140–2; confidential commercial
  (business) information and, 152;
  direct-to-consumer advertising
  and, 150–1; discomfort with
  transparency, 153; drug approvals
  and, 142–6; drug promotion
  and, 148–51; drug safety
  and, 146–8; explanations for
  communication style, 151–3;
  Innovative Medicines Canada
  and, 150; inspections of drug
  manufacturing facilities and,
  147–8; neoliberal relationship
  with industry and, 151–2;
  Notice of Compliance with
  conditions (NOC/c) and, 144;
  personnel and resource issues,
  153; Pharmaceutical Advertising
  Advisory Board (PAAB) and,

149–50; Phase IV studies and, 141–2; priority reviews and, 143–4; Public Advisories and Warnings, 147; Summary Basis of Decision (SBD) and, 142–3; Vanessa's Law and, 144–5

health-care providers, payments to, *20*, 37–9, 133, 167–8, 176, 177

health media, 40–1, 173–4

Health Products and Food Branch (Canada), 117, 264

Health Protection Branch (Canada), 116, 117, 264

Health Sector Payment Transparency Act (Canada, 2019), 39

health technology assessment (HTA), 29

health technology assessment (HTA) agencies, 6

Healy, David, 237

Heintzman, R., 14–15

Heller, M.A., 170

Heneghan, Carl, 75

hepatitis C, 36, 101

Herder, Matthew, 96, 146, 204

hidden power, 46–7

Hobbes, Thomas, 46

Hoffman, J.R., 34–5

Hoffmann-La Roche, 175

hormone replacement therapy, 166

Hospital for Sick Children (Toronto), Motherisk Program, 130

Hróbjartsson, A., 34

human papilloma virus (HPV) vaccines, 81, 122

human research participants, 184, 185, 189, 192–3. *See also* privacy, and rare diseases

Humira (adalimumab), 169

Huntington disease, 188, 200

ignorance, selective production of, 166, 176

IMPACT Observatory, 197

independent researchers, 166–7

independent review panels, 202–3, 205–6

Industry Practices Review Committee (IPRC), 150

influence, political economy of, 161. *See also* ghost-management; politics; power

influenza pandemics: European Medicines Agency's guidelines for vaccines, 222–3, *223*, 224; narrative of, 221–2, 271; registration process for vaccines, 237–8. *See also* H1N1 influenza pandemic and vaccine

informed consent, 198–202, 205

Inland Revenue Act (Canada, 1874), 115

Innovative Medicines Canada (IMC), 32, 150, 264

Innovative Medicines Initiative, 256

inspection reports, 141, 142, 148

Institute of Medicine, 36, 39, 202

institutional membership, *20*, 35–7

institutions and structures, 266–8

intangible assets, 163, 164–5. *See also* ghost-management

intellectual property rights, 152, 169–70, 255, 267. *See also* confidential commercial (business) information; open access; patents

InterMune, 80

International Clinical Trials Registry Platform (ICTRP), 26, 119

International Committee of Medical Journal Editors (ICMJE), 26, 33, 119, 196

International Committee on Harmonization (ICH), 103

International Society of Drug
  Bulletins (ISDB), 68
Intervet International, 80
invisible power, 47
Ioannidis, J.P.A., 36
Ireland, 43
ISRCTN registry, 26
Italy, 249–50, 251, 252, 253, 255

James Lind Initiative, 73
Janssen Pharmaceutical, 120
Japan, 186
Jefferson, A.A., 36
Jefferson, Tom, 25, 75, 79, 80, 81, 82
*Journal of the American Medical
  Association (JAMA)*, 5
journalism, 174. *See also* media
journals: articles and clinical trial
  data, *24*, 25; conflicts of interest
  and, *19*, 33–5; ghostwriting, 165–6;
  open access, 253; publication bias
  and "missing data" issues, 71–4,
  219–20; transparency initiatives,
  26, 196

Kaiser Health News, 33
Kanter, G., 52
Kefauver amendments (US, 1962),
  9, 97
Kelsey, Frances Oldham, 4, 97
Know the Lowest Price Act (US,
  2018), 42
Krimsky, S., 36
Krleža-Jerić, K., 202

Landefeld, C.S., 39
Lane, Síle, 77
Lehmann, L.S., 52
Lemmens, Trudo, 201–2, 204
Lexchin, Joel, 29, 146, 194; *Private
  Profits vs Public Policy*, 151
Liberati, Alessandro, 245

licensing, drug, 5, 81, 118
Lipworth, W., 51
lobbying, *19*, 31–2, 171, 174, 176
Löblová, O., 268
Loewenstein, G., 52
Lönngren, Thomas, 69, 70
Lundh, A., 34
Luxembourg, 43
lysine, 172

Mario Negri Institute: approach
  to, 12, 243; clinical trial registry,
  244; collaborative and public-
  oriented research values, 245,
  248, 252; commercialization
  concerns and, 256; *Gruppo Italiano
  per lo Studio della Sopravvivenza
  nell'Infarto Miocardico* (GISSI) trials,
  249–50
market capture, 171–3
Marketed Health Products
  Directorate (Canada), 119, 146,
  149, 153, 263
Mauss, Marcel, 251
Mayes, C., 51
McKee, C., 52
McKee, M., 266
McLean, J., 141
MCM Research, 174
media, 40–1, 173–4
Mediator, 72
medical education, *20*, 39–40
medical education and
  communication companies
  (MECCs), 39
Medicine Evaluations Board (MEB),
  81
Medicines & Healthcare products
  Regulatory Agency (MHRA), 81
Medicines in Europe Forum (MiEF),
  67–8, 77, 268–9, 272
Meijer, A., 16

Mello, M.M., 52
Merck, 14, 166–7
mergers and acquisitions, 172
Merton, R.K., 252
Michols, Dann, 117
Miller, D., 164, 173–4
Mintzes, Barbara, 75
Moss, D.A., 165, 170
Motherisk Program, 130
MSD Animal Health Innovation, 80
Multi-Regional Clinical Trials Center, 197
muraglitazar, 63–4
myocardial infarction, 249–50

Naclerio, Nicholas, 170
narcolepsy, 220, 232–3, 234, 238n1
National Press Foundation, 40
National Vaccine Advisory Committee (NVAC): *Dose Optimization Strategies for Vaccines: The Role of Adjuvants and New Technologies*, 225
Natural Sciences and Engineering Research Council of Canada, 253
Nelson, G.S., 193
neoliberalism, 151–2
Netherlands, 39, 43, 81
neuraminidase inhibitors (NIs), 72–3, 80
Nevada, 42
New England Journal of Medicine (*NEJM*), 34
New York Times, 5, 35
"No Forced Switch" campaign, 33
non-approved pharmaceuticals, *17*, 27, 83n1, 108
Nordic Cochrane Collaboration, 70–1, 219, 269
Nordic Pharmaceutical Forum, 43
Nordic Trial Alliance, 196

Notice of Compliance with conditions (NOC/c), 144
Novartis, 175, 227

Obama, Barak, 52
Office of Consumer and Public Involvement (Canada), 114
Olivieri, Nancy, 167
Ontario, 33, 39
Ontario Medical Association, 43
open access, 170, 252–4
Open Government Act (US, 2007), 99
openness, and public-oriented research, 245–6
OpenPrescribing.net, 136
OpenSecrets.org, 30–1
opioids, 36, 129, 131
Oregon, 42
orphan drugs, 189–91
oseltamivir (Tamiflu), 63–4, 71, 73, 80, 81, 122, 129, 130
Ottawa Statement, 118–19, 196
Oxford Centre for Evidence-Based Medicine, 71–2, 73

pan-Canadian Pharmaceutical Alliance, 43
Pandemrix: adjuvants and, 226, *226*; adverse events from, 232–3, *235*, 235–6, 238n1; approach to and conclusion, 11–12, 221, 237–8; "impending doom scenario" and data-free registration, 220, 233; problems from rushed development and lack of transparency, 234–7; roll out, 232; testing program, 227, *228–31*, 232. *See also* H1N1 influenza pandemic and vaccine
PARI Pharma, 80
paroxetine (Paxil), 130, 166, 244
Partnership to Fight Chronic Disease, 31

Passarani, Ilaria, 75
patents, 115, 163, 168, 169–70, 255
patient (advocacy) organizations, *19*,
    32–3, 175, 176. *See also* advocacy
    and advocacy coalition framework
Patient Right to Know Drug Prices
    Act (US, 2018), 42
Paxil (paroxetine), 130, 166, 244
payments, to health-care providers,
    20, 37–9, 133, 167–8, 176, 177
Pearson, S.D., 36
periodic safety update reports
    (PSURs), 69
Persaud, Nav, 122, 153
Pfizer, 14, 163–4, 165–6, 174
Pharmaceutical Advertising Advisory
    Board (PAAB), 30, 149–50
pharmaceutical industry: benefits
    from data transparency, 82;
    campaign financing and, 30–1;
    capital accumulation, 163–4,
    176; ghost-management by, 161,
    164–77; influence on regulatory
    agencies, 5; information
    requirements from FDA and
    Health Canada, 103–4, 108;
    lobbying and, 31–2, 171, 174, 176;
    medical education sponsorship
    and payments, 39–40; neoliberal
    relationships with government,
    151–2; patient organizations
    and, 32–3, 175, 176; payments
    to health-care providers, 37–9,
    133, 167–8, 176, 177; pushback
    against European Medicines
    Agency's transparency regulations,
    78–80; transparency policies and
    initiatives, 191, 195–6
pharmaceutical regulations: access
    to information and, 64–5;
    accountability vs. transparency,
    7, 14–15, 52, 262; in Canada, 95,
96, 97, 115–18, 119–20; corporate
    influence on regulators, 5;
    critiques of, 5–6, 263; process
    of, 3–4, 125; role of, 262–3;
    transparency and, 139; in US, 4–5,
    95–7. *See also* European Medicines
    Agency (EMA); Food and Drug
    Administration (FDA); Health
    Canada; transparency
Pharmaceutical Research and
    Manufacturers of America
    (PhRMA), 31, 40, 42, 78, 196, 272
pharmaceuticals: adverse events, 4,
    25, 27–8, 29, 104, 108; licensing,
    5, 81, 118; prevalence of, 3; prices,
    6, *20–1*, 41–3, 172; spending
    on, 133–4; supply, *21*, 43–5;
    withdrawals of, 4, 27, 69, 108, 132.
    See also clinical trial data; drug
    approval; drug promotion; drug
    safety; pharmaceutical industry;
    pharmaceutical regulations;
    transparency
pharmacogenetics, 189–90
pharmacy benefit managers (PBMs),
    42–3
PharmaWatch, 202
Phase IV studies, 141–2
Physician Payments Sunshine Act
    (US, 2010), 37, 167–8
physicians, payments to, *20*, 37–9,
    133, 167–8, 176, 177
PLoS Medicine, 71–2, 73–4, 196
policy-making: evidence-based, 270;
    and politics and power, 16, 45–7,
    49–52; revision process, 125
politics: advocacy and organization,
    67–8, 77–8, 80, 219–20, 268–9;
    capital accumulation and, 162–4,
    176; and power and policy-making,
    16, 45–7, 49–52; transparency and,
    272–3. *See also* ghost-management

Portugal, 38
power: capital accumulation and, 162–4, 176; commercial interests and, 46; discursive techniques for, 50; and politics and policy-making, 16, 45–7, 49–52; types of, 46–7
Prepulsid (cisapride), 102, 120
"Prescriber Checkup" (website), 38
prescription drugs. See pharmaceuticals
Prescrire (La Revue Prescrire), 68, 69, 269
prices, drug, 6, 20–1, 41–3, 172
priority reviews, 143–4, 265
privacy, and rare diseases: approach to and conclusion, 11, 184–5, 187, 204–6, 271; benefits for individuals from data sharing, 189; breach of privacy concern, 191–8; context, 185–6; corporate transparency policies and, 191; independent review panels and research ethics committees/boards (RECs/REBs), 198, 202–3, 205–6; informed consent and, 198–202, 205; orphan drugs and, 189–91; overstatement of privacy-related fears, 193–4; proportionality and, 194–5; reasons for increased transparency, 187–91; research participants on sharing data, 192–3; suggestions for, 198–204; terms of use agreements and, 198, 203–4, 206; transparency-enhancing projects and, 195–8; and understanding and treatment of rare diseases, 188
Privacy Commissioner of Canada, 191
procedural and administrative oversight, 18, 29–30
professional capture, 167–8, 176–7
Project Data Sphere, 195

promotion. See drug promotion
proportionality, 194–5
Proprietary and Patent Medicine Act (Canada, 1908), 115
ProPublica, 31, 35, 38
Protecting Canadians from Unsafe Drugs Act (2014). See Vanessa's Law
protocol document, 22, 23
PTC Therapeutics International, 80
Public Health Agency of Canada, 263
public relations (PR), corporate, 173
publication bias, 71–4, 219–20
Purdue Pharma, 40
Pure Food and Drug Act (US, 1906), 96

Randall, James, 172
randomized controlled trials (RCTs), 246. See also clinical trials; clinical trial data
rare diseases, 185–6, 188. See also privacy, and rare diseases
rationality, bounded, 270
registries, clinical trials, 6, 25–6, 118–19, 243–4
Regulatory Advertising Section, 149
regulatory agencies, 5, 15. See also European Medicines Agency (EMA); Food and Drug Administration (FDA); Health Canada; pharmaceutical regulations; transparency
regulatory capture, 170–1, 177
Relenza (zanamivir), 71, 80
Report of the Committee of Inquiry on the Case Involving Dr. Nancy Olivieri (Thompson, Baird, and Downie), 167
reporting guidelines, 247
reports, inspection, 141, 142, 148

research: academic research, 82,
  170, 244–5, 246–7, 249, 254–5;
  better vs. more research, 257;
  collaborative research, 248, 250–1;
  human research participants, 184,
  185, 189, 192–3; independent
  researchers, 166–7; openness
  and, 245–6; researchers, role in
  transparency, 256–7; research
  waste, 134; spending on, 245. *See
  also* clinical trials; clinical trial data;
  privacy, and rare diseases
research ethics committees/boards
  (RECs/REBs), 142, 198, 202–3,
  205–6
Restoring Invisible and Abandoned
  Trials (RIAT), 74
reviews. *See* expedited reviews
Revue Prescrire, La (*Prescrire*), 68, 69, 269
rimonabant (Acomplia), 69, 70
Ringrose, Peter, 169
risk, 29–30, 52, 140
Roche, 175
rofecoxib (Vioxx), 117, 166–7
rosiglitazone (Avandia), 63–4, 167
Rubinstein, I.S., 194

S-3 Group, 31
safety, 125. *See also* drug safety
Sah, S., 52
Schaaber, Jörg, 75
Scharpf, Fritz, 268
Schneider, L., 36
Schnier, A., 51
Schroter, S., 35
scientific capture, 165–7, 176
scientific evidence, 3–4, 13
selective serotonin reuptake
  inhibitors (SSRIs), 153, 166
Senate Standing Committee on
  Social Affairs, Science and
  Technology, 141–2

Sense About Science, 73
Sentinel, 6, 28, 29
sertraline (Zoloft), 165–6
Sismondo, Sergio, 161
Smith, R., 34, 35
social determinants of value, 160,
  164–5. *See also* ghost-management
Social Issues Research Centre
  (SIRC), 173–4
social media, 41
Social Sciences and Humanities
  Research Council of Canada, 253
Southern European Initiative, 43
specialty drugs, 41
stakeholders: advocacy coalition
  framework and, 269; Health
  Canada and, 117, 145–6; and
  independent review panels and
  research ethics committees/boards
  (RECs/REBs), 202, 206
stakeholders, and Health Canada,
  145–6
statins, 35, 81
Steinman, M., 39
Stiglitz, Joseph, 170
Structural Genomics Consortium,
  195–6
structures and institutions, 266–8
sulfanilamide, 8, 96
Sulston, John, 170
Summary Basis of Decision (SBD),
  103, 117, 118, 142–3, 265
supply, drug, *21*, 43–5
"SUPPORT" Act (US, 2018), 37
surrogate markers, 5, 144

Tamiflu (oseltamivir), 63–4, 71, 73,
  80, 81, 122, 129, 130
technological capture, 168–70
terms of use (ToU) agreements, 79,
  198, 203–4, 206
thalidomide, 4, 9, 14, 97, 116

Therapeutic Access Strategy
    (Canada), 264
Therapeutic Products Directorate
    (Canada), 9, 119, 153
Therapeutic Products Program
    (Canada), 264
think tanks, 173–4
Thompson, J.: *Report of the Committee of
    Inquiry on the Case Involving Dr. Nancy
    Olivieri* (with Baird and Downie), 167
time, 132
Toronto Star, 141, 146, 147, 148, 149
trade agreements, international, 267
Transatlantic Trade and Investment
    Partnership (TTIP), 267
TransCanada Corporation (now TC
    Energy Corporation), 159–60, 173
Trans-Pacific Partnership (TPP), 267
transparency: accountability and,
    7, 13–15, 52, 262; achievements
    and barriers, 47, *48–9*; advocacy
    and organization for, 67–8, 77–8,
    80, 219–20, 268–9; approach to,
    6–12, 15, 45, 52, 129, 136, 257,
    261–2, 266; Banzi's changes in
    perspective on, 247–9; bounded
    rationality and, 270; career
    promotion and, 254–5; clinical
    trial data and, 16, *17*, 22–9;
    vs. commercialization, 255–6;
    conflicts of interest and, 16,
    19–20, 22, 30–41, 52; cultural and
    institutional changes for, 273–4;
    definitions, 16; drug prices and,
    20–1, 41–3; drug supply and, *21*,
    43–5; essential medicines lists
    and, 134–6; failures to improve
    health, examples, 129–31;
    failures to improve health,
    reasons, 52, 131–2; framing and,
    271; implementation from the
    beginning, 246–7; for improved

health, 129, 136; incentives for,
    252–6; non-health benefits of,
    132–4; open access, 170, 252–4;
    openness and public-oriented
    research, 245–6; pharmaceutical
    regulations and, 139; politics and,
    272–3; and power, politics, and
    policy-making, 16, 45–7, 49–52;
    and procedural and administrative
    oversight, *18*, 29–30; relationships
    of, 16, *17–21*; researchers'
    role, 256–7; and structures and
    institutions, 266–8; time and,
    132; windows of opportunity,
    271–2. *See also* Canada; clinical
    trial data; European Medicines
    Agency (EMA); European Union;
    Food and Drug Administration
    (FDA); ghost-management; H1N1
    influenza pandemic and vaccine;
    Health Canada; privacy, and rare
    diseases; United States of America
Transparency International: *Clinical
    Trial Transparency* (2017), 203
TranspariMED, 246
Tri-Council Policy Statement, 196
trust, in government and medical
    profession, 133
Turner, Chris, 146

unapproved pharmaceuticals, *17*, 27,
    83n1, 108
United Kingdom, 26, 32, 74, 81, 136
United States of America: access to
    information legislation, 9, 97–9,
    108–9, 267, 272; approach to,
    8–9, 265; campaign financing,
    30–1; drug pricing, 41, 42–3;
    drug supply, 43–4; lobbying, 31;
    medical education sponsorship
    and payments, 39–40; patient
    organizations, 32–3, 175; payments

from industry to health-care providers, 37–8; rare diseases, 186; structures, institutions, and transparency, 267; technological capture and, 170; user fees, 263. *See also* Food and Drug Administration (FDA)
user fees, 263

vaccines. *See* H1N1 influenza pandemic and vaccine
Valletta group, 43
Vanessa's Law (Protecting Canadians from Unsafe Drugs Act, 2014): access to information and, 102–3; clinical data transparency and, 27, 28, 114, 197–8; communications by Health Canada and, 144–5; implementation of transparency provisions, 122–3, 124; inclusion of transparency provisions, 7, 9, 120–1, 269; post-market requirements in, 108
Veblen, Thorstein, 160, 161, 162–4, 177nn1–2
Vigilance Adverse Reaction online database, 28
Vijayaraghavan, M., 36
Vioxx (rofecoxib), 117, 166–7
vitamins, 172
Vivli project, 197

Waechter, F., 35
We Work for Health, 31
Weber, Max, 13
Wilkes, M.S., 34–5
Willmott, Glenis, 76–7, 79
Wilson, M., 52
Windels, Catherine, 174
windows of opportunity, 271–2
Wismar, M., 52
withdrawals, of pharmaceuticals, 4, 27, 69, 108, 132
World Health Organization (WHO): on adjuvants, 225, 227; clinical trial registration and, 26, 119, 244; essential medicines lists and, 134–5; H1N1 influenza pandemic and, 221; on influenza pandemics, 221–2, 224; "Joint Statement on Public Disclosure of Results from Clinical Trials," 196, 207n18
Wyeth, 31, 166

Yale University Open Data Access (YODA) Project, 27, 195
Young, Terence Hart, 102, 120, 124. *See also* Vanessa's Law

zanamivir (Relenza), 71, 80
Zoloft (sertraline), 165–6

www.ingramcontent.com/pod-product-compliance
Lightning Source LLC
Chambersburg PA
CBHW030238030426
42336CB00009B/150